Workbook

Egan's
Fundamentals of Respiratory Care

Ninth Edition

Stephen F. Wehrman, RRT, RPFT, AE-C
Professor/Program Director
Respiratory Care Program
Kapi'olani Community College
University of Hawaii
Honolulu, Hawaii

with 48 illustrations

MOSBY
ELSEVIER

11830 Westline Industrial Drive
St. Louis, Missouri 63146

WORKBOOK FOR EGAN'S FUNDAMENTALS OF RESPIRATORY CARE   ISBN: 978-0-323-05188-0

Notice

Knowledge and best practice in this field are constantly changing. As new research and experience broaden our knowledge, changes in practice, treatment, and drug therapy may become necessary or appropriate. Readers are advised to check the most current information provided (i) on procedures featured or (ii) by the manufacturer of each product to be administered, to verify the recommended dose or formula, the method and duration of administration, and contraindications. It is the responsibility of the practitioner, relying on their own experience and knowledge of the patient, to make diagnoses, to determine dosages and the best treatment for each individual patient, and to take all appropriate safety precautions. To the fullest extent of the law, neither the Publisher nor the Author assumes any liability for any injury and/or damage to persons or property arising out of or related to any use of the material contained in this book.

The Publisher

Previous editions copyrighted 2003, 1999

Library of Congress Control Number 2007940787

Managing Editor: Billi Sharp
Senior Developmental Editor: Mindy Hutchinson
Publishing Services Manager: Pat Joiner-Myers
Senior Project Manager: Rachel E. Dowell
Design Direction: Maggie Reid

Printed in the United States of America

Last digit is the print number: 9 8 7 6 5 4 3

Working together to grow
libraries in developing countries

www.elsevier.com | www.bookaid.org | www.sabre.org

ELSEVIER   BOOK AID International   Sabre Foundation

Dedication

This book is dedicated to my son, James Forest Wehrman, Sgt. United States Air Force, Manhattan Community College Respiratory Care Program Class of 2008

The next generation of respiratory therapists—I am proud that he is following me into this wonderful career of saving life and breath.

Preface

EAGER FOR EGAN!

"Anyone who keeps learning stays young."
Henry Ford

Dear Student:
The year was 1977. I had just started school to become a respiratory technician. My first textbook was *Egan's Fundamentals of Respiratory Therapy*. I have to confess that I had to read everything three times to understand it. Egan's really bent my brain out of shape! I was really glad to graduate and be done with the difficult task of understanding that book. When I began teaching, there was Egan's waiting for me. A new edition and a new challenge to help students make the most of a book that is full of everything you need to know to prepare for this exciting career.

The problem for all health students is information overload. This is just as true for teachers as it is for anyone else. It is just as true for you today as it was for me 30 years ago. This workbook will help you learn and help you sort out some of the important information you will need to succeed in practice and to pass your board exams. If you want to get the most out of this book and the textbook, here's what you should do. First, read the assigned chapter in *Egan's*. I read lightly and quickly using a highlighter to touch on key points. Next, open the workbook and *Egan's* and go through the chapter answering the questions. I suggest you get in the habit of noting the page numbers where you find answers. I have provided an answer key (located on the Evolve site) so you can check your work. The answer key is **not** a substitute for hard work (yours) or a way to copy someone else's work (mine). When you get stuck and have to use my answer, you should indicate your choice is from the answer key and not pretend that you got it! That way you and your teachers will know which concepts are not clear.

At the end of the chapters you will find questions written in the same style as your NBRC examinations. You'll also find cases, exercises, and Internet tools. When you graduate and prepare for your boards, you'll find *Egan's Fundamentals* and this workbook waiting to help you succeed.

Learning how to be a Respiratory Therapist is a challenging, fun, difficult, and sometimes painful experience. Don't ever give up along the way. Your instructors, textbooks, and clinical faculty are all there to help you succeed. You've chosen a dynamic and exciting field that will always keep you on your toes and give you a feeling of pride and satisfaction in helping people breathe better.

A team of people made it possible for you to have a book like this to help you in your studies. My wife, Cathy, spent many hours helping me with the manuscript. My faculty, Abby and Ed, encouraged and supported my efforts. Mindy Hutchinson and Rachel Dowell did an amazing job of organizing and fixing my mistakes, and the reason for writing—my students, who are always the best inspiration.

Aloha,
Stephen

P.S. Want to talk? Your feedback, questions, or comments are always welcome at wehrman@hawaii.edu.

ADDITIONAL LEARNING AIDS

Mosby's Respiratory Care Online
New to this edition of *Egan's Fundamentals of Respiratory Care* is *Mosby's Respiratory Care Online,* a Web-based course designed to supplement the textbook. This Web-delivered course supplement, available as a separate purchase, has been carefully designed to reinforce the learning and synthesis of the concepts presented in the text through a range of visual, auditory, and interactive elements.

This unique program offers additional learning opportunities while accommodating different learning styles and environments. The online course features:
- Animations, slideshows, videos—With audio narration!
- Image enlarge function
- Interactive learning activities
  - Labeling
  - Fill-in
  - Sequencing
  - Short answer
  - Matching
  - Image association
  - And more!
- Mini Clini Challenges with representative patient photos and simulated medical records
- Formulas—Organized by content area and printable
- Glossary—With audio pronunciations
- Breath sounds—Included in some activities
- Ventilator graphics
- Branching logic case studies

- Module assessments—Written in NBRC exam format; automatically scored and reported to the instructor grade book
- And much more!

This online course supplement is only accessible with purchase of an access code. For more information, visit http://evolve.elsevier.com/Wilkins/Egans.

Evolve Resources—http://evolve.elsevier.com/ Wilkins/Egans

Evolve is an interactive learning environment designed to work in coordination with *Egan's Fundamentals of Respiratory Care*. It contains the following:
- The answer key for all of the exercises found in this workbook.
- For students, Evolve features a detailed cross-reference of the content in *Egan's* to the National Board for Respiratory Care (NBRC) matrices for the certified respiratory therapist (CRT) and registered respiratory therapist (RRT) examinations. This handy reference will help students use *Egan's* to prepare for the certification exams.
- Instructors may use Evolve to provide an Internet-based course component that reinforces and expands the concepts presented in class. Evolve may be used to publish the class syllabus, outlines, and lecture note; set up "virtual office hours" and e-mail communications; share important dates and information through the online class calendar; and encourage student participation through chat rooms and discussion boards. Evolve allows instructors to post exams and manage their grade books online.

For more information, visit http://evolve.elsevier.com/Wilkins/Egans.

Contents

1 History of Respiratory Care

It is history that teaches us to hope.
General Robert E. Lee

In 1977, I learned to do something called "T-piece" weaning to help a patient get off the life support machine. The process was uncannily similar to the spontaneous breathing trials for weaning from mechanical ventilation found on the national board examinations today. There are also differences after more than three decades of *Egan's*. We are getting a lot more evidence to help guide us toward effective and efficient practice. The rapid shallow breathing index, for example, makes it easier to identify which patients are ready to breathe again on their own.

In Chapter 1, we take a look at the past with an eye toward the future. The topic is so important that there is a course in my program that covers the material in this foundational chapter along with the ethics and professionalism covered in Chapter 5. Pay special attention to the descriptions of the profession, our basic areas of care, and milestones that mark the path to our expanded role in disease management and acute cardiopulmonary care.

WORD WIZARD

Getting to know the terminology of medicine can be a real challenge. Each chapter in this workbook starts off with some word work to get those neurons firing and help you learn to talk the talk of a professional respiratory therapist.

Match the following terms to their definitions.

Definitions	Terms
_____ 1. caregiver who acts as a physician extender after receiving additional education	A. AARC
	B. CoARC
_____ 2. national professional association for respiratory care	C. NBRC
	D. cardiopulmonary system
	E. respiratory care
_____ 3. health care discipline that specializes in the promotion of optimum cardiopulmonary health	F. respiratory therapy
	G. respiratory therapist(s)
	H. oxygen therapy
_____ 4. name suggesting increased involvement in disease prevention and management and promotion of health and wellness	I. aerosol medications
	J. mechanical ventilation
	K. airway management
	L. pulmonary function testing
_____ 5. one of the primary treatments for asthma uses this method of delivery	M. physician assistant
	N. respiratory care practitioner(s)
_____ 6. widely prescribed in hospitals by the 1940s and still a mainstay of respiratory care	
_____ 7. organization responsible for the respiratory credentialing examinations	

Continued

1

_____ 8. iron lung is an example of this therapy that helps patients who cannot breathe

_____ 9. professional organization that accredits respiratory care schools and programs

_____ 10. heart and lungs working together is the "bread and butter" of our profession

_____ 11. method to test the ways that height, age, obesity, and disease alter lung function

_____ 12. another name for the RT is this more formal term

_____ 13. individual trained to deliver care to patients with heart and lung disease

_____ 14. relieving obstruction is the key to this respiratory procedure

MEET THE OBJECTIVES

Chapter 1 presented four main objectives for learning. Test how well you understand these mysteries of history by providing short answers.

15. Define the respiratory care profession in your own words. Include at least three main concepts.

16. Respiratory care has three main professional associations. Describe the role and write out the full name for
    A. CoARC
       Full name _____

       Role _____
    B. NBRC
       Full Name _____

       Role _____
    C. AARC
       Full name _____

       Role _____

17. Describe current trends in respiratory care education in the United States.

18. The future of the profession is based on demand for our services. Explain why we have such a bright future and how we can ensure appropriate care for our patients.

KEY POINTS

19. Respiratory therapists apply scientific principles to _____, identify, and _____ dysfunction of the cardiopulmonary system.

20. The _____ is the professional organization for the field.

21. The iron lung was used extensively during the _____ epidemics of the 1940s and 1950s.

22. In the future, there will be an _____ in demand for respiratory care due to advances in _____ and increases in and _____ of the population.

CASE STUDIES

Your book provides you with two good case studies called Mini-Clinis. Our students all participate in Respiratory Care Week at the college. We also ask our students to serve on our advisory committee just like the example in the text. I recently ran into a graduate whose boss had just asked him to make a presentation as part of his clinical promotion ladder. That's when it struck me that one of the great things about *Egan's* is the Mini-Clinis and cases, which reflect real practice.

WHAT DOES THE NBRC SAY?

The subject of history does not come up on the board exams. If you like to play our national pastime, Sputum Bowl, however, you will find this chapter invaluable!

FOOD FOR THOUGHT

The associate degree is the entry point into our profession, as the authors make clear. These days, if you want to advance your career and be competitive with similar medical professionals, you will need more education.

23. Describe at least four careers that would open up for you as a result of baccalaureate or graduate education.

    A. _____

    B. _____

    C. _____

    D. _____

INFORMATION AGE

You do not have to look far to find the best Web site for respiratory care. www.aarc.org is the home of our national organization and the best repository of respiratory history on the internet. Imagine a billionaire pharmacist with a cabinet of curiosities and you'll want to go to http://www.ucl.ac.uk/histmed/ to find the Wellcome Trust Centre for the History of Medicine.

2 Quality and Evidence-Based Respiratory Care

Mediocrity killed the cat.
Forrest Gump

Everyone expects quality, from the goods we buy to the services we receive. Health care is no different. You want to work for a quality-oriented organization. You try to deliver quality care to your patients. The patients expect to be treated by qualified providers, and to get the best care at all times! In Chapter 2 we look at what quality means in the health care setting and at specific ways we can monitor and achieve quality in the respiratory care profession. We also look at the trend toward using evidence-based methods for determining best practices in our profession.

WORD WIZARD

Before you can understand quality care, you need to know the specific terms that are used to describe quality. After reading the second chapter of the text, try your hand at completing this crossword puzzle.

ACROSS

1. _____ director. The physician who helps manage your department
4. Body that reviews health care companies such as hospitals
8. Recognition
11. Characteristic reflecting excellence
13. Credentializing organization for respiratory care

DOWN

2. Original author of your textbook
3. Permission to practice
5. Someone like you ...
6. Informal training in the workplace
7. Agency that regulates drugs
9. Therapist _____ protocols
10. Improvement that is ongoing in nature
12. College of chest doctors

MEET THE OBJECTIVES

Chapter 2 presented five main objectives for learning. How well do you understand these important ideas about delivering the best care? Fill in your answers in the space provided.

1. Providing quality care to the patient involves many dimensions. Name at least three elements that are part of quality respiratory care.

   A. _____

   B. _____

   C. _____

5

2. Quality must be monitored to ensure it is being obtained. State the two basic monitoring strategies, and give one example of each.

A. _____

B. _____

3. How can protocols enhance the quality of respiratory care services? Support your answer with evidence from the text.

4. What are the four essential components of disease management program?

A. _____

B. _____

C. _____

D. _____

5. Evidence-based medicine specifies precise methods for analyzing data and making decisions. Give a brief explanation of the three main components of this process.

A. _____

B. _____

C. _____

CHAPTER HIGHLIGHTS

Identify eight key points from Chapter 2. Complete the following questions by writing the correct term(s) in the blank(s) provided.

6. The _____ director is professionally responsible for the clinical function of the respiratory care department.

7. Ordering too many respiratory care services is called _____ and hinders delivery of quality care.

8. Specific guidelines for delivering appropriate respiratory care services are called _____.

9. The _____ respiratory therapist is the highest credential in the profession.

10. Respiratory care credentialing examinations are administered by the _____.

11. Personnel _____-_____ is the method most frequently cited as the optimal strategy for decreasing redundancy of patient care activities.

12. An ongoing form of quality assurance that puts emphasis on quality and cost-effectiveness is called _____ quality _____.

13. The two major forms of credentialing in health fields are state _____ and voluntary _____.

CASE STUDIES

Case 1

A 25-year-old woman has returned to a medical/surgical nursing unit following an appendectomy. She has no history of lung disease and is wearing a nasal cannula at 3 L per minute. She is alert and oriented, with a respiratory rate of 18 and a heart rate of 82 beats per minute. Her SpO_2 (pulse oximeter reading) is 99% on the nasal cannula. Her physician orders "respiratory therapy protocol," and you are asked to assess this patient.

Use the protocol found on page 23 (Figure 2-1) in the text to help you answer the following questions.

14. What are the clinical signs of hypoxia/hypoxemia? Name at least three.

    A. _____

    B. _____

    C. _____

15. Using the oxygen therapy protocol, determine if the oxygen therapy is appropriate for this patient. Support your answer with information from the textbook.

16. What action would you recommend at this time?

A 54-year-old man with a history of asthma and cigarette smoking was admitted to the hospital for a hernia repair. Following the procedure, his chest radiograph shows elevated diaphragms with bilateral atelectasis. Vital capacity is acceptable but the patient is unable to hold his breath. The pulse oximetry reading is 95% on room air. His heart rate is 84, blood pressure 110/78, respiratory rate 17, and temperature 36.8° C. Breath sounds are decreased bilaterally with apical wheezes. He has a weak nonproductive cough. The patient is alert and oriented.

17. Use the algorithm in Figure 2-1 to determine how to give this patient his meds. If you've never used an algorithm before, it may be useful to write out the steps in your path. Start with "Is the patient alert and put your answer in Step 1.

   Step 1 _____

   Step 2 _____

   Step 3 _____

   Step 4 _____

   Respiratory therapists routinely plan, deliver, and assess the effects of care!

WHAT DOES THE NBRC SAY?

The National Board for Respiratory Care (NBRC) expects you to be able to participate in the development of care plans. You might expect to see five questions on this area in the Entry-Level Examination. I have written some questions that are similar in style to the ones on the boards for practice. If you are a beginner, you will need to look up the therapeutic interventions and disease management options in other parts of your text.

Circle the best answer for the following multiple choice questions.

18. A patient with chronic obstructive pulmonary disease complains of difficulty breathing when he is ambulating. His SpO$_2$ is 88% at rest. Which of the following would you recommend?
    A. oxygen therapy
    B. PEEP therapy
    C. antibiotic therapy
    D. aerosolized bronchodilator therapy

19. An alert 18-year-old patient is admitted with difficulty breathing. A diagnosis of asthma is determined, and you are asked to instruct the patient in the use of an MDI. An MDI is a device used for
    A. oxygen therapy
    B. PEEP therapy
    C. antibiotic therapy
    D. aerosolized bronchodilator therapy

20. A patient with pneumonia is receiving oxygen via nasal cannula at 2 L/min. The SpO$_2$ is 89%, heart rate 110, and respiratory rate 24. Which of the following would you recommend?
    A. Increase the liter-per-minute flow to the cannula.
    B. Intubate and begin mechanical ventilation.
    C. Initiate aerosolized bronchodilator therapy.
    D. Initiate postural drainage.

21. Incentive breathing devices are primarily used in the treatment of
    A. patients with emphysema
    B. postoperative patients
    C. adult respiratory distress syndrome
    D. pulmonary fibrosis

22. Protocol-based therapy and quality assurance efforts do not always work! Discuss some of the reasons you think these two strategies might fail.

23. Evidence-based medicine (EBM) goes hand-in-hand with protocols to help us deliver the most effective care to the right patient at the right time. In 2001, *Respiratory Care* published two editions devoted to EBM. Of course, there's much more since then, and EBM remains a hot topic in our profession. How did EBM change the way we look at alpha-1 disease?

INFORMATION AGE

Computers have become invaluable tools in the practice of respiratory care. The World Wide Web is a good place to search for information that is hot right now. Keep in mind the rules for evaluating information found on the Web (see Chapter 7); approximately 80% of this information is neither scientific nor educational in nature.

Here are a few helpful Web sites for further research:

Centre for Evidence-Based Medicine	www.cebm.net	Web site offers many free resources to help with learning and using evidence-based medicine
American Association for Respiratory Care (AARC)	www.aarc.org	Best site for respiratory care protocols and clinical practice guidelines
National Guideline Clearinghouse (NGC)	www.guideline.gov	Public resource for evidence-based clinical practice guidelines

3 Patient Safety, Communication, and Recordkeeping

So, our prime purpose in this life is to help others. And if you can't help them, at least don't hurt them.
Dalai Lama

■ Safety first. How many times have we heard that one?
■ Say the right thing at the right time. How do you do that?
■ Nobody loves paperwork. The hospital environment is swimming in it.

Chapter 3 combines a huge amount of information that can be hard to swallow all at once. I am going to break this down into bite-sized pieces, and you see if you can digest the material. It's important stuff!

WORD WIZARD

Read Chapter 3 in your textbook and see if you can fill in the missing words.

You'll Get a Charge Out of This

The medical center is filled with electrical equipment. Everything has a three-pronged plug. The third prong is the neutral

wire, or _____, which helps prevent electrocution. For this reason, no outside electrical devices are allowed in the hospital unless they are checked out by the biomedical staff. Electrocution can occur in the form of

a(n) _____ shock. This might happen if you were standing on a wet floor and a power cord fell onto the floor. Many of the power cords are detachable, so this is a potential hazard. Always clean up spills. A small

shock, or _____ shock, is a hazard to patients who have pacemakers, ECG leads, and indwelling heart catheters.

This may result in ventricular _____ and death! This could happen if the ground wire gets broken, so don't ever roll beds or other equipment over the electrical power cords. Report frayed cords and take suspect equipment out of use.

Burn, Baby, Burn

Because high oxygen concentrations are used in respiratory care, fire is a real hazard.

Even though oxygen is _____ and does not burn, it greatly speeds up an existing fire.

In fact, oxygen is necessary for fires to exist. For a fire to start, you also need _____

material, and heat. Remove any of these three and the fire will go out. You must make sure that ignition sources such

as _____ are not allowed when oxygen is in use. Most hospitals will call a "Code Red" if a fire exists, and you must respond. One of the respiratory therapist's responsibilities in a fire is to shut off the zone valve to the affected area if the fire is near a patient using oxygen. (See Chapter 37: Storage and Delivery of Medical Gases.)

KEEP IT MOVING!

Anyone who stays immobile in a bed for too long will suffer consequences. We need to ambulate the patient as soon as he or she is stable.

Here are some guidelines for safe ambulation. Number them 1 through 7 in the right order.

_____ Dangle the patient.

_____ Sit them up.

_____ Assist to a standing position.

_____ Encourage slow, easy breathing.

_____ Lower the bed and lock the wheels.

_____ Move the IV pole close to the patient.

_____ Provide support while walking.

I CAN'T HEAR YOU

Communication plays a big part in your ability to gain patient cooperation, evaluate progress, and make recommendations for care. What you do (nonverbal) is just as important as what you say (verbal). Communication will also play a role in your satisfaction on the job. Exchanging information and working out problems with other members of the health care team are an everyday part of hospital life.

MEET THE OBJECTIVES

Chapter 3 presents 14 objectives for learning. We've already covered some of them. How well do you understand safety and communication? To find the answers, just read the book! Fill in your answers in the spaces provided.

1. Name at least three risks that are common among patients receiving respiratory care?

   A. _____

   B. _____

   C. _____

2. Describe two problems of bed rest and two benefits of ambulation.

   A. _____

   B. _____

3. What is the main reason you should use good body mechanics? _____

   _____

4. State at least two factors you should monitor during patient ambulation. (There are a total of five!)

   A. _____

   B. _____

5. Name at least four of the many factors that influence the communication process.

    A. _____

    B. _____

    C. _____

    D. _____

6. The text lists five ways to improve your effectiveness as a sender of messages. Describe two of these that apply to you. Give examples of situations where you communicated well (or not!).

"I need to improve in

    A. _____"

    B. _____"

Give an example of good communication

Give an example of unsuccessful communication

7. Name four sources of conflict in health care organizations. Give an example of each.

    A. _____

    B. _____

    C. _____

    D. _____

Chapter **3 Patient Safety, Communication, and Recordkeeping**

8. What is a medical record? Who owns the record? Who is allowed to read it?

9. State one legal and one practical essential of recordkeeping.

   A. _____

   B. _____

10. One of the most common formats that respiratory therapists (and others) use in charting is the SOAP format. What does SOAP mean? (besides something you use in the shower!) Give examples of information you would chart for each category.

	MEANING	EXAMPLE
S		
O		
A		
P		

CHAPTER HIGHLIGHTS

Identify eight key points from Chapter 3. Complete the following questions by writing the correct term(s) in the blank(s) provided.

11. You should begin _____ as soon as a patient is stable.

12. A(n) _____ is a small current that enters the body through external catheters and may cause ventricular fibrillation.

13. Avoid electrical shocks by always _____ your equipment.

14. You can minimize fire hazards by removing flammable materials and ignition sources from areas where

    _____ is in use.

15. _____ skills play a key role in your ability to achieve desired patient outcomes.

16. Accommodating, avoiding, collaborating, competing, and compromising are basic strategies for handling

    _____.

17. A medical record is a _____ document.

18. You must _____ each treatment, medication, or procedure you provide.

Case 1

The physician orders ambulation for a patient who is receiving oxygen. The nurse asks you to assist. The patient is in bed wearing a nasal cannula running at 2 L/min.

19. What equipment will you need *before* you try to walk with this patient? _____

_____

After 5 minutes of walking, you notice that the patient is breathing at a rate of 24, and using his accessory muscles of ventilation. His skin appears sweaty, and he is exhaling through pursed lips.

20. What observations are important to note in this situation? What action would you take?

Case 2

You are caring for a patient who is on a mechanical ventilator. You need to transport the patient to radiology for a CT scan. The nurse unplugs the IV pump and pulse oximeter from the *back* of each unit. The pumps and the pulse oximeter are now running on their battery systems. As you prepare to leave, you notice that the power cords are still plugged into the wall outlets. The physician and the nurse are anxious to get the transport under way.

21. Describe the actions you would take if you encountered this situation.

Chapter **3** **Patient Safety, Communication, and Recordkeeping**

22. What potential conflict/communication problems exist? How will you deal with them?

WHAT DOES THE NBRC SAY?

By now you should be asking the question, "Does any of this apply to my board examinations?" The answer is yes and no. The "no" part is fire and electrical safety. Those things are just practical to know for the job of a respiratory therapist. The "yes" part is found in the content outline for the board exams in Section III, Therapeutic Procedures, with "Maintain Records and Communicate Information" including:

1. **Explain** therapy to patients in terms they can understand.
2. **Document** a treatment correctly.
3. **Note responses** to therapy—includes vital signs, adverse reactions etc, but also includes interpreting subjective and attitudinal response to therapy!
4. **Verify computations** and correct errors.
5. **Communicate clinical information** to other health care practitioners.
6. **Communicate to avoid conflicts**, maintain scheduling and sequencing of treatments.
7. **Communicate results of therapy** and alter therapy per protocols.
8. **Counsel patient and family** about smoking cessation/disease management.

Wow! That must mean they really care about this stuff! You should expect seven questions on this specific material on the certified respiratory therapist (CRT) and five harder ones about the same material on the written registry examination (WRE). (More on this subject in Chapter 15.)

Try a few problems, in board exam style. Circle the best answer for the following multiple choice questions.

23. A respiratory therapist has completed SOAP charting in the progress notes following a bronchodilator treatment. While signing the chart form, she notices that the wrong amount for the medication has been entered. Which of the following actions should be done at this time?
   I.   Draw one line through the error.
   II. Notify the physician of the error.
   III. Write "Error" and initial.
   IV. Recopy the progress notes.
      A. I and II
      B. I and III
      C. II and IV
      D. III and IV

24. An asthmatic patient has orders for albuterol by medication nebulizer every 2 hours. During the shift, the patient improves, and the order is changed to every 4 hours. In regard to the new frequency, what action should you take?
   I.   Note the change in your charting.
   II. Inform the registered nurse of the order.
   III. Frequency will change on the next shift.
      A. I and II
      B. I and III
      C. II and III
      D. I, II, and III

25. A patient's heart rate increases from 88 to 134 following a breathing treatment. After reassuring the patient, the respiratory therapist should
    A. discontinue the therapy
    B. reduce the dosage of the medication
    C. place the patient on oxygen
    D. notify the physician

FOOD FOR THOUGHT

Every year people die in work-related fires and electrocutions. The hospital can be a busy, stressful environment, and it is really easy to skip some of the steps in the safety process. That is one of the reasons the Occupational Safety and Health Administration (OSHA) requires health care institutions to train workers in fire, electrical, blood-borne pathogen, back injury, and other safety areas *every year!* We all know friends, patients, and co-workers who have been injured on the job. I hope you're not going to be one of them.

26. What do you think is the most common type of injury in health care? _____

    _____

27. On what shift do most injuries, accidents, and patient incidents occur? _____

    _____

INFORMATION AGE

A wealth of information is out on the Web that addresses safety and legal issues in health care. See the sites!

Food and Drug Administration	www.fda.gov	It might surprise you to know that the FDA has lots of information about safety as it relates to devices.
MedWatch	www.fda.gov/medwatch	You can look at MedWatch, which is the FDA's safety information and adverse event reporting site.
Occupational Safety and Health Administration (OSHA)	www.osha.gov/SLTC/respiratoryprotection	Check out this site if you want to protect your own lungs.

   Use any of the major search engines and you'll get hundreds more like these—anything from needle safety to healthy back practices. The Internet really sheds some light on the subject of medical safety!

Principles of Infection Control

The doctor is to be feared more than the disease.
Latin proverb

Nobody comes to the hospital to get sick! But let's face it, 5% to 10% of all the patients who enter a hospital get an infection while they are there. To make matters worse, up to 40% of these infections involve the respiratory system. It costs billions to treat hospital-acquired illness, and even more to pay for lost work time. Patients are not the only ones who get sick. Each year, thousands of health care practitioners are exposed to "bugs" like hepatitis, HIV, and TB (or, worse, SARS), and some of them will be infected. Fortunately, there are plenty of simple, easy ways you can protect yourself and the patients.

WORD WIZARD

Chapter 4 introduces a lot of new terms that you should know if you want to be able to beat bacteria and viruses. After you read about this timely topic, you will be able to make these key definitions match up.

Definitions	Terms
_____ infections that are acquired in the hospital	A. fomite
	B. nosocomial
_____ inanimate objects that help transfer pathogens	C. sterilization
	D. disinfection
_____ death of all microorganisms	E. standard precautions
_____ universal method of protection for health workers	
_____ death of pathogenic microorganisms	

MEET THE OBJECTIVES

Chapter 4 presented 10 objectives for learning. How well do you understand these important ideas about infection control? Fill in your answers in the spaces provided.

1. What is a health care–associated infection? How many people get sick?

   A. HAI = _____

   B. How many get sick? _____ What percent of patients? _____

2. Why are HAIs important to our profession?

3. Name the three elements that are required for these infections to take place.

    A. _____

    B. _____

    C. _____

4. A susceptible host may be elderly, have HIV, or have chemotherapy, but we can still reduce host susceptibility by focusing on employees and chemoprophylaxis. Name five vaccinations that might help you decrease the risk. (Now you see why you had to be vaccinated to be in the respiratory therapist program!)

    A. _____

    B. _____

    C. _____

    D. _____

    E. _____

5. Respiratory therapists must know about the routes of transmission of disease so we can avoid infection. What are the three **major** routes? Give an example of each.

	ROUTE	EXAMPLE
A		
B		
C		

6. Interrupting the route of transmission involves special equipment processing. What is the first step in cleaning equipment that is going to be resterilized after a critical procedure like bronchoscopy?

7. State the six methods of sterilization. For each method, give an example of applicable equipment to be sterilized. Refer to Table 4-5 (page 61) of your text if you get lost.

	METHOD	EQUIPMENT
A.		
B.		
C.		
D.		
E.		
F.		

8. You will need to decide how to clean the RT equipment. Use the Mini-Clini on "Selection of Equipment Processing Methods" of your text to help decide how to clean and sterilize these items:

ITEM	DISINFECT	STERILIZE
A. Laryngoscope blade		
B. Humidifier		
C. Mechanical ventilator		

9. List the three general barrier methods used to prevent exposure to organisms. Describe a situation or an organism where you need this type of protection as a respiratory therapist.

A. _____

B. _____

C. _____

CHAPTER HIGHLIGHTS

Identify the key points from Chapter 4. Complete the following questions by writing the correct term(s) in the blank(s) provided.

10. _____ is the best choice for high-level disinfection of semicritical respiratory care equipment.

11. Among respiratory care equipment, _____ have the greatest potential to spread infection.

12. Always use _____ fluids for tracheal suctioning and to fill nebulizers and humidifiers.

13. Thoroughly _____ your _____ after any patient contact, even when gloves are used.

14. Use standard (universal) precautions in caring for _____ patients, regardless of their diagnosis or infection status.

15. Wear _____ and _____ during any procedure that can generate splashes or sprays of body fluids.

16. The use of _____ is part of routine care when there is skin contact.

17. Ventilator circuits may be used up to _____ days before they need to be changed.

Case 1

You work in the surgical intensive care unit (ICU) of a large urban hospital. Over the past 2 days, a number of patients in the unit have developed serious *Staphylococcus aureus* infections.

18. Why do postoperative patients have an increased risk of infection?

19. What is the most common source of *S. aureus* organisms? _____

_____

20. Identify three ways to disrupt the route of transmission in this situation.

 A. _____

 B. _____

 C. _____

Case 2

During your third day of clinical, you are assigned to go with a therapist who has an extremely heavy workload on a medical floor of the hospital. The therapist puts on gloves for each patient contact, and asks you to do so also. When you go to wash your hands after the first treatment, the therapist tells you, "We don't have time for that, and besides the gloves will keep our hands clean."

21. Explain the role of gloves in protecting practitioners and preventing the spread of infection.

22. What does the CDC say about cleaning your hands in regard to washing? Are there any alternatives?

A serious tuberculosis outbreak occurs in a local prison facility. You are called to the emergency department as four of the sickest patients are being admitted together to your hospital for treatment.

23. By what route does tuberculosis spread? _____

_____

24. When transporting these patients out of the emergency department, what action should you take?

25. What kind of precautions should be taken to prevent the spread of infection once these patients are admitted?

26. What special guidelines exist in regard to cough-inducing and aerosol-generating procedures for patients with active tuberculosis?

27. What other concerns do you have in working with these patients?

28. If private rooms were not available for these prisoners, how far do they need to be for safety?

_____

WHAT DOES THE NBRC SAY?

You'd be right if you thought your board exams would place an emphasis on infection control. The Entry-Level Examination Matrix has this to say:

"Will assure selected equipment cleanliness" and
1. Choose the right method or agent for disinfection and sterilization.
2. Perform disinfection and sterilization procedures.
3. Monitor sterilization effectiveness.
4. Protect the patient from nosocomial infection.
5. Follow infection control policies and procedures.

Here are some questions like the ones you might see on the test. I have put them in the form of a single case, but they will normally be spread throughout the exam. You can expect at least two questions on infection control in your entry-level board and one on the registry.

Circle the best answer for the following multiple-choice questions.

The following questions refer to this situation:

A 72-year-old female patient with COPD has a tracheostomy tube in place following prolonged intubation and mechanical ventilation. She is currently in the medical intensive care unit. After you take her off the ventilator, you will need to set up a heated aerosol system with an FIO_2 of 40%.

29. What type of water should be placed in the nebulizer?
    A. distilled water
    B. tap water
    C. normal saline solution
    D. sterile distilled water

30. To help lower the risk of a nosocomial infection when using heated aerosol systems, the respiratory therapist should do which of the following?
    I. Label the equipment with the date and time it is started.
    II. Avoid draining condensate into the nebulizer.
    III. Use aseptic technique during the initial set-up.
    IV. Remove the capillary tube to reduce the volume of water particles.
        A. I and II only
        B. I, II, and III only
        C. I, III, and IV only
        D. I, II, III, and IV

31. The best way to prevent the spread of infection in the ICU is to:
    A. ensure that sterilized equipment is used
    B. wash your hands after every patient contact
    C. wear gloves when you come in contact with body fluids
    D. isolate infected patients

FOOD FOR THOUGHT

Because many hospitalized patients acquire respiratory infections, the respiratory therapist is really under a microscope at work. We have to maintain the highest standards of behavior, to protect ourselves, our patients, and our loved ones.

32. One of your fellow students comes to clinical with a cold. He asks you not to tell your clinical instructor, because missed clinical days are hard to make up. What is your reaction to this situation? What are the potential problems with this scenario?

33. The college recommends that you get immunized against hepatitis B prior to attending clinical. The consent form lists a number of possible side effects of the vaccine, and the vaccination is expensive. What are the pros and cons of vaccines? What will you choose?

34. What is respiratory etiquette? Can you name the five elements? If not, you'll want to check this out and ask your patients (and your children) to follow good hygiene.

INFORMATION AGE

There is one truly great Web site that can meet a lot of our needs in the infection control arena: www.cdc.gov. This is the Centers for Disease Control and Prevention (CDC) Web site. Here you will find the most current guidelines for infection control in hospitals. You may be surprised to find that handwashing with soap and water is no longer considered the best method! The CDC recommends using alcohol-based germicides. You will save time (as much as an hour per shift) and decrease the risk of spreading germs by using these products. The CDC still recommends handwashing when you are grossly contaminated by blood or any other body fluids. You can find the new guidelines at www.cdc.gov/handhygiene/.

P.S. The current board exams still emphasize handwashing. We'll see if there are any changes when the NBRC releases the new exams.

5 Ethical and Legal Implications of Practice

Ignorance of the law excuses no one from practicing it.
A. Mizner

Malpractice is a word that strikes fear into the hearts of physicians. A word that could strike fear into your heart! Let's face it; we live in a society where lawsuits are commonplace. You hear about them every day. Do respiratory therapists ever get sued? You bet they do. To make matters worse, the ethical issues that are always present in health care are crossing into the legal arena more and more. Should we terminate life support? How can health services be rationed? What if the patient cannot afford the care? Your two safeguards are knowledge and good defensive recordkeeping. Chapter 5 gives you the tools you need to provide care with confidence.

WORD WIZARD

Law, like medicine, has a language of its own that most people do not understand. (Shakespeare said, "It was Greek to me.") You will need clear comprehension of some basic legal terminology to avoid ending up in court. For these words, let's skip the ethics and go directly to legal issues on page 86 in your text. Complete the following paragraphs by writing in the correct terms in the blanks provided.

The two basic types of law in the United States are public and civil law. Public law is further divided into

administrative law and _____ law. Health care facilities operate under a mountain of regulations

set by government agencies. Private, or _____, law protects citizens who feel they have been

harmed. The individual who brings a complaint is called the _____, and those accused of wrong

doing are known as _____. A(n) _____ is a civil wrong. These cases

could easily involve a health care practitioner. There are three types. _____ is the failure to
perform your duties competently. Cases in which the patient falls, is given the wrong medication, or is harmed by equipment revolve around a provider's duty to anticipate harm and prevent it from happening.

Expert testimony, professional guidelines, or even circumstantial evidence can determine what a reasonable and

prudent respiratory therapist would have done in a given situation. The Latin term _____ ("the
thing speaks for itself") is sometimes invoked to show that harm occurred because of inappropriate care. When a profes

sional fails to act skillfully, breaches ethics, or falls below a reasonable standard, it is called _____.

Wrongdoing may be considered intentional or unintentional. Intentional acts include _____, or

placing another person in fear of bodily harm, _____, or physical contact without consent. Other

common intentional harm occurs through _____, which is verbal defamation of character, and

_____, which is written defamation of character. Finally, information about patients is considered

private, or _____, and cannot be shared with anyone who is not involved in their care.
There are two good defenses against all of these problems. The first is to show that actions were not intentional. For example, fainting during a procedure is not a voluntary act. The second defense is to obtain consent from the patient. Consent, whether verbal or written, should be obtained from the patient for most procedures. Of course you have to explain the risks and the procedure in clear language the patient can understand.

Be sure to check out the Mini-Clinis in this chapter.

Case 1

You get a chance to meet with your fellow students for lunch in the hospital cafeteria during a busy clinical day. One of your classmates is bursting with excitement as you sit down to eat. "You won't believe what I got to do today! I was taking care of Mr. Brainola patient in the intensive care unit (ICU), and he started to go bad, and we had to intubate. Then he coded and I got to do CPR! It was so cool!"

1. What's the problem with this picture? What violation has your classmate committed?

2. What are the possible consequences of this scenario?

3. What action should you take?

4. Is this situation simply a breach of ethics or a violation of law?

You receive an order to administer a bronchodilator to a 27-year-old asthmatic. The patient refuses the therapy, stating, "I just can't take any more of this today!" He appears alert and oriented.

5. Does the patient have a legal right to refuse in this case? Cite evidence from the text to justify your answer.

6. How would you respond to this situation?

7. What other action should you take at this time?

After finishing with the previous patient, you receive a stat call to the orthopedic floor. The registered nurse informs you they are having problems with a 76-year-old woman who recently had surgical repair of a broken hip. As you enter the room, you notice that she has removed her oxygen. She is breathing rapidly, and her color is not good. The pulse oximeter shows a saturation of 84%. When you try to get the patient to wear the oxygen, she screams at you to get out of the room.

8. Does the patient have a legal right to refuse in this case? Cite evidence from the text to justify your answer.

9. How would you respond to this situation?

10. Would physical restraints be an option or a possible case of battery?

WHAT ABOUT ETHICS?

No, I haven't forgotten about ethics (although this subject *is* less clear-cut than the legal issues). The law sets minimum standards that we all must try to follow. Ethics, on the other hand, are a set of guidelines for doing your job in a way that is morally defensible. The problem is not that there are a lot of people out working in health care who are immoral but rather that the presence of ethical dilemmas is one no one can avoid.

Start at the Beginning

The most famous ethical code in medicine is the Hippocratic oath. Respiratory therapist's have a code of ethics that was developed by the AARC. You can find it on page 79 in *Egan's*.

Do No Harm versus Save Lives

When two or more "right" choices are in direct conflict, an ethical dilemma exists. A hot topic in medicine and government right now involves how we end our lives, or "assisted suicide." On one hand, we don't want people to suffer needlessly. Watching a terminally ill patient suffer is a sad and demoralizing experience for respiratory therapists. On the other hand, taking someone's life is an equally difficult decision with far-ranging consequences (some of which could be legal). Reducing these issues to simple rules and formulas is not easy, perhaps not even possible. Every ethical principle involves two parts: professional duty and patient rights.

CASE STUDIES

Case 1

A 17-year-old male, is admitted for pneumonia. This young man is depressed and has expressed thoughts of ending his life if "my worst fears are true about this illness." Laboratory studies reveal that the patient is HIV positive. His physician expresses concern to the other caregivers about revealing the patient's diagnosis to him.

11. Under what circumstances can you lie (or not tell the truth) to patients?

12. What are your feelings about telling the truth to patients?

13. What would you do if the patient asks you if he has AIDS?

Ethical decision-making model

Let's apply the ethical decision-making model to Case 1 (see page 86, Box 5-2, in your text). Write your answer in the spaces provided.

14. What is the problem or issue in this case?

15. Who are the individuals involved?

16. What ethical principle(s) apply here?

17. Who should make the decision to tell the patient?

18. What is your role as a respiratory therapist who is giving treatments to this patient?

19. Are there short-term consequences to either decision? Long-term consequences?

20. Make the decision! (What would you do?)

21. How would you proceed after you made your choice?

Case 2

A respiratory therapist, is a deeply religious individual who has strong feelings about homosexuality. When he is assigned to provide therapy for an openly homosexual patient, he objects to the supervisor saying, "I do not want to take care of him. It is against my religious principles. Assign someone else."

22. What are some of the possible problems for the respiratory department that could arise out of this situation?

23. Patients are allowed to refuse even life-sustaining treatment for religious reasons. What about professional caregivers?

24. What would you do if you were the supervisor?

I would rather be the man who bought the Brooklyn Bridge than the man who sold it.
Will Rogers

CHAPTER HIGHLIGHTS

Identify seven key points from Chapter 5. Complete the following questions by writing the correct term(s) in the blank(s) provided.

25. Ethical _____ occur when there are two equally desirable or undesirable outcomes.

26. Professional codes of ethics are general guidelines to identify _____ behavior.

27. The two basic ethical theories are _____ and _____.

28. _____ law deals with the relationships of private parties and the government.

29. Professional _____ is negligence in which a professional has failed to provide the _____ expected, resulting in _____ to someone.

30. Practitioners must carry out their duties with an eye toward _____ themselves in the case of _____ action.

31. A(n) _____ act defines who can perform specified duties in health care. The purpose of _____ is to provide for the public's safety.

WHAT DOES THE NBRC SAY?

Sorry, but ethics and legal issues aren't really a part of your examinations to obtain a license to practice respiratory care. Considering the case of a respiratory therapist in California accused of so-called "mercy killings," though perhaps these areas should be on the test!

FOOD FOR THOUGHT

A relatively new law that affects all health care workers is called HIPAA. The Health Insurance Portability and Accountability Act of 1996 was not actually ready for enforcement until 2002. HIPAA provides for both civil and criminal penalties for violations. Respiratory therapist students can get into trouble in many ways besides simply breaching confidentiality, which is now a part of HIPAA.

32. You are asked to do a clinical case study by your instructor. What is PHI? What things do you think you should take out of the case to avoid identifying the patient to others?

Want more information? Visit one of the following Web sites:
www.hhs.gov/ocr/hipaa/
www.HIPAA.org

Don't worry that *Egan's* didn't spend too much time on HIPAA. We all have to receive additional training in this area each year. You'll get a lot of detailed information but the bottom line has never changed: Keep your lips zipped about the patients. Period.

Here is another thought for you. I am sure you know about the living will and the idea that people make a choice in advance about care during emergencies. We ask them when they are admitted. Here's the question, though: do you have a living will or advanced directive? Try asking around and see if your instructors have one or the respiratory therapists at clinic. You might be surprised . . .

INFORMATION AGE

Here is a helpful Web site for further research:

Karolinska Institute in Stockholm	www.mic.ki.se/Diseases/k1.316.html	This dynamic site is a storehouse of links to hundreds of others on almost every topic in medical ethics from biomedicine to malpractice. It is probably the only site you'll need to find up-to-date information on ethics.

6 Physical Principles of Respiratory Care

Mrs. Peter's Law:
Today if you're not confused you're just not thinking clearly.

Irene Peter

Physics is a subject that everyone (everyone normal, that is!) struggles to understand. The purpose of this chapter is to help you figure out what is important and how to apply the information. You don't have to be a rocket scientist to understand the physical principles of respiratory care. We are applied scientists, after all, so the secret to physics is to find examples, analogies, and experiments that help you understand the rules.

WORD WIZARD

Words are the keys that open up your mind so you can start to learn a difficult subject. After you read *Egan's*, you will be able to put the right words into the blanks. There's a lot to this chapter, so I'll emphasize the materials I think you might need to know for your examinations.

Complete the following paragraph by writing the correct terms in the blanks provided.

Yes, but It's a Dry Heat...

Without humidity, our airways get irritated and mucus gets thick and nasty. The actual amount, or weight, of water vapor

in a gas is called _____ humidity. As respiratory therapists, we compare the weight of water vapor to the amount it could hold if the gas was fully saturated. This ratio of content to capacity is known as

_____ humidity. You hear about this on the weather report every day. I'm more interested in how

much vapor gas can hold inside the airways. This amount is called percent _____ humidity. When

inspired gas has less than 100% of its capacity, a humidity _____ exists. Humidifiers are used to

make up the difference. When you get a can of icy soda on a hot day, water droplets begin to form on the outside of the can. That's because the air around the can is cooling (everyone knows cold air does not hold as much water vapor

as warm air). When air cools, and gaseous water returns to a liquid form, we say that _____
has occurred. The opposite effect occurs when the drink sits out. Water molecules escape from the liquid into the air.

This process is called _____ and adds to the humidity in the air.

Some Like It Hot...

Heat moves in mysterious ways—four of them, to be precise. Newborn babies are especially sensitive to heat loss. Keeping a preemie warm can make the difference between life and death! When babies are born, we dry them off to

prevent loss through _____.

Then the little one is wrapped in cloth to prevent _____, or loss that occurs when you are touching a cooler object. Finally, we put the tyke in an incubator. The incubator provides warmth in two ways. First, a

special light _____ heat toward the baby. Second, warm air blows into the incubator. Transfer of heat through movement of fluids (or gas) is called _____.

OBEY THE LAWS

Remember the bumper sticker: "Gravity: it's not just a good idea, it's the law!"? Gases have to follow the laws of physics, too. Because respiratory therapists work with different gases, like oxygen, nitrogen, carbon dioxide, and helium, it's important that you know the laws and how gases behave. This section provides some real examples of gas laws in action. In the space provided, identify which law is being demonstrated.

Example 1
A registered pulmonary function technologist (RPFT) is performing lung testing on a patient. The patient inhales 1.5 L from the spirometer.

1. What will happen to the volume of gas inside the patient's lungs? _____

_____

2. What is the gas law? _____

Example 2
A home care respiratory therapist places an oxygen cylinder in the van so that she can take it to a client's house. The sun is shining through the window on the cylinder.

3. What will happen to the pressure inside the cylinder as it gets warmer? _____

_____

4. What is the gas law? _____

Example 3
When you start to inhale, your diaphragm drops and your chest expands. In other words, you increase the size, or volume, of your chest.

5. What happens to the pressure inside your chest? _____

_____

6. What is the gas law? _____

TRY IT, YOU'LL LIKE IT!

Here are some safe, easy experiments you can perform in the lab at school or at home.

Experiment 1
Place a dry, empty *glass* soda bottle in the freezer for at least 15 minutes. Take the bottle out and *immediately* cover the mouth of the bottle with a balloon. Wait a few minutes and watch!

7. What happened to the balloon? _____

8. What gas law is responsible for the result? _____

Experiment 2

Cut a 1-inch strip of notebook paper. Hold one end of the paper to your chin, just below your lip. Blow steadily across the top of the paper.

9. What happened to the paper? _____

10. What principle is responsible for this action? _____

Another experiment that shows this same principle can be accomplished with balloons. Blow up two round balloons and tie them off. Attach about 1 foot of string to each balloon. Tape the string to a stick (like a ruler, or yardstick) so the balloons are about 6 to 8 inches apart. Blow between the balloons.

11. What happened to the balloons? _____

Experiment 3

Get a coffee stirrer, an ordinary straw, and a big straw (like the kind you use for a milkshake). Now get a couple of cups. Put some water in one cup. Put some honey in another. (I put a chocolate shake in the third glass!) Suck the water up through each straw. Now try the honey (and/or the shake). To make this more interesting, get a 6-foot length of oxygen-connecting tubing. Try the two fluids again!

12. Which tube is easiest to suck through? _____

13. Which fluid is easiest to suck up? _____

14. What hard-to-pronounce, French-sounding law explains all this? _____

Because gases and liquids are both fluids, the same rules apply to the inhaling!

CASE STUDIES

Case 1

A respiratory therapist decides to attend the AARC International Congress. To get there, the therapist must travel by air. Before taking off, the flight attendant explains about the oxygen system. The therapist pays attention (unlike everyone else) when he sees the partial rebreathing mask. He also knows that something interesting happens to oxygenation at 30,000 feet.

15. What is the barometric pressure (P_B) and inspired (P_{IO_2}) partial pressure of oxygen at this altitude?

P_B _____

P_{IO_2} _____

16. A properly fitting oxygen mask can deliver about 70% oxygen to passengers. What would the P_{IO_2} be while wearing the mask?

_____

17. What gas law did you use to make these conclusions?

_____

Chapter **6** **Physical Principles of Respiratory Care**

Respiratory therapists frequently draw arterial blood samples to measure the partial pressures of oxygen and carbon dioxide in the blood. Many patients have elevated or decreased body temperatures.

18. What effect does a fever have on these partial pressure readings?

_____

19. A normal arterial carbon dioxide pressure ($Paco_2$) is 40 mm Hg (torr) at a body temperature of 37° C. Estimate the new $Paco_2$ if body temperature was 40° C.

20. Why is temperature correction of arterial blood gas readings controversial?

MATHEMATICS

You must be able to perform calculations in the clinical setting and on board examinations. Chapter 6 gave several examples of problems found in both settings. Write the formula, and then solve the following problems **without using a calculator.** (Because your board examinations do not allow use of electronic calculators, only use a calculator to check your work.) I always write out the formula first and then plug in the numbers to avoid mistakes, but I am mathematically challenged. If you're good at it, just skip this step.

21. Convert 30° C to degrees Kelvin.

    Formula _____

    Solution _____

    Answer _____

22. Convert 68° F to degrees Celsius.

    Formula _____

    Solution _____

    Answer _____

23. Convert 40° C to degrees Fahrenheit.

Formula _____

Solution _____

Answer _____

24. At body temperature, gas has a saturated capacity of about 44 mg of water vapor per liter. If a gas has an absolute humidity of 22 mg/L, what is the relative humidity?

Formula _____

Solution _____

Answer _____

25. What is the humidity deficit in Question 24?

Formula _____

Solution _____

Answer _____

26. Convert a pressure reading of 10 millimeters of mercury (mm Hg) to centimeters of water (cm H_2O).

Formula _____

Solution _____

Answer _____

27. Convert a pressure reading of 10 centimeters of water (cm H_2O) to kilopascals (kPa). Hint: It's okay to round off.

Formula _____

Solution _____

Answer _____

28. Air is normally about 21% oxygen. Calculate the partial pressure of oxygen in air (PIO_2) when the barometric pressure is 760 mm Hg.

Formula _____

Solution _____

Answer _____

29. Now calculate the new P_{IO_2} that would result if the barometric pressure is 500 mm Hg.

Formula _____

Solution _____

Answer _____

FOOD FOR THOUGHT

Math may be hard for some of us (like me). Getting good at it can make the difference between success and failure on the board exams! Pay special attention to the sections "Obey the Laws" and "Mathematics" and the two case studies because this is the area you'll need to focus on for credentialing.

INFORMATION AGE

Physical principles can be hard to grasp, because you can't always see them in action. There are dozens of Web sites posted by science teachers to help students better understand gas laws and physics. Here's a good place to start:

Multimedia Educational Resource for Learning and Online Teaching (MERLOT)	www.merlot.org/merlot/index.htm	A collection of resources for teaching and learning. I used their ideal gas law simulation.
University of Oregon Department of Physics	jersey.uoregon.edu/vlab/Piston/	This one has a cool chamber where you control the variables to perform gas law experiments. "Vlab" stands for virtual laboratory, and there are very clear instructions on how to work the experiments. Pretty good fun!

7 Computer Applications in Respiratory Care

The real danger is not that computers will begin to think like humans, but that humans will begin to think like computers.

Sydney Harris

Let's face it, we are living in the "Information Age." Microprocessor technology is part of everyday life in the intensive care unit (ICU), respiratory therapists use computers to chart at most clinical sites, and you can download medical podcasts to keep up to date. If you can learn to use these tools effectively, you will be a more effective respiratory therapist. Will this give you more free time? Probably more free time to use the computer!

WORD WIZARD

Most of the words that describe computers are not even in the dictionary yet. If you want to travel the information highway, you will need to be able to talk the talk. Let's get started with a few key terms.

Complete the following paragraphs by writing the correct term in the blank provided.

Computereze

The most common computers in use today are personal computers. Desktops, laptops, and handhelds are all commonly

used. In each case you need software applications. We write a procedure using _____

processing programs. My students learn to make presentations using _____. When a manager

wants to make a budget, a(n) _____ program like Excel is useful. Your state respiratory

society might keep member records in a _____ base program for easier retrieval of information in organized chunks.

Talk to Me!

Computers can talk to each other through local network inside the hospital, or they can go outside the institution. The

global network of computer networks is called _____. Inside the hospital, a similar network called the

_____ serves as a conduit for information. If you want to go surfing, you've got to come to

Hawaii or you can navigate using the _____.

COMPUTERS IN HEALTH CARE

Clinicians use computers to help interpret data, reach a diagnosis, and automate certain aspects of patient care. Now you need to open your textbook and look up some information about this subject. Fill in your answers in the space provided.

1. Give five examples of patient data that might be stored in the HIS and useful to the respiratory therapist.

    A. _____

    B. _____

    C. _____

    D. _____

    E. _____

2. In addition to staffing and billing, how do respiratory therapists use the RCMIS?

3. What are the advantages of wireless handheld systems? List three.

   A. _____

   B. _____

   C. _____

4. What is the difference between an open and a closed loop in a mechanical ventilator's software?

5. In the near future, health care providers will expand into several emerging areas. Tell us a little more about these four emerging applications of information technology. How will respiratory therapists use technology to better care for patients?

   A. Tobacco cessation: _____

   _____

   _____

   B. Telemedicine: _____

   _____

   _____

   C. Electronic health records: _____

   _____

   _____

   D. Disease management: _____

   _____

   _____

GARBAGE IN, GARBAGE OUT

Fill in your answers in the spaces provided.

The ability to find information and sort out the good from the bad is one thing that identifies the best medical practitioners in our modern age. Evidence-based medicine is our best tool to improve practice and we find the evidence using information technology.

6. Who was Cochrane and what did he collect? _____

_____

7. Google may be lovely for routine stuff, but you can get more from Google Scholar. Give one pro and one con for this site.

   A. Pro _____

   B. Con _____

8. What happens to a search engine like Google when you

   A. Use the term "AND"? _____

   B. "Define"? _____

   C. "Refine" _____

   D. "..." _____

9. Ovid was a Greek philosopher, or something like that! What is OVID and why would you use it?

   A. What is it? _____

   B. Why use it? _____

CASE STUDIES

Case 1

A technical director for a respiratory department in a large urban medical center knows that asthma mortality is on the rise. He wants to find out information about patients admitted to the emergency department with asthma and what happened to them. He wants to develop a report on the subject to present to administration and plans to develop an asthma education program that will require a budget for equipment, personal, and training materials.

10. What type of software program is most useful for gathering specific information on patient populations?

_____

11. What program will the director use to help prepare the budget for his project?

_____

12. What kind of software will he use to prepare the written report for administration?

_____

13. When the technical director decides to present his findings to the board of directors, he'll probably want to use some presentation software. What is the most common one?

_____

Case 2

A respiratory care student is asked by her instructor to locate the URL for the American Association for Respiratory Care (AARC) so she can access information on Clinical Practice Guidelines (CPGs).

14. What does the term URL mean? _____

_____

15. What are the three major components of an URL?

A. _____

B. _____

C. _____

16. Identify the three components of the URL for AARC.

A. _____

B. _____

C. _____

17. What action can you take to avoid having to write down or remember the URL for sites you wish

to revisit? _____

_____

PRACTICE MAKES PERFECT!

It isn't good enough to just talk the talk. Now you have to walk the walk!

You will need a computer with access to the World Wide Web so you can practice some of the skills discussed in the text. Most colleges will provide a free e-mail account for students and have wireless hot spots and computers with Web access. If your college does not, you can try your local Internet café, or go to the public library!

Activity 1: Information Search

Access

You will need a computer that has a Web browser like Netscape Navigator or Microsoft Explorer to get started. After you open the browser, enter Yahoo's URL. Select the top heading "Health." Pick one of the topics that relates to respiratory care and spend some time browsing.

Conduct a search

Start up your browser and go to www.google.com. Of course, you can go to competing sites like ask.com or use Yahoo, Netscape, AOL, or any of the others. Now you can enter a keyword or phrase to look for information on a specific topic. Initially, it is alright to use natural language such as "asthma causes" or "what causes asthma" as a keyword. You may find too much information and need to narrow your search. Box 7-1 on page 127 of your text contains examples of Boolean operators, or special ways to refine searches. For example, try "asthma AND causes." When you find a site or an article that looks worthwhile, bookmark the URL for future reference.

Personally, I like to use Google (www.google.com), now considered the top search engine, for ordinary stuff. But watch out because Internet-savvy librarians estimate that between 80% and 90% of all the information on the Web is NONSCIENTIFIC and NONEDUCATIONAL! The first few things that pop up are usually provided by paying sponsors, but that's the price of the Web, so move on and refine your search.

Activity 2: Evaluate!

Not all the information on the Internet is reliable. There is a lot of "junk science," amateur material, and sales and marketing you will have to sort through to get worthwhile information. Once you have found a Web site that contains the information you want, you can test it!

Find a Web site now, and answer these simple questions:

Site: _____

- Is it clear who is sponsoring the page? Look at the URL. Does the address end in "edu" or "gov"? These sites tend to be more reliable than the ".com" URL sites. In any case, it should be very clear who is sponsoring the page.
- Can you verify the legitimacy of the sponsor? Look for a telephone number or address for more information, not just an e-mail address.
- Is it clear who wrote the material (and the author's qualifications)?
- Is the information free of spelling, grammar, and typographical errors?
- Is the information free of advertising?
- Are there dates on the page to indicate when the material was written or revised?
- Is it clearly stated when data or statistical information was collected?

The more "YES" answers you got, the more reliable is the information! Refer to Table 7-3 on page 130 for more information on evaluating Web sites.

Activity 3: Respiratory Care!

In this exercise, you will locate a specific document from the AARC's web site.
- Open the AARC home page (www.aarc.org).
- Click on "Resources" and find the section on Clinical Practice Guidelines (CPGs).
- Open the guideline on pulse oximetry.
- Print this guideline and use it as a study reference. Why? One reason is the reliability of this material. Another good reason is that the National Board for Respiratory Care says in its newsletter: "CPGs" are a valuable tool for preparing for board examinations.

How about that! I think the AARC Web site is the single most useful resource for students and practitioners on the World Wide Web.

Portions of the AARC Web site are only accessible to members of the association. You can gain full access by joining. All respiratory students are eligible for free AARC memberships if their faculty belong and sign you up. If you do not have a free membership, you can join up for less than the cost of French fries—about $0.20 per day.

Copyright © 2009, 2003, 1999 by Mosby, Inc., an affiliate of Elsevier Inc.

FOOD FOR THOUGHT

It is easy to learn how to use the computer for more than just games. Besides the activities listed earlier, you may want to try the following:

- Locate the home page for your college.

- If your program has a Web site, locate it and print the home page or find some specific information from the page. If you do not have a page, find one from another program. These sites are easily accessed from the AARC Web site. (You can find my program at www.kcc.hawaii.edu. Click on "programs" and then "Respiratory Care Practitioner.")

- If you do not have a program Web site, design one as a class project. Ask your media or learning center to provide skills and access to the campus server. With the new software available, anyone can learn to make a Web site.

- If your college offers e-mail accounts for students, get the entire class to sign up. Create an address list for the class, and send messages via e-mail. Ask your instructors to e-mail assignments, class syllabus, etc. (Save the trees!)

- Search any of the Web sites in Table 7-1 on page 126 in the textbook. Find a specific article, protocol, practice guideline, or other information that can be linked to a class activity or a personal need. For example, GOLD has diagnostic criteria and treatment plans for COPD. You could use this to help write a report or complete a journal assignment. The NBRC, www.nbrc.org, has your examination blueprint and practice board exams! For free!

- Visit the Evolve site available with *Egan's:* http://evolve.elsevier.com/Wilkins/Egans. Evolve is an interactive learning environment designed to work in coordination with your text. Your instructors may use Evolve to provide an Internet-based course component that reinforces and expands the concepts presented in class. Even if your instructor hasn't incorporated Evolve into your course, you may access a list of helpful weblinks to sites of interest on the Web. You can also access an NBRC exam cross-reference of the content in *Egan's* to the exam matrices for the CRT and RRT exams.

A FINAL THOUGHT

PDAs, or personal digital assistants, are great tools for students and therapists alike. I have an inexpensive PDA (under $100) that has the usual calendars, games, phonebook, and all that jazz. I have added several VERY USEFUL medical applications. All of them were free downloads! For example, I have a program that allows me look up almost any drug and check doses, costs, side effects, etc. I have a blood gas calculator, Henderson-Hasselbach calculator, peak flow and PFT norms, you name it. Lots of my students buy PDAs because there is no better digital tool. Plus it fits in your lab coat pocket. Check out Table 7-2 on page 130 of your text to find out where you can get a ton of free and useful software.

8 | The Respiratory System

Anatomy is destiny.
Sigmund Freud

Remember anatomy? It was one of those required courses, the one where you memorized a lot of body parts. It turns out that structure and function have a lot to do with each other. Anatomy even has clinical applications! In this chapter, we bring anatomy back to life (sounds like Dr. Frankenstein). Before we go there, I just want to check and see if you still remember some important terms that relate to the anatomy of the respiratory system.

WORD WIZARD

Boy, *Egan's* really puts the key in "key terms" in this chapter. It's like learning a new language. Perhaps I can help you translate some of the more important words. Fill in either the key term or the definition in the space provided. The first one is completed for you.

	MEDICAL TERMINOLOGY	IN PLAIN LANGUAGE, PLEASE
A.	Alveoli	Tiny air sacs for gas exchange
B.		Place where trachea splits into R and L
C.	Cilia	
D.		Primary muscle of breathing
E.	Epiglottis	
F.		Hole that opens into your windpipe
G.	Hilum	
H		Voicebox
I.	Pharynx	
J.		Wrapping that lines the lungs
K.	Sternum	
L.		Windpipe

JUST LIKE DEAR OLD DAD

I don't know about you, but I wasn't all that happy to inherit my dad's hairline, or my mom's asthma, for that matter. You just can't hide from your family ties. Several very important pulmonary conditions find their origins in our genetics. Cystic fibrosis is the most famous example, but even emphysema and lung cancer have genetic components. Lung cancer therapies are being tailored to individual genetics. It is important for the respiratory therapist to find out about family health when making assessments or taking the pulmonary history. The National Board for Respiratory Care (NRBC) board exams agree.

47

FETAL FACTS

Respiratory therapists take care of a wide range of patients, from the tiniest preemie to elderly adults. That means you need to know about the ways in which lungs grow and develop.

1. During what stage and week of development is alveolar capillary surface area considered sufficient to support extrauterine life?

   A. Stage: _____

   B. Week: _____

2. What is the primary organ of gas exchange for the fetus? _____
   _____

3. Describe the umbilical cord blood vessels.

4. The fetus lives in a relatively hypoxic environment. What is considered to be a major factor that enables the fetus to survive under these conditions? _____
   _____

5. About half of the blood entering the right atrium is shunted to the left atrium via what structure?
   _____

6. Why is fetal pulmonary vascular resistance so high?

7. What percentage of blood entering the pulmonary artery actually flows through the lungs? Where does the rest of the blood go?

8. Describe the events that occur in the first few breaths after birth in terms of transpulmonary pressure, blood gases, and circulatory changes.

9. Compare the number of alveoli in newborns and adults.

_____

THEY AREN'T JUST LITTLE ADULTS

10. Let's compare the head and upper airway of adults and babies. Check out Figure 8-10 if you get lost.

	ANATOMY	INFANT	ADULT
A.	Head		
B.	Tongue		
C.	Nasal passages		
D.	Larynx		
E.	Narrow point		
F.	Dead space		
G.	Airways		

11. Describe the breathing pattern of a normal infant.

12. Why is the FRC of the baby different than that of the adult?

13. What is grunting and what does it mean?

14. Why do infants experience severe hypoxemia more readily than do adults?

A PICTURE IS WORTH

Rather than talk about adult anatomy, there's something else I want you to do. Identify the structures in these figures.

15. What's in a chest? Write your answers on the indicated lines in the figure.

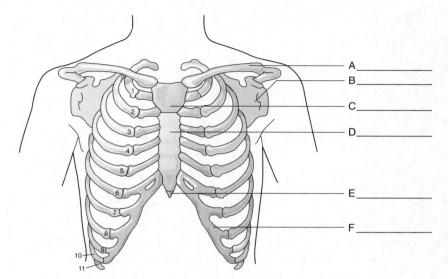

A_____
B_____
C_____
D_____

E_____

F_____

Anterior view of the bones of the thorax. (From Hicks GH: Cardiopulmonary anatomy and physiology, Philadelphia, 2000, WB Saunders.)

Pneumopnuggets

When you put your stethoscope just below the clavicle (in the front!), you are listening over the upper lobes. You can also see that the lower lobes are not really on the front of the chest at all. There's a little on the side, but mostly they are in the back. If you know your locations, your auscultation improves. If you look at the location of the apices, you will see they are *above* the clavicle. So if someone inserts a subclavian line, the lung could get punctured in the process!

16. Imagination 1

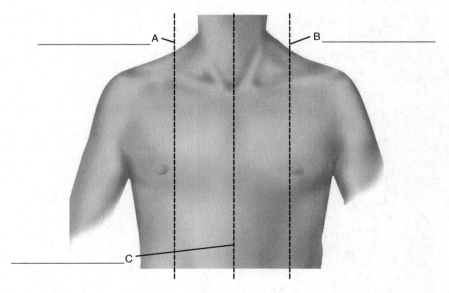

A
B _____

_____ C

Imaginary lines on the anterior chest wall.

17. Imagination 2

A _____

B _____

Posterior axillary
line

Imaginary lines on the lateral chest wall.

Pneumopnuggets

You could use these imaginary lines for a couple of things. First, when you perform a 12-lead ECG on a patient, you use the lines to line up the electrodes (plus counting the ribs). The lines are also good if you notice something unusual (like a scar or a lesion) and want to document where it is located.

18. Pump me up

A _____
_____
_____

D _____

Internal
intercostal

B _____

C _____

Sternum

Transverse abdominus

E _____

Internal obliques

F _____

G _____

The muscles of
ventilation.

Pneumopnuggets

Watch closely when someone breathes. Start with someone normal, like a kid. See the belly move out on inspiration. That's diaphragmatic breathing. See the relaxed exhalation. That's normal. A good place to see people breathe wrong (besides the hospital) is a shopping mall! Lots of people use their accessory muscles to breathe. The chest, especially the upper chest, moves on inspiration, but there is no outward excursion of the abdomen. When we get into distress or exercise really hard, you will see the abdominal group come into play to force exhalation. Sharpen your assessment skills by watching the *anatomy* of breathing.

19.   What's up, doc?

Structures of the upper airway and oral cavity.

Pneumopnuggets

Look at the nasopharynx. You'll be sticking tubes in there. It's fun if you know your anatomy. Notice that it goes straight back (a short distance) and then drops down into the oropharynx. When you insert a catheter or an airway, don't go straight back (very far)—aim downward. Stay midline along the septum or you'll ram the turbinates (ouch!). In this cross-sectional view, it's easy to see how that big fat tongue could block the airway if it falls back.

20. "Adam's apple"

Anterior view of the larynx.

Pneumopnuggets

The thyroid cartilage sticks out on guys. So find a guy, and go for the throat. Palpate the thyroid cartilage. Feel the front and the sides. Now move your finger down (just a little) from the big bump on the front. Feel the soft spot? That's the cricothyroid membrane. (You might learn how to do a cricothryotomy in school.) The cartilage just below that is the cricoid, the trachea's only complete ring. Keep going and feel the rings of the trachea. Gently (!) grasp the whole box in your fingers and wiggle it back and forth. It's supposed to be mobile! Now ask your victim, I mean friend, to swallow while you keep your fingers on the thryoid cartilage. What happened?

21. See Cilia

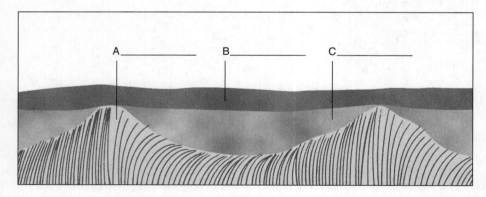

Respiratory cilia.

Pneumopnuggets

Your airway makes more than 100 ml of mucus every day. Where does it all go? Without good ciliary function, where would it go? Drugs (like smoking tobacco, for instance) can impair ciliary function. Hot or toxic gases (like smoking, for instance!) can destroy cilia. There are diseases that involve the cilia, too!

22. You can call me Al

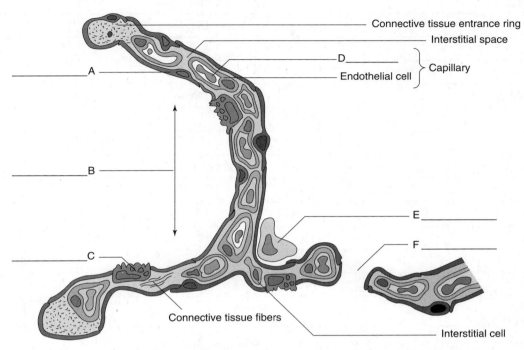

Cross-sectional sketch of the cells and organization of the alveolar septa. (From Hicks GH: Cardiopulmonary anatomy and physiology, Philadelphia, 2000, WB Saunders.)

Pneumopnuggets

These buggers are small! The distance from alveoli to blood is only about 0.2 microns. (Remember, there's 1000 microns in a millimeter!) Oxygen has less than 1 second to cross this distance and combine with the RBCs. So anything, like the fluid from pulmonary edema, that increases this distance will impair gas exchange.

There are about 300 million alveoli in an adult lung. If you flatten them out, the area would be the size of a tennis court (a pretty delicate one).

LOBES AND SEGMENTS

Students are always dismayed when they have to learn postural drainage and find out the lungs have 5 different lobes and 18 individual segments. It's not so hard when you know there are some duplicates and break the whole thing down into little pieces. Fill in the chart on the following page. You can make your own version of this and fill it in until you get them memorized. This will really help you with postural drainage. Notice that the left lung only has 8 segments, even though they are numbered 1 through 10. Refer to Table 8-8 on page 183 of your text for help.

55

	RIGHT LUNG		**LEFT LUNG**
	Right Upper Lobe		Left Upper Lobe
1			Upper Division
2		1 and 2	
3		3	
	Right Middle Lobe		Lower Division (Lingula)
4		4	
5		5	
	Right Lower Lobe		Left Lower Lobe
6		6	
7		7 and 8	
8		9	
9		10	
10			

MEET THE OBJECTIVES

We've covered most of the material in Chapter 8. Here is some more information that is important to know about the respiratory system.

23. Name the nerves that innervate the diaphragm, intercostal muscles, and larynx. State the origin of these nerves and describe what will happen if they are damaged.

   A. _____

   B. _____

   C. _____

24. Describe the pathway gas follows as it is conducted through the lower airway. Use Table 8-7 on page 181 of your text as a guide.

CHAPTER HIGHLIGHTS

Identify eight key points from Chapter 8. Complete the following questions by writing the correct term(s) in the blank(s) provided.

25. The _____ houses and protects the lungs.

26. The _____ is the primary muscle of ventilation.

27. The upper respiratory tract _____ and _____ inspired air and protects the lungs against _____ substances.

28. The lower respiratory tract _____ gases from the upper airway to the respiratory _____ of the lung.

29. The airways branch into _____, which are in turn made up of _____ in both the left and right lungs.

30. The respiratory bronchioles and _____ provide a large _____ for exchange of gases between air and blood.

31. Fetal _____ and _____ differ markedly from those functions in the postnatal period.

32. Closure of the _____ and ductus _____ are important events in the transition from intrauterine to extrauterine life.

CASE STUDIES

Case 1

A cruel respiratory instructor forces the students to learn the anatomy of the lung. Completely by coincidence, the instructor slips while running with scissors, and the sharp shears puncture his right chest. The students gather around their fallen facilitator to discuss the anatomic consequences of this tragedy.

33. What would happen to the lung on the affected side? _____

_____

34. What would happen to the pleural space on the affected side? _____

_____

35. What is this condition called? _____

36. What is the treatment for this condition? _____

A respiratory therapist is working the night shift at a large urban medical center. As he makes his rounds, he hears loud snoring coming from a patient's room. Even though snoring is a commonly heard sound at night, the respiratory therapist stops to investigate.

37. What anatomic change results in snoring?

38. What is OSA, and how is it treated?

39. What is the similarity between snorers and unconscious victims who require resuscitation?

40. How would you approach management of the airway of an unconscious person?

WHAT DOES THE NBRC SAY?

Respiratory anatomy is not on the boards, but the applications we've been using in this chapter are part of the test. For example, you'll probably see several questions about pneumothorax. But that's not all, folks. Airway management, assessment, and electrocardiography are all areas on the boards that incorporate anatomy into questions. An endotracheal tube may be seen at the level of the aortic knob on a radiograph, lead IV is placed on the midclavicular line, and the leaf-shaped cartilage seen on intubation is the epiglottis. You get the idea. I'll give you more questions in the appropriate chapters.

FOOD FOR THOUGHT

I hope you had fun with your lungs today. Lung function is pretty miraculous when you think about all the parts that have to be working together to make ventilation and respiration successful. What happens to these structures when disease is present?

41. What happens to the airways and alveoli when a patient is having an acute episode of asthma?

42. What changes to the airways and alveoli occur in emphysema?

INFORMATION AGE

A quick search of the Web produced over 80,000 hits on "pulmonary anatomy." These range from simple overviews such as www.methodisthealth.com/pulmonary/anatomy.htm to more complex information from the excellent Virtual Hospital Web site (www.vh.org). Alas, Virtual Hospital is gone, but the files live on. The anatomy files are excellent.

The National Lung Health Education Project also has lung anatomy, and this is good for beginners and patient education (www.nlhep.org).

9 The Cardiovascular System

What the heart knows today, the head will understand tomorrow.
James Stephens

Your heart beats, on average, about 38 million times in 1 year! (I wish I could get a fuel pump for my car that works that well.) No matter how well the respiratory system works to exchange gas with the blood, it would be meaningless without the heart pushing that blood out to the organs via the vascular system. Those blood vessels are the best transportation network in the world, constantly reacting to the need for more or less flow of nutrients to the tissues.

WORD WIZARD

Because the cardiovascular function is closely connected to the respiratory system, you will meet up with it again and again in the course of your training. The words you learn today will help you throughout your career. Match the terms to the definitions listed below as they apply to respiratory care.

Terms	Definitions
_____ 1. afterload	A. membraneous sac that surrounds the heart
	B. stroke volume multiplied by heart rate
_____ 2. automaticity	C. ventricular stretch provided by end-diastolic volume
_____ 3. baroreceptors	D. biological sensors that monitor arterial blood pressure
_____ 4. cardiac output	E. pathologic narrowing or constriction
	F. force against which the ventricle pumps
_____ 5. chemoreceptors	G. biologic sensors that monitor arterial blood oxygen
	H. ability to initiate a spontaneous electrical impulse
_____ 6. pericardium	
_____ 7. preload	
_____ 8. stenosis	

MEET THE OBJECTIVES

Chapter 9 presented five objectives for learning. How well do you know your cardiovascular system?

9. We all know there are four valves in the heart. Patients commonly have disorders of the mitral valve. Where is it? What is the effect of mitral stenosis on the lung?

10. Explain how specialized tissue allows the muscle cells in the ventricle to contract in a coordinated and efficient manner.

11. Compare and contrast local control of blood vessels with central control mechanisms.

12. Describe how the cardiovascular system responds to exercise and blood loss by balancing blood volume and vascular resistance.

13. Match the mechanical events to their corresponding electrical events in the normal cardiac cycle. (Hint: Take a look at Figure 9-14 on page 213 of your text.)

	ELECTRICAL EVENT	CARDIAC EVENT (MECHANICAL)
A.		
B.		
C.		

CHAPTER HIGHLIGHTS

Identify six key points from Chapter 9. Complete the following questions by writing the correct term(s) in the blank(s) provided.

14. The _____ system consists of the heart and vascular network, which maintain

_____ by regulating the distribution of blood flow in the body.

15. Cardiac _____ is primarily determined by preload, _____,

contractility, and _____.

16. Central control of the vascular system is primarily maintained by the _____ division of the

_____ nervous system.

17. The heart and vascular systems ensure that tissues receive sufficient blood to meet their

_____ needs.

18. Just as faucets control the flow of water into a sink, the _____ control blood flow into the capillaries.

19. Specialized myocardial tissue, such as the _____ fibers, conduct impulses rapidly to ensure synchronous contraction of the ventricles.

CASE STUDIES

Case 1

A 57-year-old patient, is admitted to the coronary care unit with a diagnosis of mitral stenosis. The patient is breathing rapidly and complains of shortness of breath. Her pulse oximetry readings reveal hypoxemia. Auscultation reveals inspiratory crackles in the posterior lower lobes.

20. What is mitral stenosis? _____

21. What mechanical events are occurring to cause pulmonary edema and stiffening of the lung tissue?

22. What action should the respiratory therapist take at this time? _____

_____

Case 2

A respiratory care student is giving an aerosolized bronchodilator to a 27-year-old patient with asthma. Breath sounds reveal bilateral wheezing. The pulse oximeter shows 98% saturation on room air. The student notices the heart rate rising from 82 to 98 during the therapy.

23. What are the effects of sympathetic and parasympathetic stimulation on the sinus node in the heart?

   A. _____

   B. _____

24. Describe the two ways that drugs produce bronchodilation.

A. _____

B. _____

25. Based on this information, why would you expect increased heart rate to be a common side effect of drugs that cause bronchodilation? How much can the heart rate increase before you would consider terminating the treatment?

WHAT DOES THE NBRC SAY?

Cardiac anatomy, like respiratory anatomy, does not have a particular place on the national exams. That doesn't mean it's not important; we just use this material as a foundation for clinical applications like hemodynamics and electrocardiography. Advanced cardiac life support certification course instructors expect you to know cardiac concepts before you try to understand emergency cardiovascular pharmacology. Having said that, there was one item I thought you might like to check out.

Circle the best answer for the following question.

26. A patient has a heart rate of 70 beats per minute and a stroke volume of 60 ml with each ejection of the ventricle. What is the approximate cardiac output in liters per minute?
A. 3.6 L/min
B. 4.2 L/min
C. 5.0 L/min
D. 6.0 L/min

FOOD FOR THOUGHT

27. What four mechanisms combine to aid in promoting venous return to the heart?

A. _____

B. _____

C. _____

D. _____

28. What is meant by the "thoracic pump"? What effect does positive pressure ventilation, like IPPB, have on venous return to the chest?

INFORMATION AGE

CTSnet.org is a site sponsored by the cardiac and thoracic surgical societies. It has basic and in-depth information. Like pulmonary anatomy, there are tons of other Web sites on this topic. The Internet is a good place to look for specialized information on the heart and heart disease.

10 Ventilation

Keep breathing.
Sophie Tucker

Chapter 10 is only 21 pages long; 21 pages that are loaded with heavy-duty information. Our challenge is to sort out what is important to remember, learn the basic principles, and make the knowledge connect to what is clinically important. If you're like me, you'll have to read this chapter two or three times to get the big picture!

WORD WIZARD

I want to start off by emphasizing the difference between *ventilation* and *respiration*. Complete the following paragraph by filling in the correct term(s) in the blank(s) provided.

Remember that the primary purpose of the lung is to supply the body with oxygen and remove wastes in the form

of carbon dioxide. _____ is the process of moving air in and out of the lungs.

Some of that ventilation is _____ space, or wasted ventilation. When CO_2 builds up in the body, the pH of blood decreases, resulting in a state of acidosis. We can measure the amount of air that moves in and out with a device called a spirometer. The pressure changes in the chest are measured using a body box,

or _____. Finally, the actual rate of air flow is measured using a(n) _____.

Airway _____ is a measurement of how much pressure it takes to push the gas through the

conducting air passages. _____, or the distensibility (a fancy way to say stretchiness), is the change in lung volume divided by the pressure needed to take that breath. Stiff lungs increase the work of breathing.

Much of respiratory care is aimed at reducing the work of breathing and restoring adequate ventilation. The process of respiration, on the other hand, is the exchange of gas between blood and other tissues. I'm sure that can wait until Chapter 11.

PICTURE THIS

1. Trans what? Air moves in and out of the chest because of pressure gradients. Label the following diagram to help improve your understanding of these pressure changes.

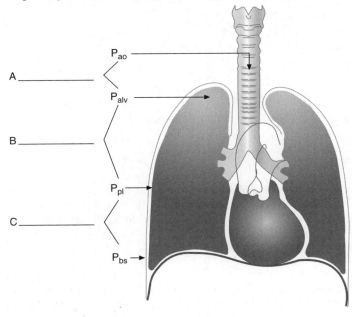

Pressures, volumes, and flows involved in ventilation. (Modified from Martin L: Pulmonary physiology in clinical practice: the essentials for patient care and evaluation, St. Louis, 1987, Mosby.)

65

Write out the definition of each gradient.

A. _____

B. _____

C. _____

Pneumopnuggets

Our ability to generate the necessary pressure changes requires muscle power. Muscles need glucose, oxygen, and nerve innervation (among other things) to work properly. Any clinical condition that requires bigger pressure gradients to move air (like asthma) makes the muscles work harder. Just like when you work out, a pulmonary patient can get muscle fatigue from increased work of breathing.

2. Where has all the ventilation gone? Fill in the missing pressures for the apex and base of the lung.

Causes of regional differences in ventilation from the apex to the base of an upright lung.

3. Where does the bulk of ventilation go during a normal breath in an upright person?

_____

Pneumopnuggets

You can use this information clinically. When a patient has serious unilateral, or one-sided, lung disease (like a bad case of pneumonia), he or she will have poor ventilation in the affected side. Positioning the patient so the good lung is dependent will preferentially increase the ventilation in that lung and away from the bad look. Remember: *Down with the good lung!*

WORK OF BREATHING

It's time to talk about the bottom line. Just like in business. Work of breathing, or WOB, has a definite energy cost. We can measure the metabolic cost in terms of oxygen consumed, and we can reduce the work for patients through our

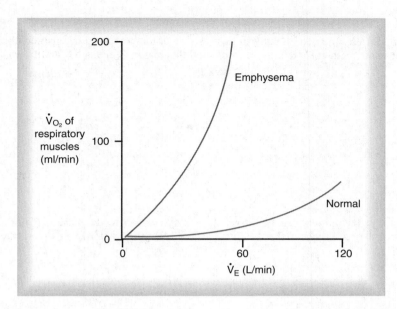

FIGURE 10-1 Relationship of oxygen cost of breathing to minute ventilation for a healthy subject and for a patient with emphysema.

interventions. A healthy person consumes about 250 ml of oxygen per minute. Only 5% of this oxygen is needed to power the muscles of ventilation. The cost goes up about 1 ml for each liter of additional ventilation. Look at what happens to this cost when a patient has emphysema (Figure 10-1).

There are four factors that contribute to WOB: compliance, resistance, active exhalation, and ventilatory pattern. Let's look at each of these separately and talk about strategies for improvement.

Compliance

Compliance is a measure of lung elasticity, or stretchability. It is defined as:

$$\text{Change in volume (liters)} \div \text{Change in pressure (cm } H_2O)$$

A healthy lung is pretty stretchy and compliance is 0.2 L for every cm H_2O of pressure you generate.

However, the lungs sit inside the thorax, which has its own compliance. Completely coincidentally, the compliance of the chest wall is also 0.2 L/cm H_2O! You have to remember that the lung wants to recoil in and the chest wants to spring out, so they are pulling in opposite directions. Mathematically this is like a cancellation, so the net result is a compliance of 0.1 L/cm H_2O for health lungs in a healthy chest. However, if the lungs are overinflated or underinflated, the whole thing changes. You can understand this by trying a simple experiment (I know it is oversimplistic).

Experiment

- Get an ordinary balloon.
- Blow it up a little tiny bit. This is your underinflated lung.
- Blow it up some more. Hard to do, right?
- Now blow it up some more. Pretty easy.
- Now inflate the balloon until it is almost full.
- Blow in some more! Hard to do!

Lungs are a little like this balloon. A patient who has a very low lung volume has to work harder to take a breath than does a person with a normal amount of functional residual capacity. A person with air-trapping (like emphysema) is like the balloon that is overinflated.

Try this for yourself: Take a deep breath. Don't exhale. Now try to breathe in. You get the idea.

Bottom Line

You can move 500 ml of air with 5 cm H_2O pressure. Pretty good!

Questions

4. What interventions can we apply to the lung to increase the amount of residual air (and compliance) in a patient's lungs when they are underinflated? (Hint: you won't find this one in Chapter 10. Try the chapter on lung expansion therapy.)

5. What simple breathing techniques can we apply during exhalation to decrease the amount of residual air in a patient's lungs when they are overinflated? (Hint: optimal breathing patterns for obstructive airway diseases?)

Resistance

Resistance comes in two kinds: tissue and frictional. Tissues have to move when the chest expands. Obesity (outside the lung) and fibrosis (inside the lung) are examples of increased tissue resistance. The really big problem is the frictional resistance created when you move air through your pipes (80% of all resistance). Airway resistance (Raw) is defined as the driving pressure it takes to create a flow of gas. Or to put it mathematically: Raw = Change in pressure (cm H_2O) ÷ Change in flow rate (liters/min). Your upper airway causes most of this resistance. The normal value is 0.5 to 2.5 cm H_2O per liter per second of flow. Conditions like asthma narrow the airways and significantly increase resistance. You can understand this with another simple experiment.

Experiment

- Get a straw and a coffee stirrer (the hollow kind).
- Breathe in and out slowly through the stirrer. Now the straw. Which one is easier?
- Now try putting your lips together and sucking in the air really fast. Feel the work?

Bottom Line

The inner diameter of the airway determines the amount of resistance. (Remember old what's-his-name's law? The French one that is so hard to pronounce. Starts with a P.) If the bronchi decrease from 2 mm to 1 mm in diameter, the resistance increases *16 times!* Your muscles will have to generate a much higher pressure to achieve ventilation if the airway is narrow.

Questions

6. What important changes occur in the airway of an asthmatic patient to increase resistance? (Hint: This one isn't in the chapter either! You'll have to look up the pathophysiology of asthma in the chapter on obstructive lung disease.)

7. What kind of medications can respiratory therapists use to reduce airway resistance in asthma?

_____

Active Exhalation

Normal exhalation is passive. The power comes from energy you stored by stretching the lung and chest during inspiration. When you actively exhale, you have to use your abdominal muscles (and internal intercostals). Remember that additional muscle work takes additional energy. You can actually observe patients using their abdominal muscles when they are in distress and trying to get the air out quicker, or through narrowed airways. You can try this for yourself.

Experiment

- Place your hands on your belly.
- Breathe in.
- Exhale normally.
- Breathe in again. This time, push firmly in with your hands as you exhale. Air moves faster, right?
- Release your hands, and breathe in again. This time, bear down with your abs and blow out hard and fast until your lungs are empty. Feels like work!

Bottom Line

Actively exhaling has a price. When you see a patient doing this, they are either exercising or in distress.

Questions

8. What does it mean when you see active exhalation in your patient?

9. What happens to a person with a spinal cord injury who cannot use their abdominal muscles? (Hint: what other important respiratory activity uses these muscles?)

Ventilatory Pattern

The way you breathe can change the amount of work. In healthy people, a big deep breath increases the elastic part of WOB. Fast breathing increases the frictional work. Healthy people adjust their tidal volume and respiratory rate to minimize the work of breathing during exercise. Our patients exhibit altered patterns, too. Patients with fibrosis (loss of elasticity) breathe with a rapid shallow pattern to reduce the mechanical work of distending the lung. Patients with obstructive diseases like asthma and emphysema need to reduce their rate to reduce work, because they have increased frictional resistance.

Experiment

- Tie something tightly around your upper chest. I use a bathrobe tie. This will restrict chest movement.
- Try breathing faster with shallow breaths.
- Now try to breathe slowly and deeply. Which way feels better?
- Now, untie yourself.
- Get out your straw, or coffee stirrer. Breathe rapidly and shallowly through the tube.
- Now take slow, deep breaths. Which way feels better?

(This is as close as I could get to simulating these two types of conditions.)

Bottom Line

You can learn a lot by observing someone's breathing pattern.

Questions

10. What is the optimal pattern of breathing for patients with obstructive airway diseases?

_____

11. I don't have any more questions, do you?

DEADSPACE

My teachers in respiratory school always said I had cerebral deadspace. I guess they meant that things went in and out of my brain without anything vital being exchanged! Deadspace is, plainly put, wasted ventilation—gas that does not participate in exchange with the blood. You normally waste the first third of each breath, or about 1 ml per pound of ideal body weight. Alveolar deadspace occurs when gas enters the alveoli but no blood comes to pick up the oxygen. A pulmonary embolus (blood clot, fat clot, air bubble, etc.) blocks blood flow to alveoli and causes increased deadspace. Too much (50% to 60% of each breath) deadspace will result in the inability to maintain adequate ventilation through spontaneous breathing. The patient will need mechanical ventilation until the problem improves.

12. Label the types of deadspace in this diagram.

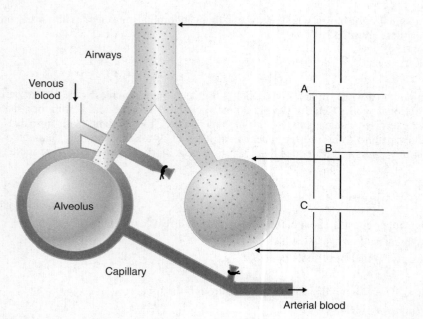

Three types of deadspace.

13. What is the normal range for anatomic deadspace? _____

_____

14. What type of ventilatory pattern will be seen with significantly increased deadspace?

_____

15. What is the difference between *hyperventilation* and *hyperpnea?*

MATHEMATICS

In Chapter 6, I mentioned that math is part of our board examination process and a clinical reality. Don't use a calculator to solve these problems!

16. Calculate exhaled minute ventilation for a patient who has a tidal volume of 800 ml and a frequency of 8 breaths per minute.

    Formula _____

    Calculation _____

    Answer _____

17. Calculate anatomic deadspace for a patient who is 6 feet tall and weighs 180 lb.

    Formula _____

    Calculation _____

    Answer _____

18. Calculate alveolar minute ventilation using the data from problems 1 and 2.

    Formula _____

    Calculation _____

    Answer _____

The NBRC (and everyone else) will expect you to be able to calculate exhaled minute volume, alveolar minute volume, and apply the information. SERIOUSLY, this is always on your boards. Here's a sample.

Circle the best answer for the following multiple-choice questions.

19. The minute volume for a 68-kg (150-lb) patient who has a respiratory rate of 12 and a tidal volume of 600 ml would be
    A. 4800 ml
    B. 5400 ml
    C. 6000 ml
    D. 7200 ml

20. The estimated alveolar minute ventilation for an 82-kg (180-lb) patient who has a respiratory rate of 10 and a tidal volume of 500 ml would be
    A. 3200 ml
    B. 3500 ml
    C. 4800 ml
    D. 5000 ml

21. Which of the following ventilator settings would provide the optimal alveolar ventilation?

	Rate	Volume
A.	10	600
B.	12	500
C.	15	400
D.	20	300

INFORMATION AGE

Strangely enough, http://training.seer.cancer.gov/ has a dynamic section on anatomy and physiology of the entire body. Included in the respiratory system pages http://training.seer.cancer.gov/module_anatomy/unit9_1_resp_intro.html is a whole section on mechanics of ventilation, as well as lots of other goodies. Of course, you can use this site to look at any body system or to learn more about cancer.

11 Gas Exchange and Transport

To Air is human, to Respire divine.
Paul Thackara, RRT

In Chapter 11, we go for it and jump in the deep end (of physiology, that is). I know this will be challenging at first, but when you have mastered the basics of gas transport, you're going to feel exhilarated! It's going to feel great to get a grasp of how gas exchange works and how respiratory therapists apply physiology to patient care.

WORD WIZARD

Let's get on the hemoglobin-oxygen train and take a little ride. First you're going to learn the different names for all those forms that hemoglobin (Hb) takes when it combines. Complete the paragraphs below by filling in the correct term(s) in the blank(s) provided.

All Aboard

It's natural for this complex molecule to want to be in a relationship. Hemoglobin meets oxygen. When they get together,

the new name is _____. Their newfound affinity is likely to end when they meet

up with the _____ effect at the tissue level. So, hemoglobin takes up with
carbon dioxide and we get carbaminohemoglobin. The fickle heme will drop CO_2 off at the lung when they run into the

_____ effect. Life could go on like this, unless our conjugated protein meets up with

a really unusual gas like carbon monoxide. This combination is called _____, and it really

lasts because hemoglobin's affinity for CO is _____ times greater than its affinity for
oxygen.

Why Be Normal?

Not all hemoglobins are created equal. Some are downright unnatural. Abnormal hemoglobins are given letter designations. Complete the paragraph below by filling in the correct term(s) in the blank(s) provided.

HbS, whose common name is _____ _____ hemoglobin, not only
carries on poorly with oxygen but also causes red blood cells to deform and clump together into thrombi. Babies are

born with _____ hemoglobin, which causes a(n) _____ shift of
the curve and makes babies more prone to cyanosis. Sometimes heme is altered in other ways. When the iron compound

is oxidized, we get _____, which causes the blood to turn a brownish color. Poisoning from
nitric oxide is one thing that can cause this transformation of our gas-loving protein.

OXYGEN TRANSPORT

Before oxygen can go to the tissues, it has to get into the alveoli. There is a useful formula for calculating the partial pressure of oxygen (PAo_2) in those little grape-like clusters. True, this equation has never won any popularity contests with students, but it is clinically useful (and can show up on those board exams). So, put on your thinking caps, and we'll show them who's in charge here! The fancy formula looks like this:

$$PAo_2 = Fio_2(Pb - P_{H_2O}) - Paco_2(Fio_2 + 1 - Fio_2/R)$$

We usually simplify this to read:

$$PAO_2 = FIO_2(Pb - 47) - PaCO_2/0.8$$

Or in English . . .

The partial pressure of oxygen in the alveoli is equal to the inspired oxygen percent multiplied by the barometric pressure minus water vapor pressure.

Why?

Dalton's law gives us the first part (partial pressure = concentration × total pressure). Because water vapor in the lung acts like a gas, it takes up space. That's space that oxygen can't occupy.

Next: Subtract arterial CO_2 × a factor.

Why?

What we want to know is how much CO_2 is in the alveoli. (CO_2 takes up space, too.) It's hard to measure; solution: Use a converted arterial value in its place. You don't really need to do this when the patient is breathing a high FIO_2, like 60% or more.

At this point, my students usually ask

Who Cares?

All of this sounds like pulmonary laboratory stuff, except for the fact that we can use this baby to find out how *efficiently* the lungs are at transferring oxygen into the blood by comparing *alveolar PO_2* with *arterial PO_2!* This relationship is called the A − a gradient. A normal A − a gradient is about 5 to 10 mm Hg on room air, or about 10%.

MATHEMATICS

1. Calculate alveolar oxygen tension for a person breathing room air. Assume that barometric pressure is 760 mm Hg, FIO_2 is 21%, and $PaCO_2$ is 40 mm Hg.

   Formula _____

   Solution _____

   Answer _____

2. If the patient in problem 1 has an arterial PO_2 of 90, what is the A − a gradient?

   Formula _____

   Solution _____

   Answer _____

3. Calculate alveolar oxygen tension for a person breathing 60% oxygen (Pb = 760, CO_2 = 40).

   Formula _____

   Solution _____

   Answer _____

4. If the patient in problem 3 has an arterial PO_2 of 90, what is the A − a gradient?

   Formula _____

   Solution _____

   Answer _____

Both patients have identical PaO_2 values of 90 mm Hg. If you only look at PO_2, or only look at oxygen saturation, they appear to be the same.

However, the A − a gradients are very different. The second patient is having serious problems getting oxygen from the lung into the blood. In fact, the patient breathing 60% oxygen should have a PaO_2 of about 340 (PAO_2 − 10%).

"By the Pricking of My Thumbs..."

Everyone loves a good rule of thumb. If you're in a big hurry and don't have a calculator at the bedside, you can try this shortcut. To estimate alveolar P_{O_2} for a patient breathing room air, multiply F_{IO_2} by 5 ($5 \times 20 = 100$). For 40% or more, multiply by 6 ($40 \times 6 = 240$). *Remember,* this only works when the CO_2 is normal. Besides, what respiratory therapist doesn't have a calculator at the bedside?

BARRIERS TO DIFFUSION

5. Do not pass "go" until you pass through the three barriers to diffusion. List them here.

   A. _____

   B. _____

   C. _____

Pneumopnuggets

The partial pressure of a gas is the main driving force across the A-C membrane. Respiratory therapists routinely increase the driving pressure of oxygen by increasing the PA_{O_2}. CO_2 has a much lower driving pressure, but is about 20 times more soluble than O_2, so it has little difficulty in making the journey. In some cases, time can limit diffusion due to increased blood flow. Fever and septic shock are clinical examples.

LET'S GET MOVING!

Once it gets into the blood, oxygen is only transported two ways. First, it dissolves in the plasma. To calculate, dissolve O_2, multiply Pa_{O_2} by 0.003.

$$\text{Dissolved } O_2 = Pa_{O_2} \times 0.003$$

The second way that oxygen is transported is as oxyhemoglobin; 1.34 ml of O_2 binds to each gram of hemoglobin (per 100 ml of blood). If all the hemoglobin carried oxygen, this would be simple, but it doesn't. Remember the anatomic shunt? Hemoglobin saturation is usually less than 100%.

$$\text{Combined } O_2 = 1.34 \times Hb \times \% \text{ saturation}$$

Put them together and what have you got?

$$O_2 \text{ content} = Pa_{O_2} \times 0.003 + 1.34 \times Hb \times \% \text{ saturation}$$

MATHEMATICS

While computers in the hospital will usually calculate content for you, the National Board for Respiratory Care (NBRC) thinks you should be able to do this yourself (and without a calculator)!

6. Calculate oxygen content for Patient 1 with an Hb of 15 g/dl, Sa_{O_2} of 97%, and Pa_{O_2} of 100 mm Hg.

   Formula _____

   Solution _____

   Answer _____

7. Calculate oxygen content for Patient 2 with an Hb of 15 g, Sa_{O_2} of 80%, and Pa_{O_2} of 50 mm Hg.

   Formula _____

   Solution _____

   Answer _____

8. Calculate oxygen content for Patient 3 with a Hb of 10 g, Sao_2 of 97%, and Pao_2 of 100 mm Hg.

Formula _____

Solution _____

Answer _____

   Now compare the results. Patient 2 has pretty crummy values but a good hemoglobin level. Patient 3 has good values but a crummy hemoglobin level. Who has better oxygenation?

The Moral of the Story

Looking at pulse oximetry values, or any other simple indices of oxygenation like Pao_2, doesn't tell the whole story. You *always* have to consider hemoglobin. A patient may need blood as a treatment for poor oxygen content. Remember that there may be enough hemoglobin, but it may not be able to combine with oxygen, like in carbon monoxide poisoning.

THROW ME A CURVE

The last piece of the oxygenation puzzle (for now at least) is to look at the relationship of oxygen and hemoglobin. This relationship is described by the oxyhemoglobin dissociation curve. Look at the curve shown on page 248 in Figure 11-9 of your text. The flat upper part of the curve means that you can have a large drop in Pao_2 and only get a small drop in saturation. In fact, Pao_2 can drop from 600 mm Hg to 60 mm Hg and the saturation will only drop from 100% to 90%! The steep part of the curve is equally cool, physiologically speaking. A small increase in Pao_2 will give you a large increase in saturation. If you raise the Pao_2 from 27 mm Hg to 60 mm Hg, the saturation will rise from 50% all the way to 90%. Normally, a given Pao_2 will produce a predictable hemoglobin saturation.

   Fill in the correct values for partial pressure of oxygen and saturation (with a normal pH) on the chart below. Use the Mini Clini on Hemoglobin Saturation if you need help.

	Pao_2	Sao_2
9.	40 mm Hg	
10.		80%
11.	60 mm Hg	
12.		97%

   But the curve doesn't always stay in the same place! Fill in the correct answers for how the curve will shift on the chart below:

	Factor	Shift
13.	Acidosis	
14.	Hypothermia	
15.	High 2,3-diphosphoglycerate (2,3-DPG)	
16.	Fever	
17.	Hypercapnia	
18.	Carboxyhemoglobin	

   The shift of the curve to the right facilitates oxygen unloading to the tissues, but a given Pao_2 will have a lower hemoglobin saturation. A left shift does the opposite.

FICK IT

Fick was a physiologist who figured out something pretty cool—how to calculate cardiac output using oxygen content data and tissue oxygen consumption. Your instructors may want you to learn this now, or later in Chapter 46. I vote for Chapter 46, but because this can show up on your NBRC exams, you may want to take a look at this old formula that keeps on working. Basically, you divide the amount of oxygen the tissues are using (average of 250 for the normal adult) and divide by the difference between arterial and venous oxygen content, and you get the cardiac output. We measure output more directly these days, but Fick's formula is a good way to explain the relationships. More in Chapter 46!

CARBON DIOXIDE TRANSPORT

CO_2 is transported three ways in the blood. Just like oxygen, it dissolves right into the plasma. This factor is more important than dissolved oxygen, because it transports a fair amount of CO_2. Just like oxygen, CO_2 is carried by hemoglobin. Unlike oxygen, this is a relatively small amount. The majority of the CO_2, about 80%, is transported in the form of bicarbonate. Sorry, there are no math problems for you to do right now. But do remember this equation:

$$CO_2 + H_2O = H_2CO_3 = HCO_3^- + H^+$$

This reaction is called hydrolysis, because it involves combining CO_2 with water. First, carbonic acid is formed, but this quickly ionizes into bicarbonate and hydrogen ions. Remember, the reaction can move in both directions. Most of the hydrolysis occurs inside the red blood cell because of the presence of an enzyme (carbonic anhydrase) that speeds up the reaction rate.

Carbon dioxide levels are inversely proportional to alveolar ventilation. If you increase alveolar ventilation, the CO_2 will decrease. A normal Pa_{CO_2} is 35 to 45 mm Hg. A high CO_2 level means that the patient is not ventilating adequately. We draw arterial blood gases when we want to accurately assess ventilation. A high CO_2 in the blood indicates hypoventilation. Because CO_2 has an acidifying effect on the blood, the pH of the blood will decrease when the CO_2 rises. The normal lower limit of pH is 7.35. The normal upper limit is 7.45. Low values reflect acidosis, while increased pH represents an alkaline state.

BAD GAS EXCHANGE

Oxygen delivery and CO_2 removal are where it's at, physiologically speaking. The following questions will test your knowledge of the causes of poor gas exchange.

Fill in the correct term(s) in the blank(s) provided.

19. Inadequate delivery of oxygen to the tissues is known as _____.

20. _____ is the medical name for a low level of oxygen in the blood.

21. Physiologic _____ occurs when blood passes through areas of the lung that have no ventilation.

22. Ventilation-_____ imbalances are the most common cause of low blood oxygen in patients with lung disease.

23. Patients with pulmonary fibrosis have a(n) _____ defect that results in low blood oxygen levels.

24. A low blood pressure results in _____ and poor tissue oxygen delivery.

25. Myocardial infarction is an example of _____, a localized reduction in blood flow to tissues that can result in tissue death.

26. Increased _____ space ventilation may result in increased levels of carbon dioxide in the blood.

27. Drug overdose may result in an inadequate _____ ventilation due to central nervous system depression.

28. Patients with severe COPD are unable to maintain adequate ventilation due to ventilation-_____ imbalances.

WHAT DOES THE NBRC SAY?

The NBRC thinks you should be good at assessing gas exchange and treating abnormalities.
Circle the best answer for each of the following multiple-choice questions.

29. A room air blood gas reveals the following results:
    pH   7.50
    $Paco_2$ 30 mm Hg
    Pao_2 110 mm Hg

    In regard to these data, the respiratory therapist should
    A. report the results to the physician
    B. redraw the sample due to air contamination
    C. report that the patient is on oxygen
    D. place the patient on oxygen

30. Calculate oxygen content for a patient with the following data:
    Hb   10 g
    Pao_2 80 mm Hg
    Sao_2 95%

    A. 12.73 ml O_2/dl
    B. 12.97 ml O_2/dl
    C. 13.40 ml O_2/dl
    D. 13.64 ml O_2/dl

31. Calculate PAo_2 for a patient with the following data:
    Pb   747 mm Hg
    Fio_2 0.21
    Pao_2 95 mm Hg
    $Paco_2$ 40 mm Hg
    Sao_2 97%

    A. 97 mm Hg
    B. 103 mm Hg
    C. 107 mm Hg
    D. 117 mm Hg

Case 1

A 29-year-old housewife is brought to the emergency department following exposure to smoke during a house fire. She is breathing at a rate of 30 per minute. Her heart rate is 110. Blood pressure is 160/110. The patient complains of headache and nausea. The pulse oximeter is reading a saturation of 99%.

32. Why are pulse oximetry readings unreliable in this setting? _____

_____

33. What is wrong with this patient?

34. What action would you take at this time? _____

_____

Case 2

A patient is brought back to the unit following major surgery after a motorcycle accident. He was given a massive transfusion of blood to replace loss from both the trauma and the surgical procedure. The pulse oximeter is reading 96% on room air, but the nurse has requested you to evaluate due to the patient's clinical condition. You find him sitting up and breathing 32 times per minute. He has tachycardia and tachypnea and complains of difficulty breathing. Breath sounds are clear on auscultation.

35. The patient's clinical signs are consistent with what gas exchange abnormality?

_____

36. What is one of the potential problems with banked blood? _____

_____

37. Name some of the other possible causes of the patient's distress.

38. What diagnostic procedure could you recommend? _____

   _____

A woman is admitted with a diagnosis of pneumonia. Arterial blood gases reveal a pH of 7.55, $Paco_2$ of 25 mm Hg, Pao_2 of 75 mm Hg, and an Sao_2 of 94%. She complains of feeling short of breath. Lab data reveal a hemoglobin level of 8 g/dl.

39. Interpret this blood gas in terms of gas exchange.

40. What other laboratory information plays a key role in helping determine oxygen content?

   _____

41. What is absolute anemia, and how is it treated?

Case 4

A young man has been brought by paramedics to the emergency department after an accidental overdose of narcotics at a party. The patient is unconscious and has a respiratory rate of 8. The pulse oximeter shows a saturation of 85%.

42. Why would carbon dioxide be elevated in this patient?

43. Why is the patient's oxygen saturation so low?

FOOD FOR THOUGHT

Dysoxia

Is your brain full yet? Dysoxia is a form of hypoxia where cells do not uptake oxygen properly.

44. What is the classic example of dysoxia? _____

_____

45. When does tissue oxygen consumption become dependent on oxygen delivery? _____

_____

46. Why does lactic acid form when tissues are hypoxic?

Food for Thought Part Deux

This next idea is so important that I had to make another section for you. A new technology has been developed that allows pulse oximeters to look beyond the usual oxygen-hemoglobin relationship. Masimo is currently the only company that offers a pulse oximeter that can detect carboxyhemoglobin and tells you how much CO you have without drawing blood. A second oximeter allows you to assess methhemoglobin or sulfhemoglobin or whatever you want. It is a non-invasive co-oximeter. This will become a standard of care in emergency medicine in the near future, so you'll want to check out these important new-generation pulse oximeters.

Chapter **11** **Gas Exchange and Transport**

REMEMBER: When new devices come out, they may not appear in your board exams right away. Currently, the answer is "pulse oximeters can't detect carbon monoxide" and we don't know if that will change in the next revision of the boards, but we'll all be watching.

INFORMATION AGE

Check out this site: ventworld.com. Ventworld claims to be the Internet's premier site on mechanical ventilation. It certainly has a wealth of information. It is sponsored by a corporation but has extensively used expert respiratory therapists. Ventworld is a good example of an exception to our rule about using .edu and .gov sites on the Internet.

I don't usually recommend corporate Web sites, but in the case of understanding unique technologies, they are a boon to the therapist. Try www.Masimo.com if you want to find out about the unique pulse oximeter technology that has produced devices that measure COHb noninvasively. The Web site explains that the technology is rich with case studies and research findings.

12 Solutions, Body Fluids, and Electrolytes

If you can't convince 'em, confuse 'em.
Harry S. Truman

Imagine yourself swimming in a warm ocean lagoon. The salty water is filled with life. Currents move you and waves propel you through this complex ecology. Now think about the inside of your body. Warm, wet, and filled with salts. An intricate environment where life depends on the relationships of fluids and electrolytes. Chapter 12 reviews various types of solutions, the mechanisms that control fluid movement, acid-base basics, and the role of major electrolytes in body function. I've focused your attention on the second half of the chapter first. Then we'll wrap up with a look at solutions.

WORD WIZARD

You'll need to have some new vocabulary to keep you afloat in the sea of salts and solutions. You could look each word in the "key terms" up in the glossary, but this time I did that for you. See if you can match the definitions to the terms. BTW, one of the rules of *Egan's* is that you'll find the key terms in the glossary and in bold print in the text. You might have trouble with a chapter like this if you don't understand these fundamental phonemes of body chemistry.

Write your answer in the spaces provided.

Definitions	Terms
1. _____ A compound that gives off H^+ in water. Vinegar is a good example in the kitchen.	acid active transport normal solution
2. _____ The opposite of inactive transport; movement across membranes	solvent solute base
3. _____ Negatively charged ion; Cl^- and HCO_3^- are common in the body.	cations hypertonic isotonic
4. _____ A compound that gives off OH^- in water. Sodium bicarbonate is an example in the kitchen.	solution diluent colloid
5. _____ Minimizing the change in pH. Think of how pleasant it is to buffer your stomach acids after eating chili!	dilute solution hypotonic buffering
6. _____ Positively charged ion. Na^+ and K^+ are common in the body.	saturated solution anions
7. _____ A substance with big molecules that hold water (among other things). Like milk in the kitchen or albumin in the blood. Also an evenly dispersed mixture or gel.	
8. _____ Something you use to water down a medication or solution.	

Continued

9. _____ The medium you dissolve something into, like your coffee.

10. _____ The stuff that gets dissolved, like sugar.

11. _____ A stable mixture of two substances, like the sugar when it is stirred (dissolved) into the coffee. Heat helps make this happen.

12. _____ A really weak solution. The soup needs more salt.

13. _____ A solution holding as much as it can. The soup is fine.

14. _____ The standard solution with 1 mEq/L. I was never like this, myself.

15. _____ Has the same amount of salt as your body fluids. A good solution in your nebulizer.

16. _____ Saltier than your body fluids. Good for inducing sputum.

17. _____ Low salt or no salt, and okay to nebulize, too.

Boy, that was tiring. It will be worth it when you get to the chapters on acid-base and pharmacology. Many of these terms come up again and again.

WATER, WATER EVERYWHERE

The human body is mostly water. Water makes up as much as 80% of your weight.

Because water is relatively heavy, the easiest way to track gain and loss is by weighing the patient! Clinicians also monitor intake and output (I and O) of water very closely.

Now you need to open your textbook (check out Table 12-3 on page 270 in your text) and look up some information about this subject.

18. Rank the relative amount of water in the following individuals. Put "1" by the lowest amount of water, and "5" by the people with the largest percentage of body water.

_____ males

_____ newborns

_____ children

_____ females

_____ obese individuals

19. Name the two major compartments for body distribution of water. List subdivisions and give the relative amount (%) of water in each area.

COMPARTMENT	% H$_2$O
A.	
B.	
1.	
2.	
3.	Normally tiny, potentially a long

WHERE HAS ALL THE WATER GONE?

A lot of water leaves your body every day through sensible and insensible losses. Give examples of these water losses and an average daily amount. I'll be incensed if you don't check out Table 12-4 on page 271 in your text to satisfy your thirst for knowledge.

	SOURCE	AMOUNT
20.	Sensible A. B. C.	
21.	Insensible A. B.	

You can also lose water through additive losses like sweating, diarrhea, and vomiting. The insensible loss that interests us the most is water lost through breathing. A tracheostomy patient with poor humidification can lose 700 ml/day or more. This results in dried-out secretions that clog the patient's lungs. If your tracheostomy patient has a fever, the problem is worse.

22. Describe the loss of water that occurs through fever.

23. Lost water is regained by two main methods. List these sources of liquid and give amounts.

SOURCE	AMOUNT/DAY

A. Ingestion
  1.
  2.	

B. Metabolism	

ACID-BASE BASICS

If your body was a playground, acids and bases would be the see-saw ride! You don't have to be a chemistry major to play. Acids are substances that release hydrogen ions (H^+) when placed in a watery solution. Another definition states that acids are substances that are proton donors. Bases release hydroxyl ions (OH^-) or accept protons. Pure water is the reference point for determining acidity or alkalinity. Any solution with more H^+ ions than water is considered an acid. A solution with less hydrogen ions is considered alkaline, or basic. A logarithmic scale, called the pH scale, is used to indicate the relative amount of acidity or alkalinity of a substance. Water is assigned a value of 7.0 on the pH scale. Because the scale is logarithmic, a pH of 6 is 10 times more acidic than water. The human body exists in a narrow range of pH values. Normally, our arterial blood has a pH of 7.35 to 7.45. A prolonged pH below 7.0 or above 7.60 is usually fatal! In Chapter 13, we'll get into clinical applications and interpretations of acid-base balance.

ELECTRIFYING INFORMATION

Electrolytes are chemicals that dissociate into ions when placed into solution, thus becoming capable of conducting electricity. Positively charged ions are called cations, and negative particles are called anions. There are seven major electrolytes in the body that are essential to life. Electrolytes are naturally regulated by the kidney (mostly), and can be manipulated by oral or intravenous intake in the health care setting. Let's see if you know your electrolytes. If I were you, I'd look at the end of the chapter around page 273 for this information.

24. List the seven major electrolytes and their primary purpose in the body.

	ELECTROLYTE	SYMBOL	PURPOSE
A.			
B.			
C.			
D.			
E.			
F.			
G.			

You will also need to know the average normal plasma value for these babies. Match the value to the chemical in the list below. Seriously, learn these values if you want to pass "go" with the NBRC.

25. _____ bicarbonate   A. 140 mEq/L

26. _____ calcium   B. 24 mEq/L

27. _____ chloride   C. 4.0 mEq/L

28. _____ magnesium   D. 5.0 mEq/L

29. _____ phosphorus   E. 100 mEq/L

30. _____ potassium   F. 2.0 mEq/L

31. _____ sodium   G. 140 mEq/L

Electrolytes are so important that a patient will exhibit some pretty interesting signs and symptoms if these powerful substances become too high or low. Complete the chart below to match up disorders, causes, and symptoms of electrolyte disturbances. Use Table 12-5 to help you get going.

	IMBALANCE	CAUSE	SYMPTOM
32.		Sweating	
33.	Hypokalemia		
34.		Starvation	Diaphragmatic weakness
35.	Hypercalcemia		
36.		Chronic renal disease	

Notice the similarities in the symptoms of many of these imbalances. When you see muscle weakness, abnormal fatigue, or ECG disturbances or metabolic acid-base disorders, take a look at the electrolytes!

CASE STUDIES

Case 1

A 68-year-old man with congestive heart failure (CHF), is being treated with a combination of diet and diuretics. He returns from a trip to New Orleans complaining of difficulty breathing and swollen ankles. He is admitted to the coronary care unit for observation and treatment. Auscultation reveals bilateral inspiratory crackles in the lung bases. His respiratory rate is 28 with a heart rate 110 with arrhythmias. *Hint:* Check out the Mini-Clini in the electrolyte section.

37. Patients with CHF are usually placed on what special type of diet? Why?

38. Diuretics commonly cause loss of what specific electrolyte that affects cardiac function? How will this electrolyte be replaced in the hospital? The home?

   A. Electrolyte: _____

   B. Hospital replacement: _____

   C. Home replacement: _____

39. As a respiratory therapist, what action will you take to further assess cardiopulmonary status? What is likely to be your initial treatment of this patient?

Chapter **12** **Solutions, Body Fluids, and Electrolytes**

40. What is the cause of this patient's lung crackles?

Case 2

A 68-year-old homeless alcoholic is found in respiratory distress by the paramedics and brought to your emergency department. The patient is malnourished. Auscultation reveals bilateral inspiratory crackles in the lung bases. His respiratory rate is 28 with a heart rate of 110. Hint: Look at the section on Starling equilibrium. We'll get back to these two cases again and again because pulmonary edema is such a common clinical problem. So common that Chapter 27 is devoted to this topic. Now is a good time to get your feet wet in the area of flooded lungs.

41. What protein accounts for the high osmotic pressure of plasma? Why is the patient lacking this

substance? _____

42. Explain why this patient has crackles.

43. As a respiratory therapist, what action will you take to further assess cardiopulmonary status? What is likely to be your initial treatment of this patient?

MATHEMATICS

Respiratory therapists frequently work with weight/volume solutions and perform dilution calculations. Dilution calculations are used in drug preparation and in the pulmonary laboratory. You will be expected to perform some of these calculations on the NBRC board examinations. Remember . . . no calculators . . . on the boards. My students always use theirs to check their work.

44. Albuterol is prepared in a 5% solution (weight/volume). How many grams of albuterol are dissolved in 100 ml to make this solution?

    Formula _____

    Solution _____

    Answer _____

45. Respiratory therapists do not usually administer 100 ml of drugs to their patients. Instead, they give 1 ml or less. How many milligrams of albuterol would be found in 1 ml of the 5% solution in problem 20?

    Formula _____

    Solution _____

    Answer _____

46. After drawing up 1 ml of a 5% solution of albuterol into a syringe, the respiratory therapist places the bronchodilator into a nebulizer along with 2 ml of saline for dilution. The total solution is now 3 ml in the nebulizer. What is the new concentration of the drug?

    Formula _____

    Solution _____

    Answer _____

Excuse me, do you mind if I help out here?

$$\text{Formula: } C_1 \times V_1 = C_2 \times V_2$$

Where C_1 = stock strength in the bottle, 5%; and V_1 = the amount you need to draw up, or 1 ml. C_2 is what we want to find out. V_2 is the 1 ml of drug and the 2 ml of saline, or 3 ml.

$$\text{Solution: } 5\% \times 1 \text{ ml} = C_2 \times 3 \text{ ml}$$

Answer: 0.16%. You can check this out in the Mini-Clini on methacholine dilution found on page 268 of your text where they apply this formula to making a new formula of a stronger drug that is safe to give to asthmatics.

WHAT DOES THE NBRC SAY?

The National Board for Respiratory Care (NBRC) would give this chapter an "E" for "emphasis of important test material." Here are more sample questions in the same format as your tests. Other items you'll need for the boards from Chapter 12 include electrolyte values and some of those calculations.

47. A patient with severe hypokalemia is receiving an intravenous infusion of potassium to correct this serious disorder. What should you monitor?
    A. Spo_2
    B. respiratory frequency
    C. mental status
    D. ECG rhythm

48. Which of the following signs and symptoms would you expect to observe in a patient with hypokalemia?
    I. metabolic acid-base disturbance
    II. muscle spasms and tetany
    III. ECG abnormality
       A. I only
       B. I and II only
       C. I and III only
       D. II and III only

49. All of the following would be consistent with administration of a large amount of IV fluid *except*
    A. increased pulmonary vascular markings on the chest x-ray
    B. presence of crackles on auscultation
    C. increased urine output
    D. increased hematocrit

50. A respiratory therapist delivers isotonic saline to a patient via nebulizer. What concentration of saline is the therapist delivering?
    A. 0.0%
    B. 0.45%
    C. 0.90%
    D. 1.0%

FOOD FOR THOUGHT

Administration of fluids with varying tonicities by both intravenous and aerosol routes is common.

51. What happens to cells in the presence of a hypertonic solution? _____

_____

52. What happens to cells when a hypotonic solution is given? _____

_____

53. What name is given for the movement of water across a semipermeable membrane? _____

_____

Here's another one for you. Once upon a time a physician asked me if the saline in my nebulizer treatment would hurt his patient, who was on a sodium restriction for his heart. "No problem," I said. Use this scenario to answer the following question.

54. If you give 3 ml of normal saline by nebulizer, how much sodium chloride is being delivered to the airway in theory? Do you think the whole thing goes into the patient?

INFORMATION AGE

- Here's a popular site that provides simple, understandable explanations of . . . everything: www.howstuffworks.com
- If you want something a little more scientific: www.nlm.nih.gov/medlineplus/fluidandelectrolytebalance.html. This is a great site from the .gov folks!

13 Acid-Base Balance

The formula for success is simple: practice and concentration, then more practice and more concentration.

Babe Didrikson Zaharias

If our bodies are factories that use oxygen and glucose to manufacture energy, then they are also producers of waste in the form of water, heat, and carbon dioxide. A respiratory therapist must understand the role that the lung and the kidney play in removing waste, how buffering systems work, and how to interpret the results of arterial blood gases. Drawing, analyzing, and, most of all, interpreting blood gas findings are hallmarks of our profession. Learning this skill will require some memorization and lots of practice!

WORD WIZARD

There's no point in building your knowledge without a foundation. Before you can learn to use acid-base information clinically, you will have to know your terminology.

Match the following terms to their definitions:

Terms	Definitions
1. _____ acidemia	A. acid that can be excreted in gaseous form
	B. decreased hydrogen ion concentration in the blood
2. _____ volatile acid	C. ventilation that results in decreased CO_2
	D. respiratory processes resulting in increased hydrogen ions
3. _____ anion gap	E. acid that is excreted by the kidney
4. _____ hyperventilation	F. abnormal ventilatory pattern in response to metabolic acidosis
5. _____ metabolic acidosis	G. nonrespiratory processes resulting in decreased hydrogen ions
6. _____ alkalemia	H. difference between electrolyte concentrations
7. _____ Kussmaul's breathing	I. respiratory processes resulting in decreased hydrogen ions
8. _____ hypoventilation	J. increased hydrogen ion concentration in the blood
9. _____ fixed acid	K. nonrespiratory processes resulting in increased hydrogen ions
10. _____ respiratory alkalosis	L. chemical substance that minimizes fluctuations in pH
11. _____ metabolic alkalosis	M. plasma concentration of HCO_3^- corrected to a normal CO_2
12. _____ standard bicarbonate	N. difference between normal and actual buffers available
13. _____ base excess	O. ventilation that results in increased CO_2
14. _____ respiratory acidosis	
15. _____ buffer	

WHERE HAS ALL THE ACID GONE?

The lungs excrete more acid each day than do the kidneys! Answer the following questions to find out if you understand the buffering process.

16. Draw a diagram of the process called isohydric buffering.

17. Explain how the lungs can compensate for increased production of fixed acids.

18. Buffers are composed of what two components? _____

_____

19. What happens when you add the acid hydrogen chloride to base sodium bicarbonate?

20. Describe the two general types of buffering systems in the body, and give examples of each system and what general type of acid (fixed or volatile) they buffer in the body (check out Table 13-2 on page 283 of *Egan's* for an example).

Blood Buffers   **Acid Buffered**

A. _____   _____

B. _____   _____

21. What does ventilation remove from the body to help eliminate acid? Support your answer with information from the text.

22. Why are buffers in the kidney essential for the secretion of excess hydrogen ions (why can't the lung do it alone)?

BALANCING ACT

When you're healthy, the lungs, kidney, and buffers work together to keep your pH normal so that enzyme systems can function and homeostasis is maintained. The system responds pretty rapidly to local or systemic changes. As long as the ratio of bicarbonate buffer to dissolved CO_2 is 20:1, your pH will be about 7.40. A variety of conditions can cause the balance to shift. Increases in ventilation will result in respiratory alkalosis. Increases in bicarbonate (or other base buffers) will result in metabolic alkalosis. These changes are referred to as acute if they take place over a short period of time. If they become chronic, the body will try to compensate to bring the pH back to normal. Of course, the respiratory system responds rapidly to metabolic disturbances, but the kidney takes time to adjust the bicarbonate. Answer these questions to test your understanding of simple acid-base disturbances.

23. List the normal range of values for pH, Pa_{CO_2}, and HCO_3^-. (You HAVE to memorize these values!)

	Low Normal	High Normal
A. pH	_____	_____
B. Pa_{CO_2}	_____	_____
C. HCO_3^-	_____	_____

24. Write out the Henderson-Hasselbach equation.

Chapter **13** **Acid-Base Balance**

25. Complete the primary acid-base and compensation chart below. Try Table 13-3 if you get stuck.

Disorder	Primary Defect	Compensation
A. Respiratory acidosis	_____	_____
B. Respiratory alkalosis	_____	_____
C. Metabolic acidosis	_____	_____
D. Metabolic alkalosis	_____	_____

26. What is the *Rule of Thumb* for determining the expected increase in bicarbonate for any acute increase in carbon dioxide?

27. How much will bicarbonate increase with a chronic increase in carbon dioxide?

A METHOD TO THE MADNESS

There is a simple 4-step method for interpreting blood gas values.

Step 1: Determine the pH first.
    1. >7.45 = alkalosis
    2. <7.35 = acidosis
    3. 7.35 to 7.45 = normal (or fully compensated)

Step 2: Evaluate respiratory status ($Paco_2$) to see if it agrees with the pH.
    1. <35 = alkalosis
    2. >45 = acidosis

Step 3: Evaluate metabolic status (HCO_3^-) to see if it agrees.
    1. >26 = alkalosis
    2. <22 = acidosis

Step 4: Evaluate compensation.
    1. Complete: pH is normal with abnormal CO_2 and HCO_3^-. (Even with complete compensation, the pH will tend to be on the primary disorder's side of 7.40.)
    2. Partial: pH is abnormal, but not as much as expected.

Interpret the following blood gas results. I'll help you with the first one.

pH	7.30
$Paco_2$	60 mm Hg
HCO_3^-	26 mEq/L

The pH is below 7.35, so the overall state is acidosis. The $Paco_2$ is above 45, which represents *acidosis*. The pH and the $Paco_2$ agree! We have *respiratory acidosis*. The bicarbonate has risen 2 mEq/L above normal. This elevation is most likely due to the increased CO_2 (remember, bicarb goes up 1 for each 10–mm Hg acute increase in CO_2). So, we have **acute (uncompensated) respiratory acidosis.**

28.
pH	7.34
$Paco_2$	60 mm Hg
HCO_3^-	31 mEq/L

29.
pH	7.36
$Paco_2$	60 mm Hg
HCO_3^-	33 mEq/L

Stop right there! We're going to continue interpreting blood gas results in our case studies and board exam review questions, but I hope you can see how the bicarbonate will be creeping up as the CO_2 rises and the pH returns to low normal to achieve compensation.

WELCOME TO THE GAP!

When a patient has a metabolic acidosis, it can be life threatening, so we need to try to establish the cause. One way to do this is through history. For example, we know the patient took an aspirin overdose. Another method for determining the type of metabolic acidosis is by looking at the difference between our positive and negative ions. Of course, you need the electrolyte values to do this calculation. Here's how you do it:

$$Sodium (Na^+) - chloride (Cl^-) + bicarbonate (HCO_3^-) \text{ or } 140 - (105 + 24) = 11$$

A normal range for the gap is 9 to 14 mEq/L. Usually, potassium is ignored. When the body loses bicarbonate through diarrhea, chloride increases and the gap remains normal. When bicarbonate is used to buffer excess fixed acids, the gap will increase.

30. Name the three common causes of anion gap metabolic acidosis.

A. _____

B. _____

C. _____

31. What are the signs of respiratory compensation for metabolic acidosis?

_____

_____

32. What are the neurologic symptoms of severe acidosis?

_____

_____

MATHEMATICS

There have been several math calculations in this chapter. You will have to use a calculator to solve some of them—probably a scientific one. I personally find the steps of the H-H tricky, so I have to pay close attention and DO THE STEPS EXACTLY IN ORDER.

Bicarbonate Blues

Calculate the new bicarbonate (assume 24 as the starting point) level for an acutely elevated $Paco_2$ of 50 mm Hg (assume it started at 40). You could use the *Rule of Thumb* like this:

Formula predicted $HCO_3^- = 24 + $ (measured $Paco_2$ − normal CO_2)/10

Solution predicted $HCO_3^- = 24 + (50 − 40)/10$

Answer predicted bicarbonate $= 24 + 1$

You try.

33. Calculate the new bicarbonate (assume 24 as the starting point) level for an acutely elevated $Paco_2$ of 70 mm Hg (assume it started at 40).

Formula _____

Solution _____

Answer _____

34. Calculate the new bicarbonate (assume 24 as the starting point) level for a *chronically* elevated $Paco_2$ of 70 mm Hg (assume it started at 40, use the other *Rule of Thumb* to make the new formula).

Formula _____

Solution _____

Answer _____

Hassle? Use the H-H Equation for This

35. Calculate pH if HCO_3^- is 30 mEq/L and $Paco_2$ is 40 mm Hg.

    Formula _____

    Solution _____

    Answer _____

36. Calculate pH if HCO_3^- is 24 mEq/L and $Paco_2$ is 40 mm Hg.

    Formula _____

    Solution _____

    Answer _____

37. Calculate pH if HCO_3^- is 24 mEq/L and $Paco_2$ is 60 mm Hg.

    Formula _____

    Solution _____

    Answer _____

Gap?

38. Calculate anion gap if Na^+ is 144, Cl^- is 100, and HCO_3^- is 22.

    Formula _____

    Solution _____

    Answer _____

39. Calculate anion gap if Na^+ is 135, Cl^- is 105, and HCO_3^- is 26.

    Formula _____

    Solution _____

    Answer _____

CASE STUDIES

The following case studies will systematically take you through the major acid-base disorders. Let's start with some simple, acute states. Remember to evaluate using the four-step process.

Case 1

A woman took too much Valium and is found shortly thereafter in a coma breathing slowly and shallowly. ABG results reveal pH of 7.28, $Paco_2$ of 60 mm Hg, and HCO_3^- of 26 mEq/L.

40. How would you interpret this ABG? _____

    _____

41. What is the primary cause of the disorder? _____

The husband of the previous patient is very worried about her condition. He complains of dizziness and tingling in his hands. ABG results reveal pH of 7.58, $PaCO_2$ of 25 mm Hg, and HCO_3^- of 23 mEq/L.

42. How would you interpret this ABG? _____

43. What is the primary cause of the disorder? _____

Case 3

The couple's young child has been sick with the stomach flu. ABG results reveal pH of 7.60, $PaCO_2$ of 40 mm Hg, and HCO_3^- of 38 mEq/L.

44. How would you interpret this ABG? _____

45. What is the primary cause of the disorder? _____

Case 4

The couple's diabetic teenage daughter has not been taking her insulin. ABG results reveal pH of 7.25, $PaCO_2$ of 40 mm Hg, and HCO_3^- of 17 mEq/L.

46. How would you interpret this ABG? _____

47. What is the primary cause of the disorder? _____

Of course, blood gases don't stay simple for long. Partial or complete compensation may occur.

Case 5

The teenage patient's grandfather has smoked for years, and now he has COPD. ABG results reveal pH of 7.37, $PaCO_2$ of 50 mm Hg, and HCO_3^- of 28 mEq/L.

48. How would you interpret this ABG? _____

49. What is the source of compensation? _____

Case 6

As soon as the Case 1 patient's brain realizes the acute nature of her illness, compensation begins. ABG results now reveal pH of 7.35, $PaCO_2$ of 25 mm Hg, and HCO_3^- of 13 mEq/L.

50. How would you interpret this ABG? _____

51. What is the source of compensation? _____

Case 7

A grandmother has congestive heart failure. She takes Lasix to reduce extra water in her body. ABG results now reveal pH of 7.46, $PaCO_2$ of 45 mm Hg, and HCO_3^- of 31 mEq/L.

52. How would you interpret this ABG? _____

53. What is a possible cause of the primary disorder? _____

WHAT DOES THE NBRC SAY?

Blood gas (acid-base) analysis is one of the largest areas in all of the exams. The Entry-Level examination will focus on simple interpretations, while the Registry Examinations will ask you for higher order thinking. Here are some examples.

Circle the best answer to the following multiple-choice questions.

54. A 17-year-old girl is brought to the emergency department by paramedics. Her mother states she is a diabetic. Room air ABGs reveal the following:

    pH   7.26
    $Paco_2$ 16 mm Hg
    HCO_3^- 8 mEq/L
    Pao_2 110 mm Hg

    This information indicates which of the following?
    I.   Partly compensated metabolic acidosis is present.
    II. This Pao_2 is not possible on room air.
    III. Respiratory alkalosis is present.
        A. I only
        B. III only
        C. I and II only
        D. I and III only

55. Interpret the following ABG results:

    Fio_2 0.21
    pH   7.36
    $Paco_2$ 37 mm Hg
    HCO_3^- 22 mEq/L
    Pao_2 95 mm Hg

    A. acute respiratory alkalosis
    B. acute metabolic alkalosis
    C. compensated respiratory alkalosis
    D. normal ABG

56. During CPR, blood gases are drawn. The results are as follows:

    Fio_2 1.0
    pH   7.15
    $Paco_2$ 55 mm Hg
    HCO_3^- 12 mEq/L
    Pao_2 210 mm Hg

    What action should be taken to correct the acid-base abnormality shown here?
    A. Increase the rate of ventilation.
    B. Decrease the Fio_2.
    C. Administer sodium bicarbonate intravenously.
    D. Add positive end-expiratory pressure (PEEP) to the ventilation system.

57. The results of an arterial blood gas are shown.

    Fio_2 .21
    pH   7.55
    $Paco_2$ 25 mm Hg
    HCO_3^- 24 mEq/L
    Pao_2 105 mm Hg

    These data indicate which of the following?
    A. metabolic acidosis
    B. metabolic alkalosis
    C. uncompensated hyperventilation
    D. uncompensated hypoventilation

58. A 72-year-old man with a history of renal failure is seen in the emergency department. The respiratory therapist notes that the patient is taking 28 very deep breaths per minute. Which of the following accurately describes this breathing pattern?
    A. Cheyne-Stokes breathing
    B. ataxic breathing
    C. Kussmaul's breathing
    D. eupnic breathing

EXERCISE YOUR MENTAL MUSCLES

In later chapters, you will be called on to use your newfound blood gas interpretation skills to make many clinical decisions about patient care. *If you are having difficulty interpreting the acid-base status, you should take time to solidify these skills now!*
    Here are some suggestions.
- **Get access to blood gas interpretation software.** Your instructors probably have a program that will give you sample after sample to interpret.
- **Make flash cards.** Take some 3 × 5 inch cards. Write high, normal, and low values for pH, $Paco_2$, and HCO_3^-. Make two extra cards for pH that will represent compensation. Use 7.36 for compensated acidotic states and 7.44 for alkalotic states. On the back of each card write out the name of the state. For example, on the $Paco_2$ 50 mm Hg card, write "respiratory acidosis." You get the idea? Now proceed to go through the combinations using the four-step method of interpretation. Pretty soon you will be an ace!
- **Drill, drill, drill until you have mastered basic blood gas interpretation!**

FOOD FOR THOUGHT

Blood gas disorders can get really complicated at times. Just like life. In some cases, a patient will have one disorder superimposed on another. Take the continuing saga of the following older patient. . . .

The older man discussed in Case 5 acquired a lung infection after visiting his daughter in the hospital. ABG results now reveal pH of 7.46 (previously 7.37), $Paco_2$ of 55 mm Hg (previously 50), Pao_2 of 57 mm Hg, and HCO_3^- of 38 mEq/L (previously 28).

59. How would you interpret this ABG?

_____

60. Why did the blood gas values change from those in case?

_____

INFORMATION AGE

Acid-base tutorial	www.acid-base.com	Seems like a logical place to start!
Tulane University	www.anaesthesiamcq.com/AcidBaseBook/ABindex.php	This acid-base tutorial was reviewed in 2006 by the American Thoracic Society (ATS) for their "Best of the Web" series.
American Thoracic Society	www.thoracic.org/sections/clinical-information/best-of-the-web/pages/critical-care/online-acid-base.html	You can get a seemingly endless parade of information on the internet when you ask your search engine for "blood gas interpretation." So the ATS came up with this solution—a review of all the online sites available.

14 Regulation of Breathing

The brain is a wonderful organ. It starts working the moment you get up in the morning and doesn't stop until you get to the office.

Robert Frost

You are getting sleepy, very sleepy . . . you didn't stop breathing did you? In just one year as an adult, you will breathe more than *seven million times!* Most of those breaths will be automatically initiated by your brainstem. Just like clockwork. Good thing, eh? (I have trouble remembering where I put my car keys . . .) It makes sense that respiratory care practitioners would need to know how this system works and what happens when it doesn't. Chapter 14 is a fitting end to the section on anatomy and physiology, because it summarizes the control mechanisms that regulate the respiratory system.

WORD WIZARD

The brain and nervous system have a language all their own. Learning these terms will make it easier to understand concepts in this chapter. (And you can impress your friends with your linguistic abilities!)

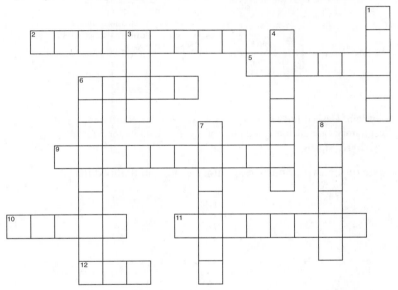

ACROSS

2. Chemo _____ , respond to changes in oxygen and pH to signal the need to breathe
5. + Breuer = parasympathetic inflation reflex
6. Absence of breathing
9. Receptors in the carotid bodies
10. 5 deep breaths ... apnea ... five deep breaths ... apnea?
11. Coughing, sneezing, laryngospasm, bronchospasm, and more when you stimulate these receptors!
12. Fluid that bathes the brain instead of blood

DOWN

1. Important cranial nerve involved in sensory and motor reflexes
3. The other center in the brainstem
4. Big Boss of the brainstem
6. Breathing pattern characterized by prolonged inspiratory gasps
7. Primary chemoreceptors
8. + Stokes = gradually increasing, then decreasing volumes with apneic episodes

Input into how we breathe comes from many areas. Conscious thought, receptors throughout the body, and reflexes all play important roles. The medulla's job is to organize the information and send messages to the motor fibers that innervate the muscles of the airway and chest (sort of a mental air-traffic controller). The medulla is located in your brainstem just above your spinal cord. If you cut the brainstem (don't try this at home) below the medulla, all ventilatory effort ceases. Another structure, the pons, sits on top of the medulla.

1. Label the parts of these central controlling bodies.

■ Inspiratory neurons
■ Expiratory neurons
□ Inspiratory and expiratory neurons

Nucleus parabrachialis medialis
Nucleus Kölliker-Fuse

(nucleus tractus solitarius, NTS)

Botzinger's complex
Nucleus retroambigualis
(caudal and rostral portions)
Nucleus ambiguous

Dorsal view of the brainstem. Dashed lines I to IV refer to transections at different levels. (From Beachey W: Respiratory care anatomy and physiology: foundations for clinical practice, ed 2, St. Louis, 2007, Mosby.)

2. Briefly explain the role of the two primary respiratory groups in the medulla.

3. Compare and contrast the two primary centers in the pons.

4. What diseases or conditions might affect the performance of brainstem's respiratory controllers?

AUTOMATIC PILOT

Respiratory reflexes are involuntary nervous responses located in airways, muscles, and tissues that influence breathing by sending information directly to the medulla (mostly via the vagus nerve). You'll need to be able to identify the most important reflexes, so here goes. Each reflex goes with a particular stimulus and has a response from receptors in a specific location.

Later on, let's apply some of these reflexes to the clinical setting and bring 'em to life.

	REFLEX	STIMULUS	RESPONSE	LOCATION
5.	Hering-Breuer			
6.	Deflation			
7.	Head			
8.	Vagovagal			
9.	C fiber			
10.	Proprioceptors			

BETTER LIVING THROUGH CHEMISTRY

Regulating ventilation ensures that tissues are exposed to just the right amount of oxygen, carbon dioxide, and hydrogen ions. Blood carries these substances to specialized nerve structures called chemoreceptors that are strategically placed in the brainstem, carotid bodies, and arch of the aorta. All these chemoreceptors will respond in some way to decreased levels of oxygen and pH or increased carbon dioxide in the blood (or vice versa).

Central Chemoreceptors

Central chemoreceptors sit in the medulla, taking a bath in the cerebrospinal fluid (CSF). They are not in direct contact with the blood because of the blood-brain barrier, a semipermeable membrane that surrounds the brain.

11. Explain the process that allows carbon dioxide to stimulate the central receptors.

12. Describe the stimulating effects of CO_2 on the receptors in terms of the immediate response to increased carbon dioxide in the blood. What happens when this goes on for 1 or 2 days?

Peripheral Chemoreceptors

Someone thought it would be a good idea to monitor the chemical composition of blood leaving the heart and heading toward the brain. Pretty smart!

13. Describe the peripheral receptor response to decreased arterial oxygen levels. What do the receptors actually respond to when oxygen levels drop?

14. What specific range of Pao_2 values causes the greatest response when CO_2 and pH are normal?

15. How does altitude modify the receptor's response to hypoxemia?

16. Describe the peripheral receptor response to increased arterial CO_2 and H^+ ions. How is it different than the central chemoreceptor response?

NO ONE UNDERSTANDS ME!

I want to introduce you to one of the most misunderstood concepts in the pathophysiology of lung disease. When you understand this one, you'll really be able to amaze the physicians, nurses, and respiratory instructors (not to mention your mom and dad).

Here goes something . . . Some patients, especially those with chronic obstructive pulmonary disease (COPD), become chronically hypoxic and hypercapnic. This happens when a high arterial carbon dioxide level persists over time. The kidneys compensate, which restores pH. Some of the bicarbonate diffuses into your head and corrects the pH in the CSF. The central receptors are fooled into thinking everything is fine. Because they are low on oxygen, the hypoxic stimulus drives their ventilation.

So far, so bad. When someone intervenes and administers oxygen to this special type of patient, the patient may experience an *acute rise in arterial CO_2*. The simple explanation is that the patient is no longer driven by the peripheral receptors to breathe because of low oxygen levels. While this is true, it is too simple of an explanation. We're not sure exactly what happens, but I follow the theory that increased oxygen also worsens the ventilation/perfusion ($\dot{V}/\dot{Q}$) relationship in the lung by increasing blood flow to poorly ventilated areas and through absorption atelectasis. Ventilation is decreased in the low-$\dot{V}/\dot{Q}$ areas and increased in the high-$\dot{V}/\dot{Q}$ regions. The drive to breathe is probably also blunted. It helps if the patient is exhausted or had medications that further depress the CNS. The result is an increased arterial P_{CO_2} in any case. (My students always ask "so what?" at this point!)

The point is that CO_2 in high concentrations in the blood is bad for you. It further decreases drive to breathe by depressing the central nervous system. So, don't give the patient too much oxygen, but **never withhold oxygen from a hypoxic patient!**

17. What concentration of oxygen is usually given to chronically hypercapnic patients? _____

_____

18. What is the best way to monitor oxygenation in these patients?

19. Why do low concentrations of oxygen usually result in adequate improvement?

OUCH!

Obviously if the brain is physically or physiologically injured, abnormal breathing patterns will occur. When you observe these patterns, you know something is wrong with the controller.

20. Describe Cheyne-Stokes breathing (use words or draw a picture). State two important causes of this distinctive pattern.

21. How does Biot's breathing differ from Cheyne-Stokes in terms of pattern and origin?

22. Describe apneustic breathing. What does this pattern indicate?

23. What are the two central neurogenic breathing patterns. State three events that could cause these patterns.

Case 1

Your patient rode his motorcycle without a helmet. He sustained a closed head injury during an accident that results in a subdural hematoma. He is intubated by the paramedics with an endotracheal tube.

24. Hyperventilation may lower the intracranial pressure of a patient with traumatic brain injury. What rules should you follow if you decide to do this procedure?

    A. When:

    _____

    B. Lowest safe CO_2 value:

    _____

    C. Length of time you can safely hyperventilate:

    _____

25. Why is lowering the carbon dioxide level controversial in traumatic brain injury?

The COPD patient from Chapter 13 is back in the hospital. He became short of breath at home and his family increased his oxygen from 2 L to 6 L per minute. When he arrives at the hospital, he is somnolent (sleepy) and difficult to arouse. ABG results reveal pH 7.25, $PaCO_2$ 75 mm Hg, PaO_2 90 mm Hg, and HCO_3^- 37 mEq/L on 6 L by nasal cannula.

26. What changes should you make in the patient's therapy? Why?

27. What target PaO_2 would be more appropriate for this patient? (I don't think *Egan* really tells you right out in this chapter—consider the PO_2 where the receptors kick in... .)

WHAT DOES THE NBRC SAY?

The NBRC won't exactly ask you direct questions about the information in this chapter, but they do love COPD patients with carbon dioxide retention and problems with hypoxic drive. See below for example variations on this theme.

Circle the best answer for each of the following multiple-choice questions.

28. A patient who has had COPD for many years is admitted for an acute episode of dyspnea. An arterial blood gas is drawn on room air with these results:
    pH   7.50
    $PaCO_2$ 48 mm Hg
    PaO_2 44 mm Hg
    HCO_3^- 36 mEq/L
    SaO_2 84%

What therapy do you recommend at this time?
A. 28% Venturi mask
B. 35% Venturi mask
C. nasal cannula delivering 5 L/min
D. simple mask delivering 10 L/min

29. A cooperative elderly patient with chronic asthma presents at her pulmonologist's office. You observe the following findings:

Pulse | 94
RR | 28
Temperature | 36.5° C
BP | 135/90
F_{IO_2} | 0.21
pH | 7.33
Pa_{CO_2} | 70
Pa_{O_2} | 35
HCO_3^- | 34 mEq/L

What action would you take at this time?
A. Administer bronchodilator therapy via MDI.
B. Administer oxygen via cannula at 2 L/min.
C. Administer oxygen via cannula at 6 L/min.
D. Administer oxygen via nonrebreathing mask.

30. A patient with COPD and a history of hypercapnia is receiving oxygen via simple mask at 10 L/min in the recovery room following admission for pneumonia. Upon transfer to the medical floor, he is noted to be increasingly drowsy and difficult to arouse. The nurse requests that you give him a breathing treatment with a bronchodilator. The most appropriate action would be to
A. Administer the breathing treatment as requested.
B. Obtain an arterial blood gas sample.
C. Change the oxygen to 2 L/min via nasal cannula.
D. Change the oxygen to 40% via Venturi mask.

There are many variations of this type of question regarding chronic hypercapnia and oxygen administration on both the Entry-Level and Registry examinations!
You may also expect:

31. A patient is being mechanically ventilated following craniotomy. During a suctioning procedure, the intracranial pressure monitor shows a sudden increase in intracranial therapist. The patient becomes restless and agitated. What is the most appropriate immediate action for the respiratory therapist in this situation?
A. Increase the F_{IO_2} on the ventilator to deliver 100% oxygen.
B. Recommend administration of a sedative.
C. Increase rate and volume of ventilation with a resuscitation bag.
D. Ask the registered nurse to page the physician "STAT."

This type of question about head injuries is a hot topic right now clinically. We'll have to keep a close watch on the NBRC to see what they say on the subject in our next revision of the tests. Currently, the boards still favor reducing the carbon dioxide to lower intracranial pressure.

EXPERIMENT

This exercise will seem simple, but it will help you understand control of breathing. It's even better if you have a pulse oximeter, some oxygen, and a nonrebreathing mask.

REMEMBER SAFETY! Sit down when you do this and have a partner! You could lower your cerebral blood flow!

- Put the oximeter probe on your finger.
- Breathe normally.
- Now inhale deeply and hold your breath.
- Time how long you can hold your breath.
- Next, inhale and exhale deeply several times. Fill your lungs and time how long you can hold your breath.
- Answer the questions below.

32. How long could you hold your breath the first time? _____ What about the second try?

_____

33. What were the pulse oximetry readings before _____, during _____,

and at the end of breath holding? _____

34. Compare the results and explain the differences in the breath-holding time and why you had to breathe. What is the meaning of the pulse oximetry readings?

- Now, breathe 100% oxygen for several minutes.
- At the end of the time, hyperventilate while breathing the oxygen.
- Now hold your breath.

35. What happened to the time of breath-hold?

36. Given a vital capacity of 5 L and an oxygen consumption of 250 ml/min, what is the theoretical maximum breath-holding time of a normal adult?

If you really want to try this experiment at its best, see your instructor about breathing from a high-flow CPAP system at 100% oxygen or use a ventilator!

The reflexes and receptors that control breathing are important. So is the input of conscious thought. The higher brain centers have a definite impact on how we breathe.

37. Why do we take the patient's respiratory rate without telling them we are doing it?

38. Name as many factors as you can that involve the higher brain centers increasing the rate of ventilation. (Hint: How do you breathe when a police car pulls up behind you and turns on the flashing lights?)

INFORMATION AGE

I didn't find anything on the Internet to get excited about. The AARC Clinical Practice Guidelines for oxygen administration do refer to the topic of hypoxic drive. Otherwise, *Egan's* has summarized this tricky little number quite nicely!

15 Bedside Assessment of the Patient

As I grow older, I pay less attention to what men say. I just watch what they do.
Andrew Carnegie

Patient assessment is the compass we steer by in the clinical setting. Chapter 15 helps you learn the fundamentals and help you identify the basics of the boards. Only bedside practice will give you mastery, and I think you'll have a lot of fun learning assessment. Your ability to evaluate using your senses will make all the difference in your career. The role of the respiratory therapist (RT) is evolving as we play an increasingly important part in critical response teams. Assessment skills are the KEY to everything from passing your boards to making lifesaving interventions at the bedside. Before you can go out and do that you need to learn the material in this chapter. This material is so important; I've packed this chapter full of questions, cases, and more questions!

WORD WIZARD

Chapter 15 starts off with an impressive list of nearly 40 new words for you to learn. Power up your medical terminology by reading the chapter and solving the crossword puzzle on the following page.

START AT THE BEGINNING

Successful assessors develop a systematic way of evaluating patients. Except in life-threatening emergencies, most practitioners begin by interviewing the patient. The interview may be short or long depending on the situation. The increasing use of protocols requires us to conduct more in-depth interviews. There is some evidence that clinicians who are trained in interpersonal communication are better able to gain valuable information from patients. Let's review the essentials of interviewing and history-taking.

1. What information would you gather prior to entering the patient's room? Hint: *Egan's* doesn't get to this for several pages, so use your common sense to come up with an answer then check Boxes 15-3 and 15-4 in "Format for Medical History."

2. Describe how to *start* the ideal interview. Be sure to discuss space, privacy, and introductions. Now you can go back to "Structure and Technique for Interviewing" on page 321 of your text.

   A. Space: _____

   B. Privacy: _____

   C. Introductions: _____

ACROSS

3. Bluish discoloration of the skin
4. Mucus from the tracheobronchial tree
8. Discontinuous abnormal breath sounds
12. Prefix for rapid
13. _____ emphysema is air under the skin
14. Look for distended veins here
15. Mucus that comes out the mouth
16. Medical term for slow
18. Extra, or abnormal sounds
22. _____ pressure, the difference between systolic and diastolic blood pressure
24. Level of consciousness (abbr)
25. Designed to expel mucus
27. _____ alternans occurs when you go back and forth between the diaphragm and the accessory muscles!
28. You have this if your breathing is labored when you lie down
29. Auscultation reveals breath _____
30. Body temperature below 32° Celsius
31. Stay at least 2-4 feet away to give the patient a personal _____ during the interview
32. Sweaty stuff

DOWN

1. _____ pressure, when the heart contracts
2. Dys, ortho, hypo, tachy—are all prefixes that go with this one lung suffix
4. Abdominal _____, occurs when the diaphragm is tired and the belly sinks in with each breath
5. Abnormal voice sounds heard over consolidation
6. Slow respiratory rate
7. _____ of monkeys (also a chest shape associated with air trapping)
8. Treasure, pigeon, or barrel
9. High-pitched continuous upper airway sound
10. Patient's perception of difficult breathing
11. Foul smelling
15. Another name for fainting
16. Heart rate below 60
17. Got pus?
18. Pattern of end-stage muscle fatigue
19. _____ signs
20. Rapid breathing pattern
21. Coughing up blood
23. Primary organ of gas exchange
26. I've got the fever

3. Circle the *best approach* from each set of choices in the following list:
   A1. "Hi, Bob, good morning"
   A2. "Good morning Mr. Johnson."

   B1. Stand at the foot of the bed.
   B2. Sit in a chair at the bedside.

   C1. Make room for your notes on the bedside table.
   C2. Keep your clipboard on your lap.

   D1. "Do you need anything right now?"
   D2. "I'll tell your nurse to check on you."

   E1. "I'll be back to see you in one hour."
   E2. "I'll return in a while to check on you."

ARE YOU ASKING THE QUESTIONS RIGHT?

The way you ask questions will determine your relationship with the patient and the amount and quality of the information you gather.

4. Circle the best approach from each set of choices in following list:
   A1. "What are you coughing up?"
   A2. "You didn't cough up blood, did you?"

   B1. "I understand you don't like your breathing treatments."
   B2. "Why don't you like these treatments?"

   C1. "How is your breathing today?"
   C2. "Is your breathing better today?"

5. When are "closed" questions most useful? Give an example.

SIGNS AND SYMPTOMS OF CARDIOPULMONARY DISEASE

I don't know about you, but five things come to mind when I think of common symptoms of heart and lung disease. I am sure there are more, but if these symptoms stand out in your mind, you can use them to your benefit as part of the interviewing process.

"I Feel Short of Breath..."

6. Describe the dyspnea (Borg) scale. Try to think of several reasons why this would be useful?

7. How else can you identify the degree of dyspnea a patient feels?

Dyspnea is the worst symptom of all and is disabling for many of our patients.

"Cough It Up!"

8. What are the possible causes of these common types of cough?

Cough	Cause(s)
A. Dry cough	_____
B. Loose, productive	_____
C. Acute, self-limiting	_____
D. Chronic	_____

9. What is the difference between mucus and sputum?

10. What are the three characteristics of sputum that should be documented and reported to the physician?

_____

_____

_____

11. Define *nonmassive* hemoptysis and give three common causes.

12. Define *massive* hemoptysis and give three possible causes.

"It Hurts When I Take a Deep Breath!"

13. What is the most serious (and famous) kind of nonpleuritic chest pain? _____

_____

14. How does pleuritic chest pain differ from nonpleuritic pain?

"Hot Stuff!"

15. Significant elevation of temperature will have what result on metabolic rate, oxygen consumption, carbon dioxide

production, and breathing pattern? _____

_____

16. Along with fever, what are two signs that are highly suggestive of respiratory infection?

A. _____

B. _____

MEDICAL HISTORY

Whether you personally take medical histories or not, you will need to be familiar with the standard format used in this process that is *always* conducted at some point (usually early on) during a patient's admission to the formal health care setting.

17. What do the initials "CC" and "HPI" stand for? List at least five important areas described in the HPI.

A. CC = _____

B. HPI = _____

    1. _____

    2. _____

    3. _____

    4. _____

    5. _____

18. What do the initials "PMH" stand for? List at least five important areas described in the PMH.

A. PMH = _____

    1. _____

    2. _____

    3. _____

    4. _____

    5. _____

General appearance is assessed during the first few seconds of *every* encounter with a patient. During the first encounter, I always look at their body as a whole, facial expression, anxiety level, positioning, and personal hygiene. (You may smell and hear information, too!)

19. Describe the significance of the findings for each of the areas of general appearance listed below.

	FINDING	SIGNIFICANCE
1.	Weak, emaciated, and diaphoretic	
2.	Appears anxious	
3.	Sitting up, leaning with arms on table	

LEVEL OF CONSCIOUSNESS

What's the difference between stuporous and lethargic? Obtunded and comatose? Alert and confused? These aren't completely subjective terms and you will see them used frequently in the medical record. After taking a look at the overall appearance, you need to determine the level of consciousness. For starters, the patient is either obviously conscious or not. If he or she is conscious, you have to find out the level of alertness. If the patient does not seem to be obviously conscious, you need to find out how depressed the sensorium is and describe this with commonly accepted terms.

20. What does the phrase "oriented × 3" mean?

_____

21. Compare and contrast the terms "lethargic" (your classmate) and "obtunded."

22. What is the difference between a "stuporous" patient and a "comatose" patient?

23. What is the first thing a respiratory therapist should evaluate in cases of a depressed level of consciousness?

_____

There are special rating systems like the Glasgow Coma Scale to help further identify the degree of coma. You also need to keep in mind that there are special circumstances that may make assessment more difficult, such as a hearing-impaired patient.

VITAL INFORMATION

Temperature, pulse, respiratory rate, and blood pressure are the traditional vital signs. These are cheap, useful, and easy to obtain. (People are starting to call pulse oximetry the "fifth vital sign" because it is taken so often.) Vital signs offer great clues about response to therapeutic interventions, but they're not as simple as you might think considering how often they are measured. Let's start with the basics.

24. Fill in the correct normal adult values (or terms) in the chart below.

	SIGN	AVERAGE NORMAL	LOWEST NORMAL	HIGHEST NORMAL
A.	Temperature			
B.	Heart rate			
C.	Respiratory rate			
D.	Systolic blood pressure			
E.	Diastolic blood pressure			

25. Name the four common sites for temperature measurement. Give a disadvantage of each site.

A. _____ _____

B. _____ _____

C. _____ _____

D. _____ _____

26. Match these pulsating terms to their throbbing definitions

Terms	Definitions
A. _____ tachycardia	1. palpable vibrations in pulse
B. _____ bruits	2. strength of pulse
C. _____ amplitude	3. pulse rate below 60 beats/min
D. _____ paradoxical pulse	4. drop in amplitude with inspiration
E. _____ pulsus alternans	5. pulse rate greater than 100 beats/min
F. _____ bradycardia	6. alternating strong and weak pulses

27. Match these flowing respiratory patterns to their whooshing definitions! (Hint: When in doubt, cheat—Try the glossary in back of the book!)

Terms	Definitions
A. _____ tachypnea	1. difficulty breathing in a supine position
B. _____ eupnea	2. abnormally low respiratory rate
C. _____ orthopnea	3. deep breathing
D. _____ platypnea	4. normal breathing pattern
E. _____ hyperpnea	5. abnormally high respiratory rate
F. _____ bradypnea	6. labored breathing in an upright position

28. How can you prevent the patient from becoming aware (and consciously altering) that you are taking their respiratory rate?

29. What condition may result in syncope in the hypovolemic patient? How can you prevent this from happening? How is it treated medically?

A. Condition: _____

B. Prevention: _____

C. Treatment: _____

30. What does it mean when patients show larger (>6 to 8 mm Hg) than normal drop in systolic pressure during inspiration?

EXAMINING THE CHEST AND LUNGS

The Big Four
- Inspect the chest!
- Palpate the chest!
- Percuss the chest!
- Auscultate the chest!

Sounds so easy when you put it that way, doesn't it? Before you start to assess, make sure you have enough **light,** enough **privacy,** enough **time,** and enough **quiet.** Chapter 15 describes the *ideal* evaluation of a patient. You will have to modify to meet the circumstances every time!

Inspection (See Me)
There's a lot you can see when you take a quick look at the patient. Practice looking. Let's find out if you know what to look for in a patient with respiratory problems.

31. Write a description for the following 6 abnormal chest shapes.

Bad Chests	Description
A. Barrel	_____
B. Kyphosis	_____
C. Kyphoscoliosis	_____
D. Pectus carinatum	_____
E. Pectus excavatum	_____
F. Scoliosis	_____

32. Breathing patterns are important, too. Describe the pattern that goes with these 6 conditions.

Condition	Pattern of Breathing
A. Asthma	_____
B. Atelectasis	_____
C. Chest trauma	_____
D. Epiglottitis	_____
E. Increased ICP	_____
F. Metabolic acidosis	_____

Experiment

To get good at this, you might try the mall. Yes, the mall. If you sit with a nice cup of espresso, you can see chest shape, breathing pattern, and all the rest. Compare adult patterns with those of children. Compare the chest shape of an elderly person to that of a young adult. After you try this exercise, answer the following questions.

33. Did you observe anyone breathing with their diaphragm? How could you tell? _____

_____

34. Did you observe the use of accessory muscles? How could you tell? _____

_____

35. How does the chest shape of a young adult differ from that of a senior? _____

_____

36. What unusual chest shapes did you observe? Anyone on portable oxygen? _____

_____

Palpation (Feel Me)

Palpation is the art of touching the chest wall. Palpation is an art (and a useful one) because it's so subjective. You have to get a feel for it. Don't practice this at the mall, please!

37. Explain the difference between vocal, tactile, and rhonchial fremitus.

38. Describe the difference in fremitus between emphysema and pneumonia.

39. How does subcutaneous emphysema form? What is the feeling of air under the skin called?

Experiment

You should learn palpation in the laboratory setting of your program. Because disrobing may be necessary, gowns, privacy, and professionalism are needed.

- Assess tactile fremitus by asking your classmate to repeat the word "ninety-nine" while you palpate under the clavicles, between the shoulder blades, along the sides, and over the lower lobes.
- Measure chest expansion as demonstrated in Figure 15-5 on page 333 in your text. Now answer these questions:

40. Describe the temperature of your partner's skin. _____

_____

41. Were there any areas of abnormal fremitus? Why (why not)?

42. Estimate the amount of chest expansion in centimeters. What is normal adult expansion?

Percussion (Touch Me)

Or tap me. Diagnostic percussion of the chest is another art form that is rarely practiced these days. Still, it can be useful in detecting some important abnormalities, and the NBRC expects you to be able to interpret the results of percussion findings!

43. Complete the chart below by identifying the percussion notes for these conditions.

Condition	Percussion Note
A. Emphysema	_____
B. Atelectasis	_____
C. Pleural effusion	_____
D. Pneumothorax	_____
E. Pneumonia	_____

44. What are the limitations of percussion? What can't you feel? _____

_____

Experiment

You should do this in the lab while you are performing the palpation and auscultation (see following section) exercises.

- Place your left middle finger on the intercostal space on the side of the chest.
- Rapidly strike it with your index finger or middle finger of your right hand. Do this on both sides of the chest.
- Repeat over the lower lobes in the back.
- Have your partner take a really deep breath and hold it while you tap.
- Have them exhale fully, then tap.
- Try tapping over something solid like the scapula.
- Try tapping over the abdomen.
- Tap on your own head.
- It takes practice to get good at percussion.

> Don't include this procedure in a routine examination of a patient unless other observations suggest an appropriate problem. Have an expert present when you try this in the clinical setting!

45. What happened to the resonance when your partner inhaled deeply? On exhalation?

Auscultation (Hear Me)

This is it. This is the big one. Auscultation seems so easy, and identifying breath sounds so difficult. Follow these 10 steps to improve your technique.

I. Sit the patient up whenever you can.
II. Turn off the TV, radio, or other external sources of noise.
III. Ask the patient to breathe slowly and deeply through their mouth.
IV. Listen to skin whenever you can.
V. Listen to the lower lobes first.
VI. Listen to one full inspiration and exhalation in each spot.
VII. Listen to both sides in each spot.
VIII. Auscultate lower, middle, and upper portions of the lung.
IX. Listen to front and back of the chest.
X. Compare right and left lungs/Compare upper and lower lobes.

Experiment

You should try this in the laboratory before going to the bedside. You can listen at home too. The more normal sounds you auscultate, the better you will be at recognizing abnormal sounds. All you need is your stethoscope, a partner (you can even start on yourself), and a quiet place to listen. Adjust the earpieces on your stethoscope so they are pointing slightly forward, not straight into your ears. (Check to make sure the diaphragm is "on" not the bell if your scope is adjustable.) Now, listen.

- Place your partner in a sitting position (or high Fowler's).
- Ask your partner to breathe in and out slowly through the mouth.
- Listen on skin over the posterior lower lobes (below the shoulder blade).
- In and out, right side and left side!
- Listen on the side of the chest (still lower lobes).

124

- Listen between the shoulder blades (not over the spine!).
- Listen on the front to the middle lobe and lingula (anterior, below nipple).
- Listen on the front below the collar bone (above nipples).
- Listen over the trachea.

Look in your text on page 335 at Figure 15-7. You can auscultate 20 or more places on the chest, but we don't usually do this much auscultation in the clinical setting. It takes too long for a routine evaluation. Always listen to upper, middle, lower, front, and back. I count 10 spots that MUST be listened to in the routine screening of breath sounds. When you hear abnormal sounds, or have a critically ill patient, you should expand your assessment.

Now that you've read the chapter and practiced, try answering these questions:

46. Fill in the chart below with descriptions of your favorite breath sounds.

	BREATH SOUND	PITCH	INTENSITY	LOCATION
A.	Vesicular			
B.	Bronchial			
C.	Bronchovesicular			

47. Compare the mechanisms and causes of coarse, low-pitched crackles and fine end-inspiratory crackles.

48. Contrast monophonic and polyphonic wheezes in terms of mechanisms, phase of ventilation, and conditions that produce these different musical sounds.

49. What's up with that rhonchi thing?

You will almost always want to take a look at patient's fingers. For one thing, it goes hand in hand with pulse oximetry. Cardiopulmonary disease may alter the fingers and other extremities.

50.   How do you test for capillary refill? (Test your own while you're at it.) What is a normal capillary refill time?

51.   Where should you check for edema caused by heart failure? Why?

_____

52.   Cyanosis is a bluish discoloration of the skin. Answer the following questions about cyanosis.

      A.   What is the specific cause of cyanosis? _____

      B.   What is peripheral cyanosis? _____

      C.   What is the main cause of peripheral cyanosis? _____

CASE STUDIES

Case 1

An alert 67-year-old politician is admitted for dyspnea and hemoptysis. While interviewing the patient you discover that he has been coughing up small amounts of thick, blood-streaked mucus several times per day for the last few days. He has a history of 100 pack-years of cigarette smoking. Physical examination reveals a barrel chest, use of accessory muscles, and digital clubbing.

53.   The patient's history and chest configuration suggest what primary pulmonary disorder?

_____

54.   Along with enlargement of the ends of the fingers, what sign helps you recognize clubbing?

_____

55.   What does the presence of clubbing suggest in this case?

_____

A 47-year-old homemaker is admitted for a systemic infection 3 days after cutting herself in the kitchen while preparing some chicken. She complains of dyspnea and has a fever. Her vital signs are pulse 110, respiratory rate 28, and blood pressure 76/58 mm Hg. The nurses notes reveal that the patient was alert on admission, but she is now confused and anxious. Her extremities are warm and capillary refill is normal.

56. Why do you think the patient's mental status has deteriorated?

57. What other "vital sign" should be evaluated? _____

58. Which abnormal vital sign has the most clinical significance in this case?

_____

You are called to the medical ward to evaluate a 29-year-old medical student who was admitted for shortness of breath and is now complaining of chest pain. The patient tells you that the pain came on suddenly and is worse when he inhales. Your interview reveals that this pain is on the right side and feels like a sharp, stabbing sensation. His temperature is normal, but blood pressure, heart rate, and respiratory rate are elevated. Palpation reveals crepitus over the right lateral chest wall.

59. What other physical assessments would be useful in determining the nature of the problem?

_____

60. What immediate treatment should you initiate in this situation? _____

_____

61. What diagnostic test would be helpful in determining the cause of the pain? _____

_____

62. What does the finding of crepitus on palpation indicate? _____

_____

Harry Garcia, a 59-year-old rock star is recovering from open heart surgery performed 2 days earlier. He is alert and oriented × 3. He complains of dyspnea (a lot of people seem to complain about that) and a dry cough. Vital signs reveal a pulse of 104 and a respiratory rate of 32 with a shallow pattern. The patient tells you that his difficulty breathing started yesterday and has been gradually getting worse. Auscultation reveals decreased breath sounds in both bases with end-inspiratory crackles.

63.	What is the most likely cause of the dyspnea? _____

_____

64.	What diagnostic test is indicated to confirm the diagnosis? _____

_____

65.	What respiratory care intervention(s) are indicated?

WHAT DOES THE NBRC SAY?

Killer. What more can I say? Whole sections of each test are devoted to this subject.

The NBRC exam matrix is filled with "assess by inspection," "assess by palpation," "assess by auscultation," and "interview the patient." There are additional questions in the therapy section of the test where you need the results of percussion or auscultation to come up with the right procedure. The effort you put into this one chapter will pay off more than any other. I know you will be looking at this subject more closely later on as you prepare for your boards. For now, let me give you some sample questions.

66.	During a chest examination of an intubated patient, the RT palpates vibrations on exhalation over the upper chest. What action should be taken at this time?
	A.	The patient should be given a bronchodilator.
	B.	The patient should be suctioned.
	C.	The patient should be given supplemental oxygen.
	D.	The patient should be placed on mechanical ventilation.

67.	A patient's medical record indicates that he has orthopnea. Which of the following best describes this condition?
	A.	difficulty breathing at night
	B.	difficulty breathing when upright
	C.	difficulty breathing on exertion
	D.	difficulty breathing when lying down

68. A child is brought to the emergency department for severe respiratory distress. Upon entering the room, the RT

   hears a high-pitched sound when the child inhales. This is most likely _____.
   A. wheezing
   B. stridor
   C. rhonchi
   D. crackles

69. An RT is asked to evaluate a patient for oxygen therapy. She notices that the patient is sleepy but arouses when

   questioned. This level of consciousness is best described as _____.
   A. confused
   B. obtunded
   C. stuporous
   D. lethargic

70. Which of the following breath sounds is most likely to be heard during acute exacerbation of asthma?
   A. wheezes
   B. crackles
   C. stridor
   D. rhonchi

71. All of the following physical findings are consistent with pneumonia *except* _____.
   A. dull percussion note
   B. presence of inspiratory crackles
   C. bronchial breath sounds over the affected area
   D. bradypnea

72. Which of the following findings suggest that a patient is oriented?
   I.   awareness of the correct date
   II. ability to correctly state his own name
   III. awake when you enter the room
   IV. cooperation with the treatment
       A. I and II
       B. II and III
       C. I and IV
       D. III and IV

73. During an interview, the patient states he has been coughing up thick, foul-smelling sputum. This finding is most consistent with
   A. a bacterial infection of the lung.
   B. a diagnosis of lung cancer.
   C. obstructive lung disease.
   D. pulmonary tuberculosis.

74. An RT is inspecting the chest of a child with respiratory distress. The practitioner notes that the child has a large

   concave depression of the sternum. This finding should be documented as _____.
   A. barrel chest
   B. pectus carinatum
   C. pectus excavatum
   D. kyphoscoliosis

75. All of the following physical findings are consistent with complete upper airway obstruction *except* _____.
   A. inability to speak
   B. stridor
   C. supraclavicular retractions
   D. flaring of the nostrils

76. While assessing a patient who is dyspneic and tachypneic, an RT notices a bluish discoloration of the lips and oral mucosa. The practitioner should document which of the following in the medical record?
   A. presence of cyanosis
   B. presence of hypoxemia
   C. presence of increased work of breathing
   D. presence of orthopnea

INFORMATION AGE

Now, this idea doesn't really have anything to do with assessment, exactly, but here goes. There is a free source of high-quality information in a low-tech format: audio. Apple computers provides all podcasts for free. The *New England Journal of Medicine*, *Vital Signs*, National Library of Medicine (NLM), and many other outstanding sources are available. I just listened to a talk on COPD provided by the NLM. This format works on both Macintosh and PC computers and is one of the most widely distributed formats anywhere. You don't need a media player to listen, only a computer and free software. So, free high-quality stuff! Better yet, I can listen and learn while I am commuting, exercising, washing the dishes—whatever. If you've ever downloaded music you can download great stuff. The emergency medical content is a good place to start on the assessment topic. They have lots of respiratory emergencies and rapid assessment to practice. Vital signs has medical mysteries you try to solve by following the assessment clues.

16 Interpretation of Clinical Laboratory Data

A little learning is a dangerous thing, but a lot of ignorance is just as bad.
Bob Edwards

In the clinical setting, laboratory assessment directly follows the interview and physical assessment. The NBRC's Clinical Simulation Examinations often follow a similar format. So, it seems natural for Chapter 16 to follow Chapter 15! A lot of students struggle with this topic because it is outside our usual realm, but I know you'll be on it when you finish these exercises. Remember, these tests are a lot harder on the patient than on you!

WORD WIZARD

The words sound so similar, it's easy to get confused. *Leuko* means "white," *erythro* means "red," and *thrombo* means "blood clot"—at least they do in Latin. Now finish these words.

White blood cells are called _____ cytes. When the white blood count goes up in

infection, we call it _____ cytosis. If the white count goes down, the new name is

_____ penia. Hemoglobin is found in the _____ cyte and can

carry oxygen. Your blood won't clot without the smallest formed element, the _____ cytes.

A condition of _____ penia may result in bleeding if you suction or draw a blood gas!

LAB TESTS

Certain laboratory test results are very useful to the respiratory therapist (RT). You will need to learn the normal values and what abnormal results mean if you want to pass your boards or get the big picture in the hospital. Let's start with complete blood counts.

White

1. What does a large elevation in white blood count (WBC) suggest?

   A. _____

   B. _____

   C. _____

2. Name three common causes of low WBC count.

   A. _____

   B. _____

   C. _____

3. What specific type of WBC is elevated in bacterial pneumonia? Viral?

    A. Bacterial: _____

    B. Viral: _____

Remember this one. We want to know if we need to give antibiotics. Also, watch for bands and segs.

4. Which WBCs are involved in problems like allergic asthma?

Red

5. What term describes a low RBC count? What is the treatment for this disorder?

    A. Term: _____

    B. Treatment: _____

         _____

6. What is a normal hemoglobin level, and why are RTs especially interested in hemoglobin levels?

    A. Normal: _____

    B. Respiratory role: _____

         _____

7. What blood abnormality is caused by chronic hypoxemia? _____

         _____

Anyone with this RBC count either has a lung problem or lives at altitude. Pumping this thick blood through the lung contributes to right heart failure.

8. Prior to performing an arterial blood gas (ABG), you would be wise to check what two *specific* laboratory values?

    A. Blood count _____

    B. Blood chemistry test _____

ELECTROLYTES

RTs are interested in electrolyte values because they affect acid-base balance and muscle function. We covered electrolytes in Chapter 12. See how much you remember.

9. What is the normal range for serum potassium? _____

_____

10. Why is potassium of particular interest in patients being weaned from mechanical ventilation?

11. Give at least one clinical example of how a patient develops a very high or very low potassium level.

    A. Hyperkalemia _____

    B. Hypokalemia _____

12. What value on the venous chemistry panel represents bicarbonate? _____

_____

13. Low chloride levels occur for what two primary reasons?

    A. _____

    B. _____

14. Why is the chloride level in sweat so important? What is the critical value?

    A. Importance: _____

    B. Value: _____

Sweat-chloride, an older test, is still useful, but genetic testing is able to give a better picture of the disease.

15. What other test is indicated when a chemistry panel shows abnormal anion gap? *This is an important idea on your board exams. If the electrolytes are off, the RT should recommend . . .*

_____

16. What are the two tests that together indicate renal function?

_____

ENZYMES

Enzymes are present everywhere in the body. They make reactions happen. (Remember carbonic anhydrase?) Specific enzymes are released when tissues are damaged. Myocardial infarction is a good example.

17. Name the two common liver enzymes that might be elevated in patients with hepatitis. Give the old names (what most people remember, like your old teachers!) and the new names.

	OLD	NEW
A.		
B.		

18. What specific enzyme found only in the heart is suggestive of a myocardial infarction?

_____

You should know that this one shows up about 3 to 4 hours after the event and is normal within about 2 days. A better one is troponin, because it spikes and peaks earlier but stays in the blood longer. Lactic dehydrogenase is an older test.

SPUTUM IS OUR BREAD AND BUTTER

You will probably be asked to obtain many sputum specimens during your career. Sputum samples are needed when lung infections are suspected. Gram stain, culture, and sensitivity are almost always performed, but only if you get the right stuff!

19. Why would the laboratory reject your beautiful sputum specimen? Give me specific reasons and include numerical values.

A. Pus _____

B. Epithelials _____

How can you improve the quality? Have the patient rinse out mouth and pharynx before you have them cough.

20. What is the purpose of growing the bacteria on a culture plate?

_____

_____

CASE STUDIES

Case 1

A patient presents in the emergency department complaining of shortness of breath, fever, and productive cough. A chest radiograph reveals pneumonia in the right lower lobe.

21. What blood test is indicated?

_____

22. What specific finding would suggest bacterial pneumonia?

_____

23. What would you like to do about the sputum?

Case 2

A 60-year-old two-pack-per-day smoker has a complete blood count ordered, and his WBC count is 9000. His hematocrit is 60%, and his hemoglobin is 20 g/dl.

24. What is the name for this elevation of red blood cells?

_____

25. What respiratory problem is indicated by the high hematocrit and hemoglobin?

_____

WHAT DOES THE NBRC SAY?

Now there aren't too many lab questions on the CRT or Written Registry Examinations. But the NBRC makes it clear you need to know every scrap of information in this chapter! Sounds confusing, but the lab values and tests will be inside the questions and especially the cases in the Clinical Simulation Examination. You may get to "order" a CBC on the exam. You'll need to be able to interpret the results. You will see some multiple-choice questions like these. Circle the best answer.

26. Sputum culture and sensitivity would be indicated for which of the following conditions?
    A. ST-segment elevation
    B. pleural effusion
    C. pneumothorax
    D. bronchitis

27. A patient presents in the emergency department with vomiting. Blood gas results reveal a metabolic alkalosis.

Based on this information, you would also suggest _____.
A. a STAT chest radiograph
B. electrolyte analysis
C. complete blood count
D. clotting time

28. A patient in the emergency department has a Chem 7 ordered and hypokalemia is present. What test should the RT recommend?
A. STAT chest radiograph
B. arterial blood gas
C. sputum culture
D. complete blood count

29. A sputum culture that is sent to the lab is likely to be rejected as saliva if _____.
A. less than 25 epithelial cells are present
B. less than 25 pus cells are present
C. more than 25 epithelial cells are present
D. more than 25 pus cells are present

FOOD FOR THOUGHT

30. A young adult male patient presents with symptoms of hypoxemia and signs of pneumonia. What are several possible reasons the white blood count is severely depressed?

INFORMATION AGE

You can learn more about troponin at http://www.labtestsonline.org/understanding/analytes/troponin/glance.html. **This is Lab Tests Online.** You want to check this out because it is made by lab professionals and written for the public to understand.

The hottest new issue in cardiac medicine is inflammation. Inflammation may cause vascular and cardiac damage in people who have normal cholesterol levels. Inflammation may result in cardiac disease in otherwise normal individuals. For more on the "C reactive protein" test of inflammation, look at labtestsonline or go to: http://focus.hms.harvard.edu/2002/Nov22_2002/pathology.html.

17 Interpreting the Electrocardiogram

There is only one thing worse than hardness of heart and that is softness of head.
Theodore Roosevelt

In the clinical setting, a lot of respiratory therapists (RTs) perform electrocardiography procedures as part of their jobs. Advanced life support certification requires knowledge of rhythms, and so do your board examinations. We discuss cardiac care in respiratory care because of the close relationship between the heart and the lungs. A lot of students struggle to learn arrhythmias, so I've tried to help you figure out what to emphasize and what the classic patterns look like on tests. The "real world" of electrocardiography is wonderfully complex and specialized so that you can spend many years learning the finer points after you graduate.

A PICTURE IS WORTH...

There are no new words that we haven't already covered, so why not go right to the picture? Label all these heart parts and conduction clues.

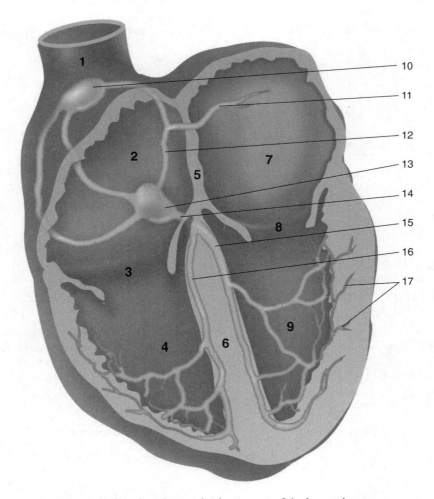

Anatomy of the impulse-conducting system of the human heart.

Heart Parts	Conduction Clues

1. _____

2. _____

3. _____

4. _____

5. _____

6. _____

7. _____

8. _____

9. _____

10. _____ natural "pacemaker" of the heart

11. _____ conducts impulses through the atria

12. _____ carries impulses across the right atrium

13. _____ "backup pacemaker"

14. _____ why not "hers"?

15. _____ carries impulse to the left ventricle

16. _____ carries impulse to the right ventricle

17. _____ fingerlike projections penetrate the ventricles

18. Let's get the basic identification perfect. Refer to the ECG waves and label the four common waves and indicate the event they represent.

Normal configuration of electrocardiographic waves, segments, and intervals. (Modified from Wilkins RL, Krider SJ, Sheldon RL: Clinical assessment in respiratory care, ed 5, St. Louis, 2005, Mosby.)

Wave   **Represents**

A. _____   _____

B. _____   _____

C. _____   _____

D. _____   _____

Now answer the following questions about ECG waves.

19. Where is atrial repolarization?

   _____

20. What is the maximum duration of the P-R Interval?

   _____

21. What pathologic abnormality results in a depressed or elevated S-T segment?

   _____

MAKING MEASUREMENTS

The ECG paper is made up of tiny boxes or grids that allow you to measure time on the horizontal axis, and millimeters of deflection on the vertical axis. A darker line occurs every five boxes.

22. What is the normal paper speed for an ECG?

   _____

23. The time (horizontal) represented by one small box is _____ seconds, and by one large

   box is _____ seconds.

24. One millivolt of electrical energy will produce a deflection of _____ small boxes or

   _____ large boxes.

START AT THE BEGINNING

Because many RTs perform ECGs on patients or take care of monitored patients, you will need to be able to evaluate the rhythms you see to maintain safe patient care. Successful assessors have developed a systematic way of evaluating the ECG.

Step 1: Evaluate the Rate
You can do this manually, or rely on the electronic data. There are time marks every 3 seconds. So, the number of QRS complexes in 6 seconds can be multiplied by 10. When the rate is regular, you can divide 300 by the number of large boxes between two QRS complexes.

Try It, You'll Like It!

Count the rate in pattern 1 by both manual methods.

Pattern 1.

25. The number of QRS complexes in this 6 second strip is _____. Multiply by 10 to get a

rate of _____.

26. There are _____ heavy lines between complex A and complex B; 300 divided by this

number is _____. That's the average rate!

   Does every P wave have a QRS that follows it? That indicates a sinus rhythm!

27. If the rate is below 60, it is called sinus _____.

28. If the rate is above 100, it is called sinus _____.

Step 2: Measure the PR Interval

Count the number of small boxes between the start of the P wave and the start of the QRS complex. Remember the normal value of less than 0.20 second (five small boxes). A P wave, followed by a QRS, but separated by a prolonged PR interval, represents a delay at the AV node. This is called a first-degree heart block. No treatment is usually needed. We just monitor for a worsening block.

Try It, You'll Like It!

Measure the PR interval in pattern 2.

Pattern 2.

29. The time from the P wave to the QRS complex is _____ second(s).

30. What arrhythmia does this represent?

_____

Step 3: Evaluate the QRS Complex

The normal QRS is no more than 0.12 second (three small boxes) in width. Wide QRS complexes are abnormal and do not result in good ventricular contractions.

Try It, You'll Like It!

Measure the QRS complex in pattern 3.

Pattern 3.

31. The duration of the QRS complex is _____ second(s).

Step 4: Evaluate the T Wave

Normal T waves are upright and rounded. Inverted T waves represent poor blood flow to the heart muscle. Strangely shaped T's may be caused by hyperkalemia.

32. The T wave in pattern 1 is (circle one)
    upright
    inverted

Step 5: Evaluate the ST Segment

A normal ST segment is basically flat-isoelectric. Elevated, or depressed ST segments are bad. They represent oxygenation problems and are seen in conditions like myocardial infarction (MI).

Try It, You'll Like It!

Evaluate the ST segment seen in pattern 4.

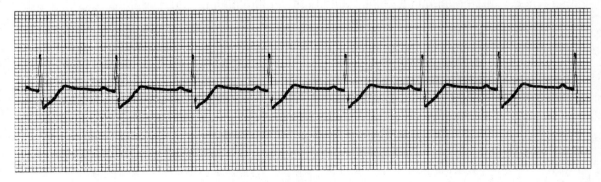

Pattern 4.

33. The ST segment in pattern 4 is (circle one)
    elevated
    flat
    depressed

141

Step 6: Identify the RR Interval

You are looking for a regular relationship. If the Rs are not the same distance apart, you have an irregular rhythm.

Try It, You'll Like It!

Evaluate the RR interval seen in pattern 5.

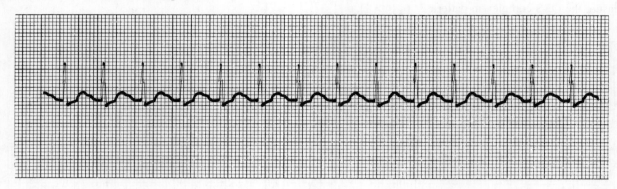

Pattern 5.

34. The RR interval in this pattern is (circle one)
regular
irregular

RECOGNIZING ARRHYTHMIAS

Now that you have the basic idea, let's take a look at the major dysrhythmias that you will encounter. This is pattern recognition, so look for the "picture" each rhythm shows.

Normal Sinus Rhythm

Pattern 6

- The P wave is upright.
- The PR interval is normal.
- Each P is followed by a normal QRS.
- RR intervals are regular and the rate is between 60 and 100 per minute.
No treatment is needed for this rhythm!

Pattern 6.

Sinus Bradycardia

Pattern 7

- Upright P wave.
- Normal PR interval.

142

- Each P is followed by a normal QRS.
- R-R intervals are regular, *but the rate is less than 60.*

This is **absolute bradycardia.** It is only a problem if the blood pressure drops. You might see this rhythm during suctioning as a result of vagal stimulation. Stop suctioning! Intravenous atropine is a treatment for this arrhythmia.

Pattern 7.

Sinus Tachycardia

- The P wave is upright.
- The PR interval is short.
- Each P is followed by a normal QRS.
- RR intervals are regular, *but the rate is over 100!*

This is sinus tachycardia. Tachycardia is the first sign of hypoxemia in most patients. Consider whether you are doing something to cause it, like suctioning. Look back at pattern 5 to see an example of sinus tachycardia.

First-Degree Heart Block

- The P wave is upright.
- The PR interval is *prolonged.*
- Each P is followed by a normal QRS.
- RR intervals are regular.

Only a problem if signs and symptoms such as low blood pressure, chest pain, and so on, come with it. It may be caused by drugs or a myocardial infarction. Look back at pattern 2 to see an example of a first-degree block.

Second-Degree Heart Block

Our block is moving lower down the conduction pathway. Not good! There are two types.

Second-Degree Type I

This one is called Wenckebach or Mobitz type I. The P waves have a progressively prolonged transmission (prolonged PR interval) followed by a P with no QRS. There is usually a repeated pattern, like three Ps and one lost QRS (pattern 8).

Pattern 8.

Second-Degree Type II

This is Mobitz type II. It is definitely not a good sign. This block is worse. You will see some Ps conducted (followed by a QRS) and some Ps with no QRS following (pattern 9).

Pattern 9.

Third-Degree Block

Also called complete heart block, this rhythm is definitely life threatening. No impulses from the SA node are conducted. Because the ventricles have their own intrinsic rate, you will see the atria paced by the SA node (P waves) and the ventricles (QRS) pacing themselves (pattern 10). These QRS complexes are often wide. Blood pressure is poor, and an artificial pacemaker is needed.

Pattern 10.

A Little Story to Help Keep It Straight

An easy way to keep the blocks straight is a love story gone wrong.

A couple gets married. At first, you have a normal sinus rhythm. She (P) is at home, and he (QRS) comes home on time. **A,** After a while, he is spending more time with his secretary after work. She (P) is at home; he is coming home late. A first-degree block. **B,** Eventually, while she (P) is at home, he (QRS) comes home later, then later, and one night, he does not come home (missed QRS)! A second-degree type one block **(C).** She (P) is rightfully furious, and tells him to mend his ways or else. He (QRS) starts coming home on time, but then he goes back to his old ways and does not come home. A second-degree type II block **(D).** AFTER this final insult, she (P) is at home, and he (QRS) is at home, but they are sleeping in separate bedrooms and have nothing to do with each other! Third-degree block! **E,** A pacemaker (or a divorce lawyer) is needed in this situation.

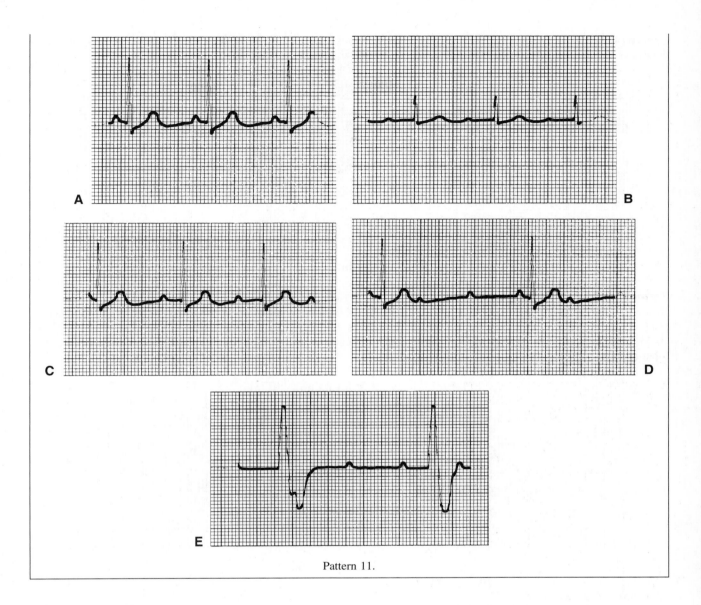

Pattern 11.

Atrial Dysrhythmias

Atrial fibrillation is an erratic quivering of the atria that does not deliver a good preload to the ventricles (pattern 11). Also, clots may form in the atria. Sometimes, the ventricle responds to fibrillation with a rapid rate as well. No P wave is seen, but the QRSs probably look OK. Drugs (like digitalis) or cardioversion are possible treatments. (Notice the RR intervals.)

Pattern 12.

Atrial flutter is a very rapid (250) atrial rate. You can spot it every time by noting the "sawtooth" or "picket fence" pattern of the atrial discharge (pattern 12). Drug or electrical treatments can help.

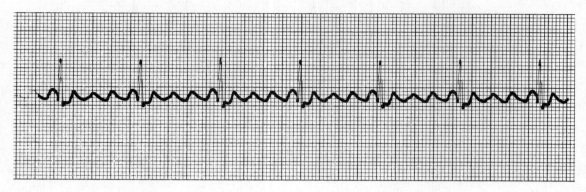

Pattern 13.

Premature Ventricular Contractions

You will want to notice these abnormal QRS complexes (pattern 13), because they are often caused by hypoxemia. In other words, if you are suctioning and the patient gets PVCs, STOP! Oxygenate the patient. There are other causes, like stress, caffeine, and nicotine. No big deal. Intravenous lidocaine is one therapy for too many PVCs (usually more than 6 per minute).

Pattern 14.

Ventricular Tachycardia

Tachycardia, of course, is a rate above 100. But this rhythm shows no P waves and shows wide QRS and does not usually have a pulse (pattern 14). **This condition is life threatening!** Stop, call for help, check for a pulse, and act appropriately. Drugs or defibrillation is needed.

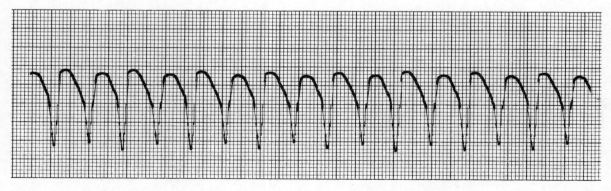

Pattern 15.

Ventricular Fibrillation

The only rhythm worse than this is a flatline (asystole) (pattern 15). There is no pulse, cardiac output, or blood pressure. Only defibrillation will really help, but you can do CPR and give oxygen and drugs as well.

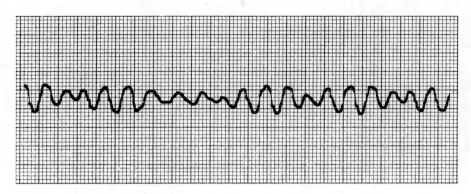

Pattern 16.

Practice recognizing the important arrhythmias. After a while, these basic patterns will be easy to spot, just like a Van Gogh painting, and you won't have to think too hard!

CASE STUDIES

Case 1

A student is suctioning a patient orally with a tonsil suction. The monitor shows sinus bradycardia. Blood pressure is falling. Alarms are alarming.

35. What should the student do?

36. What physiologic mechanism was responsible for the drop in rate?

_____

Case 2

A student is suctioning a patient via the endotracheal tube. The monitor shows sinus tachycardia with frequent premature ventricular contractions. Alarms are sounding. The patient is agitated.

37. What should Annie do? _____

38. What physiologic mechanism was responsible for the increased rate and arrhythmias?

    _____

While performing a ventilator check on a patient in the coronary care unit, a student observes the rhythm on the monitor has changed from atrial fibrillation to ventricular fibrillation.

39. What should the student do first?

40. Name at least three responses indicated to treat this rhythm.

WHAT DOES THE NBRC SAY?

Actual pictures of ECG rhythms usually appear in the Clinical Simulation Exam and occasionally on the other written exams. Cardioversion and defibrillation are on the Written Registry as well. You will need to supplement the text with more information to understand these subjects. The Advanced Cardiac Life Support material from the American Heart Association is a good resource. The Entry-Level Exam doesn't have too much on the heart ECG interpretation, but they do like to ask about performing ECGs. That isn't covered in this chapter, but you need to know about the specific lead placements for diagnostic 12-lead ECG. Here are some sample questions from Chapter 17 that you might run into on the subject of ECG interpretation. Circle the best answer.

41. An RT is suctioning a patient on a ventilator and observes the following rhythm on the monitor:

In regard to this pattern, the RT should
A. continue to suction the patient.
B. stop and administer 100% oxygen.
C. recommend atropine administration.
D. defibrillate the patient.

42. An RT is preparing to perform an arterial puncture when the following rhythm is observed on the monitor:

In regard to this pattern, the RT should
A. continue to suction the patient.
B. stop and administer 100% oxygen.
C. recommend atropine administration.
D. defibrillate the patient.

43. During a routine suctioning procedure, an RT notes the following rhythm on the cardiac monitor:

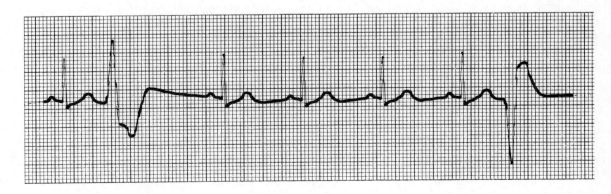

In regard to this pattern, the RT should:
A. continue to suction the patient.
B. stop and administer 100% oxygen.
C. recommend atropine administration.
D. defibrillate the patient.

44. During a routine suctioning procedure a respiratory therapist notes the following rhythm on the cardiac monitor

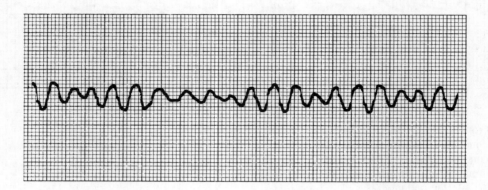

In regard to this pattern, the RT should:
A. continue to suction the patient.
B. stop and administer 100% oxygen.
C. recommend atropine administration.
D. defibrillate the patient.

FOOD FOR THOUGHT

The first time I did an ECG, it was on a woman who was my own age. I felt really embarrassed and awkward. I got over it, and so will you. Is this a good time to ask you a few personal questions?

45. Have you ever had to disrobe at the physician's office or clinic? How did you feel? How do you think patients feel when you ask them to strip?

46. How will you ensure that your patients don't feel awkward or embarrassed when you do ECGs or chest exams?

INFORMATION AGE

There is almost TOO much information about ECG on the Internet. Here are some sites that have been around a long time and are easy to use. If you are interested in this subject, you can dig pretty deep online.
- ECG Library is an excellent site from New Zealand that has been out there for more than a dozen years and has good links: www.ecglibrary.com/.
- And let's not forget the American Heart Association: www.americanheart.org.

18 Analysis and Monitoring of Gas Exchange

Vision is the art of seeing the invisible.
Jonathon Swift

Analyzing and monitoring gas exchange is one of the most important areas of the respiratory care profession. In Chapter 13 we talked about interpreting the acid-base balance of arterial blood gases. Naturally, there's more to it than that. Chapter 18 covers the equipment used to analyze blood and much more. For example, there are noninvasive methods to monitor gas exchange like capnometry and pulse oximetry. So, whether you're talking about clinical practice or thinking about credentialing examinations, you're going to need a firm grasp of this slippery subject.

WORD WIZARD

You'll have to learn the specialized terminology of invasive and noninvasive monitoring if you want to get the most mileage out of this material. Solve the crossword puzzle on the following page to test your understanding of the key terms in Chapter 18.

FIRST THINGS FIRST

First, you have to make a choice between analysis and monitoring. Analysis usually means obtaining a sample of body fluid and putting it in some type of lab analyzer to get results. Properly done, these measurements have a high degree of accuracy. Unfortunately, they are like a snapshot of a single event. Monitoring is usually done at the bedside and is a continuous process—more like watching a video. Next, you have a choice of invasive or noninvasive techniques. Invasive techniques are probably more accurate, but they also have a greater risk of harm to the patient. Good way to establish a baseline. Noninvasive methods are often used for monitoring and are especially useful when used together with invasive techniques. What is the conclusion? No one method is best. Your role as a clinician is to get the right balance. My role is to help you figure out how to do that!

MEET THE OBJECTIVES

You've read the chapter, and now you're feeling a little overwhelmed. I don't blame you. Answer the following questions and you will get a grip on the good stuff. Relax, get some coffee or soda; this is going to take a little time.

1. In your own words, explain how an electrochemical analyzer converts the number of oxygen molecules (Po_2) into a measurable reading.

2. There are two common types of electrochemical analyzers. Name them.

   A. _____

   B. _____

ACROSS

1. Oxygen analyzer that measures the flow of electrons between negatively and positively charged poles
4. _____ of care, testing blood at the bedside instead of in the lab
5. Systematic errors in measurement
6. Artery in the arm that's not your first choice
7. _____ vivo, inside the body
8. Big artery in the groin that is used for drawing blood when other choices fail
9. Allen's, for example
10. _____ vivo, outside the body
11. Never do this with a used needle
13. Pulse oximeters use this principle to detect arterial pulsation
16. Device that provides ongoing information to clinicians
18. Oxygen analyzing electrode
19. Preanalytical ones, bubble in sample for example
21. _____ invasive monitoring doesn't hurt
22. Modify this test and perform before radial puncture

23. Quality control
24. Oximeter used to measure carbon monoxide in the blood
25. Point-of-_____: method of testing blood at the bedside
26. Measure blood values in the laboratory

DOWN

2. External quality control testing program
3. Alternative to arterial sampling in infants
9. Clot buster
12. Sensor that works on optical detection instead of electrochemical properties
14. Oxygen analyzer that doesn't use a battery
15. Non-invasive oximeter commonly used to measure hemoglobin's saturation with oxygen
17. Determine the saturation of hemoglobin with a photoelectric device
20. Artery of choice for puncture or cannulation

3. Explain the differences between the two types of analyzers in terms of principle of operation and response time.

4. Describe the two-step process for calibrating an oxygen analyzer.

5. What is the gold standard of gas exchange analysis? What does this mean?

6. List four reasons why the radial artery is the preferred site for ABG sampling?

   A. _____

   B. _____

   C. _____

   D. _____

7. Describe the modified Allen test, and give the definition of a positive result.

   A. _____

   _____

   B. _____

   _____

8. Name four other sites you can use if the radial artery is unavailable or has a poor pulse.

   A. _____

   B. _____

   C. _____

   D. _____

9. How long should you wait after changing the F$_{IO_2}$ before performing an ABG on a patient with healthy lungs? A patient with COPD?

   A. _____

   B. _____

10. What technique can help prevent hyperventilation from pain or anxiety from altering the sample results?

11. AARC's ABG sampling guidelines describe several medications that may result in prolonged bleeding. These are anticoagulants (clot preventors) and thrombolytics (clot busters). Give two examples of each of these classes of drugs.
    A. Anticoagulants

       1. _____

       2. _____

    B. Thrombolytics

       1. _____

       2. _____

12. Name the four things you can do to avoid most preanalytical sampling errors. Hint: check Table 18-1 on page 371 of your text.

    A. _____

    B. _____

    C. _____

    D. _____

13. What precaution should you take when handling any laboratory specimen?

14. What are the three primary parameters measured by a blood gas analyzer?

    A. _____

    B. _____

    C. _____

154

15. If you wanted to measure actual hemoglobin saturation, what type of analyzer would be needed?

_____

16. What is the range of accuracy for most commercially available pulse oximeters?

_____

17. Describe three noninvasive ways you can determine the reliability of a pulse oximeter at the bedside.

    A. _____

    B. _____

    C. _____

18. According to the AARC guidelines, what action should you take to verify the results when pulse oximetry is unreliable or does not confirm suspicions about the patient's clinical state?

19. Describe the three main quality assurance procedures used to maintain consistently accurate blood gas results.
    A. Automated calibration

    B. Control media

C. Proficiency testing

20. For which patients is capillary sampling appropriate? _____

_____

21. What are the two most common errors committed during capillary sampling?

A. _____

B. _____

22. Explain what variables are reliable and unreliable in capillary sampling compared to arterial sampling.

23. What are the primary advantages and disadvantages of transcutaneous gas monitoring over arterial sampling?
A. Advantages

1. _____

2. _____

B. Disadvantages

1. _____

2. _____

24. When would you choose a pulse oximeter for monitoring an infant's oxygenation status over a transcutaneous monitor?

25. When would the transcutaneous monitor be preferred over the pulse oximeter?

26. Describe proper placement of a capnometer sampling chamber or adaptor for a patient who is being mechanically ventilated. _____

27. What are the normal values for end-tidal CO_2 for health individuals and how do they compare with values for arterial CO_2?

28. An end-tidal CO_2 of "0" may indicate a serious problem. Name two life-threatening causes of a "0" value for end-tidal CO_2.

    A. _____

    B. _____

29. While performing end-tidal CO_2 measurements, you notice that the baseline does not return to "0" on inspiration.

    Interpret this result. _____

Chapter **18** **Analysis and Monitoring of Gas Exchange**

30. While performing end-tidal CO_2 measurements, you notice that no real plateau is reached. Give two possible interpretations of this result.

A. _____

B. _____

CHAPTER HIGHLIGHTS

The questions you just answered covered many of the important points from Chapter 18; however, this chapter was really crammed with details. Here are a few more questions that highlight some of the main points we haven't already covered.

31. What are the three most common causes of oxygen analyzer malfunctions?

A. _____

B. _____

C. _____

32. Blood gases provide more information than other methods of gas exchange analysis. What are the three general areas that a blood gas helps to assess?

A. _____

B. _____

C. _____

33. What is the maximum ideal time between ABG sampling and analysis?

_____

34. What are the two primary benefits and hazards of indwelling peripheral arterial lines?
   A. Benefits

1. _____

2. _____

   B. Hazards

1. _____

2. _____

35. What is point of care testing, and what are the potential benefits of this method of testing blood samples?

36. What is the difference between capnography and capnometry?

Now that you have the information, let's see if you can apply it to the following scenarios.

Case 1

A 34-year-old firefighter is brought to the emergency department for treatment of smoke inhalation while fighting a house fire. His heart rate is 126, and respirations are 28 and labored. SpO_2 is 100% on 6 L via nasal cannula. Blood pressure is 145/90 mm Hg. Breath sounds are coarse with inspiratory crackles in both bases. The patient's face is smudged with soot, and he is coughing up sputum with black specks in it.

37. What clinical signs of hypoxemia does the patient display?

38. Explain why the pulse oximeter is reading 100% despite these signs?

39. What is the most probable cause of the hypoxemia?

40.   What blood test would you recommend to confirm your suspicions?

A premature infant is wearing supplemental oxygen. Her physician is concerned about the effects of hyperoxia on her lungs and eyes. The infant is being monitored by a pulse oximeter, which shows a saturation of 100%.

41.   What range of P_{O_2} is possible with an Sp_{O_2} of 100%?

42.   What type of noninvasive monitoring would you recommend in this situation?

An elderly patient is admitted for acute exacerbation of his longstanding COPD. He is wearing a nasal cannula at 2 L/min.

43.   What is the simplest way to quickly assess his oxygenation status?

44. Why would you recommend an arterial blood gas for this patient?

A patient was riding his motorcycle without a helmet when he crashed. Now he has a head injury and is being mechanically ventilated. His physician asks you to make recommendations regarding monitoring his gas exchange.

45. What are the advantages of using capnometry to monitor carbon dioxide in this situation?

46. Where would you place the capnometer probe in the ventilator circuit?

47. During monitoring, you notice that the capnograph does not return to "0" when the patient inhales.

    What does this indicate? _____

48. A few minutes later the patient's exhaled CO_2 levels begin to rise. So does his blood pressure. Jimmy becomes agitated. What action would you take?

49.	Why do rising CO_2 levels cause increases in intracranial pressure?

WHAT DOES THE NBRC SAY?

The NBRC has a strong affinity for monitoring gas exchange. So should you! You will find pulse oximeters and oxygen analyzers on the Entry-Level Exam. Capnography and transcutaneous monitoring go into the Registry Exams, so does mixed venous sampling, co-oximetry, blood gas analyzers, and quality control. Here's a baker's dozen of what you can expect. Circle the best answer.

50.	A respiratory therapist is preparing to perform pulse oximetry. Which of the following would be *least* beneficial for assessing accuracy of the device?
	A.	checking the capillary refill time
	B.	assessing skin color and temperature
	C.	performing an Allen test on the patient
	D.	assessing pulse rate

51.	Which of the following would you perform after obtaining an arterial blood gas sample?
	I.	Remove air bubbles from the sample.
	II.	Mix the sample by rotating the syringe.
	III.	Maintain site pressure for at least 1 minute.
	IV.	Add heparin to the sample.
		A.	I only
		B.	I and II only
		C.	I, II, and III only
		D.	I, II, III, and IV only

52.	A pulse oximeter is being used to monitor a patient who was rescued from a fire. The Sp_{O_2} is 90%; however, the patient is unconscious and shows signs of respiratory distress. What additional test should the RT recommend?
	A.	CT scan
	B.	electrolyte measurement
	C.	co-oximetry
	D.	hemoglobin and hematocrit levels

53.	A polarographic oxygen analzyer fails to calibrate when exposed to 100% oxygen. The first action the respiratory therapist should take would be to _____.
	A.	replace the battery
	B.	replace the membrane
	C.	replace the fuel cell
	D.	try another oxygen source

54.	An infant is placed on a transcutaneous oxygen monitor. The $Tc_{P_{O_2}}$ is reading 40 mm Hg less than the Pa_{O_2} obtained from an arterial sample. All of the following could cause this problem *except* _____.
	A.	improper calibration of the transcutaneous electrode
	B.	room air contamination of the transcutaneous electrode
	C.	inadequate heating of the skin at the electrode site
	D.	inadequate perfusion of the skin at the electrode site

162

55. Which of the following analyzers is calibrated to a value of zero when exposed to room air?
   A. Clark electrode
   B. galvanic oxygen analyzer
   C. capnometer
   D. Geisler-type nitrogen analyzer

56. Which of the following would be most useful in assessing proper tube placement following endotracheal intubation?
   A. transcutaneous monitoring
   B. arterial blood gas analysis
   C. pulse oximetry
   D. end-tidal CO_2 monitoring

57. Complications of arterial puncture include all of the following *except* _____.
   A. pulmonary embolus
   B. hematoma
   C. infection
   D. nerve damage

58. A galvanic oxygen analyzer is being used as a check of the ventilator system to measure the delivered F_{IO_2}. The set F_{IO_2} is 40%; however, the analyzer is reading 32%. Which of the following is the most likely cause of this discrepancy?
   A. The batteries in the analyzer need to be changed.
   B. The electrode membrane has water condensation on its surface.
   C. The analyzer needs to be calibrated.
   D. The ventilator requires servicing.

59. Which of the following will affect the accuracy of pulse oximeter measurements?
   I. increased bilirubin levels
   II. decreased hematocrit levels
   III. dark skin pigmentation
   IV. exposure to sunlight
       A. I and II only
       B. II and III only
       C. III and IV only
       D. II, III, and IV only

60. An arterial blood gas sample is drawn from a patient who is breathing room air. Analysis reveals the following results:

pH	7.45
Pa_{CO_2}	35 mm Hg
Pa_{O_2}	155 mm Hg

   Which of the following best explains these results?
   A. Too much heparin was added to the sample.
   B. An air bubble has contaminated the sample.
   C. Analysis of the sample was delayed for more than 60 minutes.
   D. The patient was hyperventilating during the puncture.

61. Which of the following sites would be the best for continuous monitoring of exhaled carbon dioxide during mechanical ventilation?
   A. exhalation valve
   B. inspiratory side of the ventilator circuit
   C. expiratory side of the ventilator circuit
   D. endotracheal tube connector

Chapter **18** **Analysis and Monitoring of Gas Exchange**

62. Which of the following is true concerning the use of a transcutaneous P_{O_2} monitor?
    A. Tc_{PO_2} should be checked with arterial blood samples.
    B. The skin temperature control should be maintained at 37° C.
    C. The site should be changed every 24 hours.
    D. The low calibration point is determined using room air.

FOOD FOR THOUGHT

63. How would you modify your technique if you had to perform ABGs on a patient receiving anticoagulants?

64. What problems may occur as a result of icing ABG samples?

65. Switching probes from one brand of pulse oximeter to another is strongly discouraged. What could happen if you do this?

66. Why can you use a capnometer during CPR but not a pulse oximeter?

INFORMATION AGE

You could really expand on *Egan's* review of the fundamentals of this subject by checking out these interesting corporate sites.
- I think you really MUST go to www.masimo.com. Check out the pulse oximeters that CAN measure carbon monoxide attached to hemoglobin and pulse oximeters that noninvasively measure what only co-oximeters could do with whole blood before this new technology. (Your board exams do not currently talk about these devices—you can't use a pulse ox on the boards when you have smoke inhalation.)
- Other corporate sites are equally good: www.radiometeramerica.com/ will lead you to www.deep-picture.com/, where you can learn a lot more about this topic.
- Point of care testing is super hot right now, so you could learn more at ibet.asttbc.org/poc.htm. Ibet is the Institute for Biomedical Engineering. This site also has good history on ABG analzyers in general.
- Abbott Medical now has the I-STAT, one popular point of care ABG analyzer: www.abbottpointofcare.com/istat/.

19 Pulmonary Function Testing

Most teachers would continue to lecture on navigation while the ship is going down.
James Boren

Remember when you were little, and blowing out those candles on your birthday cake was an exciting but difficult task? That was your first pulmonary function test (PFT). If you could blow out the candles, you passed and got your wish. I wish everybody liked PFTs as much as I do, but I admit it is a tough subject. In the last few years, lung testing has taken on even greater importance. Multiskilling, assessment-based protocols, increased interest in asthma, disability and legal issues, and a strong focus on the credentialing examinations are just a few reasons for the resurgence of interest in the science of diagnosing and quantifying pulmonary disorders.

WORD WIZARD

A quick glance at the key terms in Chapter 19 should leave you breathless with desire (or despair) to know what all those abbreviations mean. In fact, it would be pretty difficult to have a conversation with a pulmonary function technologist without speaking in acronyms. Match the right terms or abbreviations with the correct definition.

Terms/Abbreviations	Definitions
1. _____ DL	A. volume inspired with a normal breath
	B. greatest amount of air you can breathe in 12 to 15 seconds
2. _____ ERV	C. largest amount of air the lungs can hold
3. _____ VT	D. fastest flow rate generated at the very beginning of forced exhalation
4. _____ IRV	E. milliliters of gas the lung can transfer to the blood
5. _____ RV	F. amount of air you can exhale after a maximum inspiration
6. _____ TLC	G. ratio of volume exhaled in 1 second to total volume exhaled
7. _____ VC	H. average expiratory flow during the early part of forced exhalation
8. _____ IC	I. amount of air you can inhale after a normal exhalation
9. _____ FRC	J. amount of air you can inhale after a normal inspiration
10. _____ MVV	K. air left in the lungs after a maximum exhalation
11. _____ FVC	L. air left in the lungs after a normal exhalation
12. _____ PEF	M. amount of air you can forcefully exhale after a maximum inspiration
13. _____ $FEF_{200-1200}$	N. average expiratory flow during the middle part of forced exhalation
14. _____ FEV_1	O. volume of air you can forcefully exhale in 1 second
15. _____ $FEF_{25\%-75\%}$	P. amount of air you can exhale after a normal exhalation
16. _____ FEV_1/FVC	

As if learning all those acronyms wasn't enough, we can't really go on until you put the four lung volumes and four lung capacities into perspective with their normal values in a healthy adult. Use the box I've provided. Memorize this information! It will serve you well on your board exams!

17. Fill in the names and normal values that go with each letter in the box. See Figure 19-10 on page 418 of your text if you need help.

	VOLUME/CAPACITY	VALUE
A.		
B.		
C.		
D.		
E.		
F.		
G.		
H.		

Now see if you can draw the box and fill in the values on a separate sheet of paper without looking. Check your answers. Do this until you have it down! These are the same values the NBRC uses for normal subjects. Note the way it progresses from 1.2 to 2.4, etc., to make your memorizing easier.

Answer these questions to find out if you have grasped the important points for each area of lung testing.

Lung Volumes

Lung volume measurement is an important adjunct to spirometry and helps quantify and determine a diagnosis of restriction or obstruction. Specialized equipment is needed to perform these tests.

18. Which volumes *cannot* be measured with a spirometer?

_____

19. Which capacities *cannot* be measured with a spirometer?

_____

20. Name the three tests used to determine the volumes and capacities that cannot be measured.

A. _____

B. _____

C. _____

21. What is thoracic gas volume?

22. How will volumes or capacities for a patient with air trapping obtained by helium dilution or nitrogen washout differ from those obtained with a body plethysmograph?

23. What effect will an air leak have on the values obtained by helium dilution or nitrogen washout?

Spirometry

Spirometry is the most commonly performed pulmonary function test, and vital capacity (also known as forced vital capacity) is the most commonly obtained value. Many types of spirometers exist, but any one that meets the standards and is working properly can be used.

24. What four variables are used to calculate normal values for spirometry?

A. _____

B. _____

C. _____

D. _____

25. You must produce acceptable results that provide valid, reliable information based on how long the patient exhales, how closely multiple tests correlate, and how fast the patient starts the maneuver. Fill in the details for each of the criteria below:

A. duration _____

B. variance of two best FVCs _____

C. satisfactory start _____

D. minimum number _____

26. Which FVC should you report? Which FEV_1?

A. FVC: _____

B. FEV_1: _____

27. Which flow rate is the greatest? _____

28. Which flow rate represents large airways? _____

29. Which flow rate represents the middle range? _____

30. A spirometer is considered accurate if the volume is verified to be within what percentage of a known value? (Hint: Check out "Quality Control" in the AARC CPG on Spirometry, or look at Table 19-3 on page 404 in *Egan's*.)

31. What device is used to verify the volume of a spirometer? _____

32. What is the normal value for MVV? How is this test performed? _____

Diffusion

Diffusing capacity represents the ability of the lung to transfer gas into the blood. This test requires breathing a special gas mixture.

33. What gas is usually used to measure the lung's ability to transfer gas to the blood?

_____

34. What other special gas is used in this test? Why?

_____

_____

35. What blood test results are needed to ensure accuracy of diffusion studies?

_____

_____

INTERPRETATION FUNDAMENTALS

In a minute, we'll go to our case studies and board exam questions to test your ability to put all the information together. First, see if you have the basic ideas straight.

36. What are the two major categories of pulmonary disease classification? Fill in the chart below to compare the effects of each category. (Hint: see Table 19-1!)

	CATEGORY	ANATOMY	PHASE	PATHOLOGIC CONDITION	MEASURE
A.					
B.					

37. Fill in the corresponding percent of predicted for the degrees of impairment.

Degree of Impairment   **% Predicted Value**

A. Normal   _____

B. Mild   _____

C. Moderate   _____

D. Severe   _____

38. The original normal values for pulmonary functions were probably based on a 6-foot-tall, 20-year-old Caucasian male. How are normal values corrected for non-Caucasians?

_____

39. Compare the FEV_1/FVC ratios you would see in normal, obstructed, and restricted patients. (Hint, take a look at Table 19-2 on page 402 of your text.)

A. Normal: _____

B. Obstructed: _____

C. Restricted: _____

Now that you have the information, let's see if you can apply it to the following scenarios. Use the algorithm in Figure 19-16 on page 427 until you have the basics down pat. Remember, the LLN, or lower limit of normal, is 80% for the vital capacity, and the lower limit of normal for FEV_1/FVC is 70% for case purposes.

Case 1

Spirometry is performed on a 24-year-old woman who complains of a "tight chest" and cough. Simple spirometry shows the following:

Test	Actual	Predicted	% Predicted
FVC	3.2 L	4 L	80%
FEV_1	1.6 L	3.2 L	50%
FEV_1/FVC	50%	70%	

40. Interpretation? _____

41. What test should be performed in light of the results and the clinical information? (If you're not sure, check out PFT Report No. 2 in the Mini Clini that starts on p. 428 at the chapter's end.)

_____

Case 2

A 34-year-old respiratory care student is required by his instructor to undergo pulmonary function testing as part of a course. Here are the results:

Test	Actual	Predicted	% Predicted
FVC	3.9 L	4.8 L	81%
FEV_1	3.1 L	4.1 L	76%
FEV_1/FVC	79%	70%	

42. Interpretation? _____

43. What pulmonary function test does the algorithm suggest using now?

Case 3

A 60-year-old shipyard worker complains of dyspnea on exertion and dry cough. Here are his spirometry results:

Test	Actual	Predicted	% Predicted
FVC	2 L	4 L	50%
FEV$_1$	1.5 L	3.4 L	44%
FEV$_1$/FVC	75%	70%	
TLC	2.4	4.8	50%

44. Interpretation? _____

45. What additional test would be helpful?

46. What additional history would be helpful?

Case 4

A woman presents in her physician's office complaining of dyspnea on exertion. Spirometry and lung volume results show the following:

Test	Actual	Predicted	% Predicted
FVC	1.5 L	3 L	50%
FEV$_1$	0.75 L	2.5 L	30%
FEV$_1$/FVC	50%	70%	
TLC	2.6 L	3.8 L	68%

47. Interpretation? _____

48. What additional history would be helpful?

A 70-year-old man with a 100-pack-year smoking history complains of a dry cough and dyspnea on exertion. Results of lung tests show:

Test	Actual	Predicted	% Predicted
FVC	2.9 L	4.4 L	65%
FEV_1	1.3 L	3.7 L	35%
FEV_1/FVC	59%	70%	
TLC	6.6 L	5.5	120%
FRC	4.5 L	2.2	
RV	3.7 L	1.1 L	
D_{LCO}	16	25	64%

49. Interpretation? Be complete; what specific type of disease is suggested?

50. What disease state do the lung volumes and history suggest?

_____

51. Why is the vital capacity lower than predicted?

_____

For additional practice, be sure to check out the case studies in Chapter 19 of your textbook!

WHAT DOES THE NBRC SAY?

If you look at the board exam matrix (free at www.nbrc.com), you'll see things like "PFT studies (e.g., flows, volumes, diffusion, prebronchodilator and postbronchodilator)," and "perform FVC and FEV_1," and, of course, the equipment like body boxes, spirometers, and pneumotachometers. I guess you have to know this stuff pretty well! Try your hand at some questions in the good old NBRC style. Circle the best answer.

52. Which of the following tests would be helpful in assessing the effects on cigarette smoking on the smaller airways?
A. FVC
B. $FEF_{25\%-75\%}$
C. FEV_1
D. $FEF_{200-1200}$

53. A patient's physician asks you to recommend a pulmonary function test to help assess the effects of a possible tumor in the trachea. Which of the following would you recommend?
A. spirometry with volume-time curves
B. spirometry before and after bronchodilator
C. lung volume studies via nitrogen washout
D. spirometry with flow-volume loops

54. A pulmonary function technologist tests a spirometer by injecting 3.0 L of air from a large-volume syringe. The spirometer measures a result of 2.90 L. Which of the following is true regarding this situation?
   A. The results are within normal limits.
   B. The spirometer is not ready to use.
   C. The air was injected too slowly.
   D. The BTPS corrections were not made properly.

55. Which of the following values could be incorrectly calculated?

Test	Actual	Predicted	% Predicted
FVC	4.4 L	4.8 L	92%
FEV$_1$	3.5 L	4.1 L	80%
FEV$_1$/FVC	80%	70%	
TLC	5.2 L	5.5	
FRC	2 L	2.4	
ERV	1.2 L	1.2 L	
RV	1 L	1.2 L	

   A. TLC
   B. FVC
   C. FRC
   D. RV

56. Which of the following pulmonary measurements is usually the smallest?
   A. inspiratory capacity
   B. vital capacity
   C. functional residual capacity
   D. total lung capacity

57. The following results were obtained from spirometry of an adult female smoker with chronic bronchitis. What is the correct interpretation?

Test	Actual	Predicted	% Predicted
FVC	3.9 L	4.8 L	81%
FEV$_1$	3.1 L	4.1 L	76%
FEV$_1$/FVC	79%	70%	

   A. Results indicate a mild diffusion defect.
   B. Results are within the normal range.
   C. A mixed obstructive/restrictive defect is present.
   D. Results show obstructive lung disease.

58. What percent increase in forced spirometric volumes or flow rates after a bronchodilator is administered is the *minimum* indication that reversible airway obstruction is present?*
   A. 5%
   B. 10%
   C. 15%
   D. 20%

59. Which of the following can be measured during spirometric testing?
   A. residual volume
   B. tidal volume
   C. total lung capacity
   D. functional residual capacity

---

*On page 414 in *Egan's* you will find the answer under the topic of reversibility. Unfortunately, the new ATS standard is 12% and at least 200 ml. The boards will give a hearty increase in reversible cases so you don't get confused.

60. An increased total lung capacity combined with a decreased diffusing capacity is strongly indicative of which of the following conditions?
    A. emphysema
    B. pneumonia
    C. pulmonary fibrosis
    D. pleural effusion

FOOD FOR THOUGHT

We have just scratched the surface of a complex area of testing. Entire textbooks are devoted to pulmonary function testing! Here are a few more questions to fill up the corners of your brain.

61. What effect does smoking have on the results of a diffusion test? Why?

62. What lung volume or capacity is useful in predicting normal values for incentive spirometry?

63. Calculate your normal values for FVC, FEV_1, and $FEF_{25\%-75\%}$ using Table 19-4 on page 411 of your text. Do it using the regression equation.

    A. FVC   _____

    B. FEV_1 _____

    C. $FEF_{25\%-75\%}$ _____

    Show your work for the regression equation (be sure to use a calculator!)

    Formula: _____

    Calculation: _____

64. You should look at Table 19-2 on page 402 of your text. This is a severity rating scale based on percent predicted. You might want to know this for your boards, but it also helps when you take care of patients. Moderately severe and severe COPD might be treated with different medications than mild COPD, for example. So what would I have if my FEV_1 was 55% of predicted?

INFORMATION AGE

I have some software my students can use to practice interpretation of pulmonary function values. You can also look at clevelandclinicmeded.com/diseasemanagement/pulmonary/pft/pft.htm.

20 A Review of Thoracic Imaging

In the field of observation, chance favors the prepared mind.

L. Pasteur

Thoracic imaging provides a window for the practitioner to view structures and events inside the chest that we normally cannot see. The chest radiograph is especially important to the respiratory therapist (RT) for the purpose of confirming placement of tubes or for diagnosis of certain conditions like pneumothorax. Neck films might help diagnose croup or epiglottitis. You should also understand the usefulness of other common imaging techniques you will encounter in clinical practice such as computed tomography and magnetic resonance imaging. Perhaps you will even unlock the mysteries of the infamous Kerley B lines!

WORD WIZARD

Complete the following paragraph by writing the correct term(s) in the blank(s) provided.

The chest _____ is more commonly called a chest film, or x-ray. It is one of the most common methods for evaluating the lungs and other structures in the thorax. Air-filled lung tissue appears mostly dark

on the film because it is easily penetrated. This quality is called _____. The dense bone tissue

of ribs appears white. Dense matter that is not easily penetrated is referred to as having _____.
Soft tissues like blood vessels appear more grayish because they have an intermediate density. Abnormal conditions may be spotted through observation of certain densities in the wrong location. Accumulation of fluid in the pleural space,

or _____, appears white and may obscure the angle where the ribs meet the diaphragm. Alveoli appear white when filled with pus or blood. On the chest film these areas are called pulmonary

_____. If alveoli are filled with fluid but the airways around them are open, you will see air

_____ that may indicate pneumonia. Air in the pleural space, or _____,
is another example of an abnormal density. This condition appears as a black area with none of the usual grayish markings of blood vessels in the lung tissue.

OVERVIEW

1. Describe the four tissue densities you can see on a chest radiograph.

   A. Air: _____

   _____

   B. Fat: _____

   _____

   C. Tissue: _____

   _____

   D. Bone: _____

   _____

2. Physicians may order, but RTs recommend; we all work toward good care of the patient. The National Board for Respiratory Care (NBRC) thinks you should know when to suggest a chest film in a variety of settings. Let's call them Inpatient and Outpatient but you could use these criteria in any setting. Name three indications for a chest radiograph.

   Outpatient

   A. _____

   B. _____

   C. _____

   Inpatient

   A. _____

   B. _____

   C. _____

3. Explain lag time.

STEP-BY-STEP

Every primer on chest radiograph interpretation recommends you develop a systematic method for approaching interpretation. I remember, to this day, making an excellent evaluation of a chest film in the ICU for some students, only to realize I had interpreted the wrong film! (Still blushing!) So my first step is to make sure I am looking at the right film (patient) with the time and date I need. If you are handling an actual film, as opposed to a digitized one, make sure it is placed on the viewer correctly. The "left" side of the film (usually where the heart is) should be facing your right-hand side—as if the patient was standing facing you. A marker is normally placed on the film to indicate the left side.

4. What structures offer clues to help identify whether the patient is straight or rotated?

5. What appearance of the vertebral bodies suggests underexposure?

6. What effect does underexposure have on the appearance of lung tissue?

7. The pleura appear at the edge of chest wall (although the pleura themselves are usually difficult to see). What are the two major pleural abnormalities detected on the chest film?

   A. _____

   B. _____

ADVANCED CHEST IMAGING

Regular old radiographs are great for initial evaluation or in the ICU when you can't move the person easily, but more advanced techniques can provide vital information. RTs are often involved in the transport and management of patients to and from specialized imaging procedures like CT and MRI.

8. CT = _____

   What's the advantage over regular radiographs?

9. HRCT = _____

   Explain the thing about slices and what is this thing good for anyway?

10. MRI = _____

    What type of tissue in the chest is .imaged with this technique?

IDENTIFYING ABNORMALITIES

The second part of Chapter 20 covers evaluation of abnormalities seen in the three major anatomic portions seen in chest imaging. After you read the material, answer the following questions that highlight the important points.

Evaluation of the Pleura

11. What is the costophrenic angle? _____

12. Describe how you recognize the presence of fluid in the pleural space; what does that angle look like?

13. What view is most sensitive for detecting pleural fluid? How is the patient positioned to obtain this view?

14. When is sonography (ultrasound) indicated in the evaluation of pleural abnormalities?

15. What other imaging procedure may be helpful? _____

_____

16. Air in the pleural space is always abnormal. Name three common causes of this condition.

A. _____

B. _____

C. _____

17. What breathing maneuver will help identify a small pneumothorax on a chest film? _____

_____

18. Tension pneumothorax is immediately life threatening. Name at least two radiographic signs of tension pneumothorax.

   A. _____

   B. _____

19. What is the treatment for tension pneumothorax? _____

_____

Evaluation of Lung Parenchyma

20. What are the two components of the lung parenchyma?

   A. _____

   B. _____

21. How will alveolar infiltrates appear on the chest film?

_____

22. What is the difference between the radiographic appearance of pneumonia and pulmonary hemorrhage?

_____

23. What causes airways to become visible, and what is this sign called?

_____

24. Honeycombing, nodules, and volume loss are all radiographic hallmarks of what type of lung disorder?

_____

25. Describe the silhouette sign. Discuss the difference between a right lower and right middle lobe infiltrate as seen on a chest film.

Let's Get Wet!

26. List some of the causes of pulmonary edema
    Vascular

    A. _____

    B. _____

    C. _____

27. Describe Kerley B lines. When do you see them?

28. What are "bat's wings?" _____

Lost Volume

29. List five important indirect signs of volume loss, or atelectasis, seen on the chest radiograph. Check the Rule of Thumb on page 447 if you get lost.

    A. _____

    B. _____

    C. _____

    D. _____

    E. _____

30. You can count on your ribs to tell you about lung volumes. Fill in the chart below based on what anterior ribs you would see above the diaphragm depending on the degree of lung inflation.

	LUNG VOLUME	ANTERIOR RIBS
A.	Poor inspiration	
B.	Good effort	
C.	Hyperinflation	

31. Ribs aren't the only way to assess COPD with hyperinflation. List the two primary and three secondary radiographic signs seen with emphysema.
    A. Primary

    1. _____

    2. _____

B. Secondary

    1. _____

    2. _____

    3. _____

32. Compare the sensitivity of the chest radiograph and computed tomography for detection of obstructive airway disease.

Catheters, Lines, and Tubes

Checking placement of tubes and lines is key for RTs.

33. The endotracheal tube is made of soft plastic. How can the chest film be useful in deciding correct tube position after intubation?

34. Where is the distal tip of an ideally placed endotracheal tube in relationship to the carina?

_____

35. Where will the endotracheal tube usually end up if it is placed too far into the trachea?

_____

36. What pulmonary complication may be identified on a chest film when a CVP catheter is placed via the subclavian vein?

_____

37. A pulmonary artery catheter (Swan-Ganz) that is seen to extend too far into the lung fields of a chest radiograph may have what unwanted results?

_____

The Mediastinum

38. Where does the mediastinum lie within the chest?

_____

39. What imaging technique is most favored for assessing mediastinal masses?

_____

CASE STUDIES

Case 1

You are asked to perform postural drainage and clapping on a patient with a large right-sided pulmonary infiltrate. Evaluation of the chest radiograph shows a patchy white density with air bronchograms in the right lung. The right border of the heart is visible in the film.

40. Based on your knowledge of the silhouette sign, in what lobe is the infiltrate located?

_____

41. What diagnosis does the presence of air bronchograms suggest?

_____

42. What physical assessments could confirm the information in the chest film?

Case 2

An elderly man presents in the emergency department with acute exacerbation of his longstanding COPD. A decision is made to intubate him. It is difficult to auscultate breath sounds and chest movement is minimal; however, your impression is that breath sounds are more diminished on the left. A chest radiograph is obtained, which shows the tip of the endotracheal tube 1 cm above the carina. The left lung field is slightly smaller than the right. Both diaphragms appear flat, and you are able to count eight anterior ribs above the diaphragms.

43. Where should the tip of the tube be in relationship to the carina?

_____

44. With regard to the endotracheal tube, what action should you take?

_____

45. What is the significance of the flattened diaphragms and number of ribs seen above the diaphragm?

_____

WHAT DOES THE NBRC SAY?

I have carefully reviewed the NBRC's examination matrices and come to the conclusion that no one textbook contains all the radiograph information indicated to be part of the examinations! Chapter 20 covers some of this material, and you will find much of the rest in later chapters on lung diseases and pediatric/neonatal respiratory care.

I'll give you some sample questions based on the material covered in this chapter, but you will need to carefully review each examination matrix to identify all the areas you need to know. Both the Certification and the Written Registry Examinations require you to "Review the chest radiograph to determine the position of endotracheal or tracheostomy tube." You must also know when to "recommend a chest radiograph" and when to "review existing data in the patient record" such as the "results of chest radiographs." The examinations agree on content, including asking you to "review the chest radiograph to determine":

1. Pneumothorax or subcutaneous air
2. Consolidation or atelectasis
3. Diaphragm position
4. Hyperinflation
5. Pleural fluid
6. Pulmonary infiltrates
7. Position of chest tubes and pulmonary artery catheters are items on the Written Registry.

You will also be asked to "review the lateral neck radiograph to determine":
1. Presence of epiglottitis and subglottic edema
2. Presence of foreign bodies
3. Airway narrowing

The main difference between the two tests is the difficulty level and depth of the questions. There's more! How many questions will you see on this topic? The matrix doesn't really say, but my own review of available practice exams suggests one to three on the Certification Exam and up to five on the Registry. Each examination can vary considerably, but you are guaranteed to be tested on this material in some fashion! Try these on for size. Circle the best answer.

46. A patient has dyspnea and tachycardia following thoracentesis to treat a pleural effusion. Evaluation of this patient should include a(n) _____.
   A. CT scan
   B. MRI
   C. chest radiograph
   D. bronchoscopy

47. A pneumothorax would appear on a chest radiograph as a _____.
   A. white area near the lung base
   B. white area that obscures the costophrenic angle
   C. dark area without lung marking
   D. dark area with honeycomb markings

48. The medical record of an intubated patient indicates that the morning chest film shows opacification of the lower right lung field with elevated right diaphragm and a shift of the trachea to the right. These findings suggest _____.
   A. left-sided pneumothorax
   B. right-sided pleural effusion
   C. right mainstem intubation
   D. right-sided atelectasis

49. On a chest radiograph, the tip of the endotracheal tube for an adult patient should be _____.
   A. 2 cm above the vocal cords
   B. 2 cm above the carina
   C. at the carina
   D. 2 cm below the carina

50. A patient is believed to have a pleural effusion. Which of the following radiographic techniques would be most useful in making a confirmation?
   A. CT
   B. decubitus radiograph projection
   C. MRI
   D. AP radiograph projection

   Naturally chest film interpretation will appear as part of the information in questions that are not specifically about radiographs (same as blood gases). Remember: Chest radiographs are diagnostic, not therapeutic! If a patient is circling the drain from a tension pneumothorax, the radiograph will not be lifesaving—a chest tube will!

FOOD FOR THOUGHT

51. The author states that head position is important in assessing the tip of an endotracheal tube on a radiograph. What happens to the tube if the head moves up (extension) or the chin goes down (flexion)? How far can the tube move?

INFORMATION AGE

- The National Institutes of Health has a nice collection of radiographs to check out at www.nlm.nih.gov/medline-plus/ency/article/003804.htm.
- Virtual Hospital has lots of radiographs, too. You can download many of these pictures for free and add them to your case studies and reports at http://www.uihealthcare.com/vh/.
- Any of the search engines will give you plenty of sites to look at if you're searching for "chest x-rays."
- Another way to approach this topic is to search for "x-ray" + "emphysema" or whatever disease state you are specifically interested in at the time. You can use search engines like Google.com in "Image mode" to get more pictures.

21 Nutrition Assessment

To eat is human. To digest divine.
Mark Twain

I'm continually surprised at how little attention most of us give to what we eat. Hospitals put a tremendous effort into providing nourishing, specialized diets, with about as much public relations success as the airlines. When was the last time you heard anyone raving about the three-star meal they had after surgery? Dietary habits have far-reaching consequences in terms of overall health, so it should come as no surprise to you that nutrition plays a role in cardiopulmonary function (or that respiratory therapists would get involved).

WORD WIZARD

The language in Chapter 21 reads like a French menu—incomprehensibly. You may need to look up some of these terms before you can match them up with their definitions.

Terms	Definitions
1. _____ anergy	A. excess nitrogenous waste in the blood
	B. relationship of weight to height
2. _____ anthropometry	C. so thin that ribs stick out in persistent malnutrition
	D. daily resting energy consumption
3. _____ azotemia	E. impaired immune response
4. _____ basal metabolic rate	F. science of measuring the human body
	G. hypercatabolic form of malnutrition
5. _____ body mass index	H. hourly resting energy consumption after fasting
6. _____ indirect calorimetry	I. energy measurement based on O_2 consumption and CO_2 production
7. _____ cachexic	J. malnutrition associated with starvation
	K. calorimetry REE within 10% of predicted
8. _____ kwashiorkor	L. wasting condition resulting from a deficient diet
9. _____ marasmus	
10. _____ normometabolic	
11. _____ protein-energy malnutrition	
12. _____ resting energy expenditure	

MEET THE OBJECTIVES

13. Describe the "most helpful" technique for nutrition assessment performed by dietitians in the acute care setting.

14. What does BMI stand for, and what two variables are measured?

    A. BMI = _____

    B. Variable 1: _____

    C. Variable 2: _____

15. State the range of normal for BMI. (How is *your* BMI? What about your loved ones?)

    _____

16. State the formula for calculating ideal body weight.

    A. Males: _____

    B. Females: _____

    C. Calculate your own ideal body weight:

17. Compare starvation and hypercatabolism malnutrition. Be sure to give at least two clinical examples of each that a respiratory therapist might encounter. Check out Table 21-3 on page 460 of your text if you get lost.

    A. Kwashiorkor (starvation) _____

    B. Marasmus (kwashiorkor) _____

18. Lab studies could help restore nutrients to achieve respiratory muscle function and homeostasis. Test yourself on my meanings!

	MEANING	TEST
A.	Cheap, effective method for long-term assessment	
B.	Might help predict a compromised immune system	
C.	An acute phase protein monitored in trauma and illness	
D.	Indicator of catabolism	

19. How do patients with persistent malnutrition look? What is the funny sounding name for this appearance?

    A. How do they look? _____

    _____

    B. What is it called? _____

20. Good nourishment begins inside Mom, but that's a huge public health issue in the United States, so let's move on to children. What are the key influences that determine a child's lifetime eating habits?

21. The author suggests that teens should follow the U.S. Dietary Guidelines when choosing a meal and not go for the munchies. What approach would you take to influence a teenager with asthma or cystic fibrosis (CF) to eat a diet that helps rather than hurts their lungs?

22. Name the four diseases that now plague U.S. adults who eat too much fat and sugar.

    A. _____

    B. _____

    C. _____

    D. _____

23. Elderly patients might not eat well due to a variety of reasons. List some examples under
    A. Age-related change in senses

    B. Socioeconomic issues

C.   Health

MACRONUTRIENTS

24. Name the three macronutrients that supply your body's energy requirements. State the kilocalories per gram for each.

	MACRONUTRIENT	CALORIES PER GRAM
A.		
B.		
C.		

25. Write the Harris-Benedict prediction equation for estimating REE. Calculate yours (be sure to use the right one for your gender!).

A.   Formula: _____

B.   Calculation:

26. How many calories will an average man who weighs 80 kg need per day to maintain his body weight? Hint: use the Rule of Thumb on page 466. _____

27. State the effect of decreases in the following micronutrients through disease or malnutrition. (Just a few examples; this is a really huge subject!)

A.   Zinc _____

_____

B.   Magnesium _____

_____

C.   Hypophosphatemia _____

_____

28. What percentage of patients with acute respiratory failure suffer from malnutrition? _____

    _____

29. Give two reasons why malnourished patients are difficult to wean from the ventilator.

    A. _____

    B. _____

30. Why are COPD patients often malnourished?

31. What are the consequences of malnutrition on respiratory muscles and response to hypoxia and hypercapnia?

INDIRECT CALORIMETRY

32. List three conditions where indirect calorimetry may be indicated. (See Box 21-4 on page 466.)

    A. _____

    B. _____

    C. _____

33. What are the contraindications to indirect calorimetry in mechanically ventilated patients? (See the Clinical Practice Guideline!)

34. According to the AARC Clinical Practice Guidelines, closed-circuit calorimeters may reduce alveolar volume or increase work of breathing. Explain how these two hazards occur.

35. What actions should be taken to prepare a patient for indirect calorimetry? (See Box 21-5 on page 466.)

    A. 4 hours before the test: _____

    B. 2 hours before the test: _____

    C. 1 hour before the test: _____

36. Describe the most significant problem in performing indirect calorimetry on mechanically ventilated patients.

37. Interpret the following RQs and identify the general nutritional strategy. (See Table 21-5.)

	VALUE	INTERPRETATION	STRATEGY
A.	>1		
B.	0.9 to 1		
C.	0.7 to 0.8		

38. State the formula for calculating REE using a pulmonary artery catheter. _____

_____

39. What factors are used to adjust predicted REEs in patients? Give one example. (Go back to Box 21-3.)

RESPIRATORY CONSEQUENCES

40. How many patients in respiratory failure have malnutrition?

_____

41. COPD patients have special dietary problems. Identify four factors that lead to poor intake in these patients.

    A. _____

    B. _____

    C. _____

    D. _____

42. What is the effect of high-carborate loads on COPD patients?

_____

ENTERAL, PARENTERAL

43. What do the terms "enteral" and "parenteral" mean?

    A. Enteral: _____

    B. Parenteral: _____

44. Explain what is meant by the following tube feeding regimens:

    A. Bolus: _____

    B. Intermittent: _____

    C. Drip: _____

45. How would the respiratory therapist confirm suspected aspiration of tube feedings? How is this complication avoided?

    A. Confirmation: _____

    B. Prevention *(Give me the easy one that you can do!)*

    _____

    _____

46. Explain what happens when patients receive too much of the following substrates. Give a pulmonary example, please.

    A. Protein _____

    B. Carbohydrates _____

    C. Fat _____

47. Approximately how many people with COPD have poor nutrition? _____

48. Which disease often shows progressive severe weight loss? _____

49. In general, COPD patients eat to optimize nutrition.

   A. How often? _____

   B. Calories? _____

50. Asthmatics may greatly benefit from what specific type of fatty acids? _____

51. In addition to a lot of calories, what supplements do CF patients need? _____

CHAPTER HIGHLIGHTS

Complete the following sentences by writing in the correct term(s) in the blank(s) provided.

52. The _____-_____ equations estimate daily resting energy expenditure.

53. _____ is a state of impaired metabolism in which the intake of nutrients falls short of the body's needs.

54. For the patient with pulmonary disease, high _____ loads can increase carbon dioxide production.

55. Whenever possible, the _____ route should be used for supplying nutrients.

56. The likelihood of _____ during tube feedings can be minimized by

   _____ the head of the bed by _____ .

CASE STUDY

A thin, undernourished COPD patient tells you that he has difficulty eating because he gets tired and short of breath during meals. Besides, food just doesn't taste as good now.

57. What eating pattern should be emphasized to this patient? _____

   _____

58. Make some suggestions that would increase his nutrient intake. _____

   _____

59. What other big problem might interfere with the patient's appetite? _____

_____

WHAT DOES THE NBRC SAY?

While muscle wasting and general appearance do show up in the matrix, and while RTs are very involved in indirect calorimetry in many institutions, this information has not made it to the boards yet. No, this is just practical stuff you can use in patient assessment and patient teaching. For example, I use some of this material when I teach patient's with COPD at the Better Breather's Club.

FOOD FOR THOUGHT

60. What type of nutritional strategy may help in the weaning of COPD patients from the ventilator?

INFORMATION AGE

- I found some good material on COPD and nutrition at www.nlm.nih.gov/medlineplus/copdchronicobstructivepulmonarydisease.html.
- The Clevelend Clinic has Nutritional Guidelines for People with COPD at www.clevelandclinic.org/health/health-info/docs/2400/2411.asp?index=9451.
- And don't forget: www.yourlunghealth.org. You can ask Dr. Tom or look in the archives.

22 Pulmonary Infections

Captain of the men of death . . .
Sir William Osler

A hundred years after these words were said, pneumonia is still a leading cause of death. In fact, it is the sixth leading cause of death in the United States and the single most common cause of infection-related death in the United States. There is a tremendous clinical interest in ventilator-associated pneumonia right now. Respiratory therapists (RTs) play a key role in the research and prevention of this serious complication of life in the intensive care unit. Pneumonia is simple to understand, right? There are only two types: community and nosocomial. Or is it viral and bacterial? Acute and chronic? Typical and atypical? Ventilator associated . . . or perhaps aspiration pneumonia . . . read on, and you will meet "the old man's friend" in its many forms.

CLASSIFICATION AND PATHOGENESIS

1. What does the term "empirical therapy" mean?

2. The textbook definition of nosocomial pneumonia is now subdivided into HAP and VAP. Please describe these new terms *in depth* as they are critical to your understanding of this life-threatening illness.
    A. HAP

    B. VAP

3. How common is hospital-acquired pneumonia, and what are the costs and mortality?

    A. Prevalence: _____

        _____

    B. Cost: _____

        _____

    C. Mortality: _____

        _____

4. List two patient populations that are at special risk for fatal forms of nosocomial pneumonia.

    A. _____

    B. _____

5. Name four diseases acquired via inhalation of infectious particles.

    A. _____

    B. _____

    C. _____

    D. _____

6. List four of the patient populations at risk for aspiration of large volumes of gastric fluids.

    A. _____

    B. _____

    C. _____

    D. _____

7. State the two novel strategies mentioned in the book to reduce HAP or VAP in ventilated patients.

    A. _____

    B. _____

8. Describe the role of suctioning as a cause of lower respiratory tract inoculation.

9. Give the prime example of reactivation of a latent infection. _____

_____

10. Why is it so important to know what organisms are commonly associated with pneumonia?

11. What organism is most commonly identified as the cause of community-acquired pneumonia? _____

_____

12. Name two atypical pathogens.

    A. _____

    B. _____

13. Why is no microbiologic identification made in so many cases of pneumonia?

14. Name two viruses associated with pneumonia. What time of year are they encountered?
    A. Virus

        1. _____

        2. _____

    B. Time of year: _____

CLINICAL MANIFESTATIONS

15. Patients with community-acquired pneumonia typically have fever and what three respiratory symptoms?

    A. _____

    B. _____

    C. _____

16. What two other common respiratory problems show the same symptoms?

    A. _____

    B. _____

197

17. What is the classic, typical presentation of community-acquired pneumonia? _____

_____

_____

18. In intubated patients, VAP usually shows up as what three changes in the patient's condition?

    A. _____

    B. _____

    C. _____

19. Describe the common radiograph abnormalities associated with pneumonia.

20. Why is the chest film of limited use in diagnosing pneumonia in critically ill patients?

RISK FACTORS

21. Fill in the data for each of the following risk factors for mortality associated with community-acquired pneumonia (see Box 22-1 on page 489).

	FACTOR	DESCRIPTION
A.	Age	
B.	Gender	
C.	Vital signs	
D.	Arterial pH	
E.	High-risk causes	
F.	Comorbid illness	

22. A number of factors predispose the hospital patient to pneumonia such as poor host defenses from underlying illness. Name five such "comorbities." Hint: Table 22-5 on page 489!

A. _____

B. _____

C. _____

D. _____

E. _____

23. List four factors that expose the lung to large numbers of microorganisms.

A. _____

B. _____

C. _____

D. _____

DIAGNOSTIC STUDIES

24. Why is determining the predominant causative organism via sputum Gram stain, culture, and sensitivity so useful in pneumonia patients?

25. Describe the process for collecting a good specimen by expectoration.

26. Describe the satisfactory specimen. (This is board exam material!)

27. Name the organism identified by each of the following specialized tests:

	TEST	ORGANISM
A.	Acid-fast stain	
B.	Direct fluorescent stain	
C.	Toluidine blue	
D.	Potassium hydroxide	

28. When should HIV testing be recommended in cases of community-acquired pneumonia?

29. When should fiberoptic bronchoscopy be recommended in cases of community-acquired pneumonia?

30. Name four techniques useful in confirming the diagnosis nosocomial pneumonia.

A. _____

B. _____

C. _____

D. _____

Diagnosing VAP is a big challenge for everyone in the ICU. Regular sputum specimens just don't seem to get us the right antibiotics for those bugs. New techniques have had some success.

31. Direct visualization of the lower airway is helpful in diagnosing VAP. What are the three criteria?

A. _____

B. _____

C. _____

32. What do the initials BAL stand for, and can you please describe BAL?

   A. BAL = _____

   B. Description: _____

   _____

   _____

33. What is mini-BAL, and what health care professional performs the procedure?

THERAPY

34. What is the primary medical treatment for pneumonia? _____

   _____

35. What is the agent of choice for treating the following organisms? Hint: Table 22-8 on page 494 of your text.

	ORGANISM	AGENT OF CHOICE
A.	Pneumococcal infection	
B.	*Mycoplasma*	
C.	*P. carinii*	
D.	*Legionella*	

36. How long is a typical course of treatment for pneumonia? _____

37. How long does it take for the radiograph to show resolution of pneumonia in young individuals? What about older patients?

   A. Young patients: _____

   B. Older patients: _____

38. Immunization is one of the primary strategies for preventing community-acquired pneumonia. Individuals are immunized against what two organisms?

    A. _____

    B. _____

39. Identify three groups that should be immunized.

    A. _____

    B. _____

    C. _____

40. Identify the three "probably effective" strategies for the prevention of nosocomial pneumonia.

    A. _____

    B. _____

    C. _____

41. What positioning technique is useful in preventing pneumonia in patients? _____

    _____

42. What is the current medication for gastrointestinal bleeding prophylaxis that may be effective in preventing

    pneumonia? _____

CASE STUDIES

Case 1

A 55-year-old man arrives at the clinic complaining of chills, fever, and chest pain on inspiration. He is coughing up rusty-colored sputum. He admits to a history of heavy smoking and regular use of alcoholic beverages. Physical examination reveals a heart rate of 125, respiratory rate of 30, and temperature of 104°F. He has inspiratory crackles in the right lower lobe. Blood gases reveal a pH of 7.34, $PaCO_2$ of 50, and PaO_2 of 58.

43. What is the most likely diagnosis? Support your answer based on the clinical signs and symptoms.

44. What immediate treatment should you initiate? _____

_____

45. Give at least five reasons why the patient is at risk of dying from his condition.

A. _____

B. _____

C. _____

D. _____

E. _____

A patient is intubated and on the ventilator following a head injury. On the third day following his craniotomy, he develops a fever. During routine suctioning you notice his secretions are thick and yellow. Breath sounds are decreased in the left lower lobe.

46. What is the role of the artificial airway in development of pneumonia?

47. What test would you recommend at this time to help confirm a diagnosis?

WHAT DOES THE NBRC SAY?

Interestingly enough, they don't say much about pneumonia! Certain lung infections may appear on the boards in the context of their treatment and recognition, such as the use of ribavirin to treat respiratory syncytial virus (RSV). Or inhaled pentamidine in HIV patients with pneumonia. Isolation procedures for tuberculosis patients is a possible area of testing as well as general methods to prevent the spread of infection. You should certainly recognize when a patient has a lung infection, and *pay attention to basic microbiology*. Of course we don't know what will be added in the next test revision. The role of the RT in reducing the risk of VAP may be on the exam!

48. What is the role of the RT in educating at-risk populations about methods to prevent pneumonia?

49. Have you had your flu shot? _____

INFORMATION AGE

- A great site that I haven't mentioned yet is the American Lung Association at www.lungusa.org. Right at the top of the home page is "Diseases from A to Z." Check out their section on pneumonia; it is excellent.
- The National Institutes of Health (NIH) is a site I've mentioned before that maintains a vast online library of information via the U.S. National Library of Medicine. The pneumonia information is given at www.nlm.nih.gov/medlineplus/pneumonia.html. Of course, you can use this site to look up almost anything that pertains to medicine!

Human action can be modified to some extent, but human nature cannot be changed.

Abraham Lincoln

I first learned about obstructive lung disease by watching some of my family members develop it as a consequence of heavy smoking. The conditions discussed in Chapter 23 are so common that you probably know someone who has them too. (Famous people get chronic obstructive pulmonary disease [COPD] as well. If "honest Abe" had Marfan's syndrome, he might have developed emphysema!) Respiratory therapists spend a lot of their time working with COPD patients, and I am sure you will pay special attention to the information in this chapter, as you get to know the "pink puffers" and "blue bloaters."

WORD WIZARD

Before we start on the long dark journey into the lungs, take a shot at the COPD crossword puzzle on the following page.

CHRONIC OBSTRUCTIVE PULMONARY DISEASE

If you talk about each type of COPD as if it was "pure emphysema," you would be oversimplifying in many cases. The Venn diagram shown in Figure 23-1 on page 226 in *Egan's* demonstrates this nicely. Many patients show signs of having mixed disease states. Asthma is classified as separate from COPD, but those with longstanding poorly controlled asthma often present with signs of COPD later in life. So, while it is convenient to talk about (or test about) emphysema, chronic bronchitis, or asthma as if they were pure and separate entities, in the clinical setting you will see patients who have varying degrees of pathology that represent each of these important components of the spectrum of COPD. Remember that most COPD patients have a smoking history, so you will want to explore this issue. (You can calculate pack-years by multiplying packs-per-day by the number of years the patient smoked.)

Overview

COPD is so pervasive in the United States and worldwide that we need to start off with some definitions and demographics so you can get a clear picture of these conditions that RTs treat almost constantly.

1. *Chronic obstructive pulmonary disease* is defined by the American Thoracic Society in four key concepts. Please elaborate on:

    A. Limitation: _____

    B. Progressive: _____

    C. Inflammatory: _____

    D. Systemic: _____

2. According to the NHANES data, what percentage of the U.S. population has mild OR moderate COPD (add the two populations)?

    _____

3. How does COPD rank as a leading cause of death, and why is this condition strikingly different from heart disease or stroke?

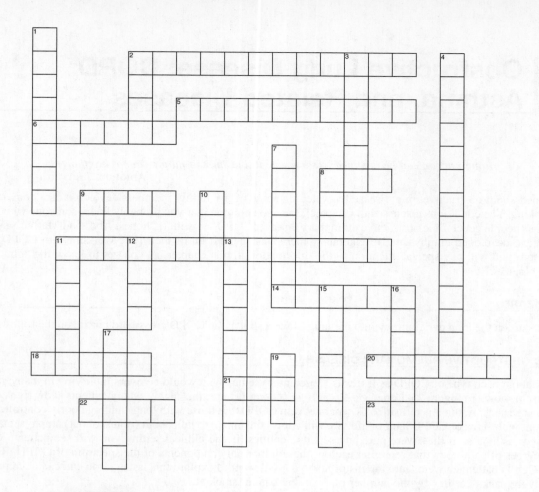

ACROSS

2. smooth muscle contraction in the airways.
5. chronic form shows productive cough for 3 months in 2 consecutive years.
6. the only thing that increases survival of end-stage COPD patients.
8. late asthma response.
9. another four letter word for COPD!
11. results in permanent dilation of the airways.
14. this fibrosis is the most frequently lethal genetic disease of white children.
18. _____ one antitrypsin deficiency, a genetic form of emphysema.
20. where COPD stands as a killer
21. asthma you get when you exercise
22. common bedside test used to manage asthma
23. these puffers really have emphysema

DOWN

1. cystic _____, known in Europe as mucoviscidosis.
2. _____ bloater, or patient with chronic bronchitis.
3. complex lung disease associated with wheezing and airway inflammation
4. drug that opens the airways
7. passed on from parents to children via DNA.
8. abbreviation for surgery that removes part of the emphysematous lung.
9. _____ pulmonale, the heart failure associated with hypoxemia.
10. most common way to deliver drugs to the airway
11. COPD chest shape
12. famous oxygen therapy study that proved increased survival with oxygen.
13. enlargement and destruction of the distal airways and alveoli
15. Stop it
16. the "C " in COPD
17. lung butter
19. early asthma response

4. What is the approximate cost of health care associated with COPD in the 2000s?

    A. Hospitalizations (1993 = $500,000): _____

    B. Office visits: _____

    C. Emergency department visits: _____

    D. Total health dollars (1993 = $24 billion): _____

Risk Factors and Pathophysiology

5. OK, so cigarette smokers get COPD. What is the other major cause of emphysema? _____

_____

6. Describe the "susceptible smoker."

7. Briefly explain the protease-antiprotease hypothesis of emphysema.

8. Describe the three mechanisms of airflow obstruction in COPD.

    A. _____

    B. _____

    C. _____

Clinical Signs

9. Name four common symptoms of COPD.

    A. _____

    B. _____

    C. _____

    D. _____

Chapter **23** **Obstructive Lung Disease: COPD, Asthma, and Related Diseases**

10. Compare the onset of dyspnea in typical cases of COPD with that of α_1-antitrypsin deficiency.

11. What physical change in the chest wall occurs as a result of prolonged hyperinflation? _____
_____

12. Name three other late signs of COPD.

A. _____

B. _____

C. _____

13. Compare chronic bronchitis, emphysema, and α_1-antitrypsin deficiency in terms of the following features.

	FEATURES	CHRONIC BRONCHITIS	EMPHYSEMA	α_1-ANTITRYPSIN DEFICIENCY
A.	Age of onset			
B.	Family history			
C.	Smoker			
D.	Lung volume			
E.	DLCO			
F.	FEV$_1$/FVC			
G.	Radiograph			

Management

Your text lists five general goals of management for COPD. In addition, we need to think about how to avoid complications when the patient has an acute exacerbation of their condition.

14. Why would it be important to differentiate asthma from other forms of COPD? List some features that favor each.

A. Why differentiate? _____

B. Features that favor COPD

C. Features that favor asthma

15. Reversible airflow obstruction is defined as an increase of what amount?

    A. Percentage: _____

    B. Milliliters: _____

16. Why is bronchodilator therapy recommended for COPD? What types of drugs are used? What is the effect on decline of lung function and survival?

    A. Why? _____

    B. Types of drugs? _____

    C. Lung decline and survival? _____

17. Discuss the role of inhaled steroids in COPD. Which group should receive glucocorticosteroids?

18. What is the primary effect of theophylline (methylxanthines) on patients with COPD? What serum blood levels are currently recommended to avoid side effects?

19. Name the four important elements of managing an acute exacerbation of COPD due to purulent bronchitis.

    A. _____

    B. _____

    C. _____

    D. _____

Chapter 23 **Obstructive Lung Disease: COPD, Asthma, and Related Diseases**

20. When hypercapnia and respiratory failure are present (and pH is <7.3) you might want to avoid intubation with noninvasive ventilation. What are some of the criteria of a good candidate for this lifesaving therapy?

21. What is the primary goal of pulmonary rehabilitation? _____

    _____

22. What is the effect of pulmonary rehabilitation programs on survival and pulmonary function?

23. A comprehensive smoking cessation program usually includes what three elements?

    A. _____

    B. _____

    C. _____

24. Only two treatments for COPD have been shown to prolong survival. Please elaborate.
    A. Oxygen:

    B. Quitting smoking:

25. What is the relationship between bronchodilator therapy and home oxygen therapy?

26. You need to know the indication for continuous oxygen. Please give the correct values for

    A. Resting Pao_2: _____

    B. Hematocrit: _____

    C. ECG: _____

27. What two vaccines are recommended for patients with COPD? Which one is given annually?

    A. _____

    B. _____

28. Describe the two surgical options for end-stage COPD. Discuss the outcomes of each of these options.
    A.

    B.

ASTHMA

All that wheezes is not asthma.
Anonymous RTs

Asthma is on the rise, and all of our drugs and technology have not been able to solve the problem. A number of interesting theories exist to explain why industrialized countries are experiencing worse problems than are underdeveloped nations. For RTs, many of whom are certified by the National Asthma Educator Certification Board (NAECB), the situation is a wonderful opportunity to apply our special expertise to help educate the public and our clients regarding prevention, treatment, and control.

Chapter **23** **Obstructive Lung Disease: COPD, Asthma, and Related Diseases**

Overview

29. What is the difference between older definitions and the more current view of asthma?

30. What percentage of people in the United States are believed to have asthma? (In 2002, it was estimated to be 5%!)

_____

Etiology and Pathogenesis

31. Airway inflammation and bronchial hyperreactivity result in airflow obstruction. Name four triggers:

   A. _____

   B. _____

   C. _____

   D. _____

32. What happens when a patient with asthma inhales an allergen to which he or she is sensitized?

33. Describe the early and late asthmatic reactions (EAR and LAR, respectively).
   A. EAR

   B. LAR

Clinical Signs

34. What factor plays a key role in suggesting and establishing a diagnosis of asthma? _____

_____

35. What are the four classic symptoms of asthma?

A. _____

B. _____

C. _____

D. _____

36. List five conditions that can mimic the wheezing of asthma.

A. _____

B. _____

C. _____

D. _____

E. _____

37. What change in values determine reversibility of airflow obstruction?

38. Bronchial provocation is the specialized test regimen used to demonstrate obstruction in suspected asthmatics that are symptom free at the time of testing. Name the drug used for this test and what response indicates hyperresponsiveness.

A. Drug: _____

B. Response: _____

39. Describe the role of arterial blood gases in the diagnosis AND assessment of asthma.
A. Diagnosis

B. Assessment

Chapter **23** **Obstructive Lung Disease: COPD, Asthma, and Related Diseases**

Management

The goal of asthma management is to maintain a high quality of life without symptoms or limitations. The goal is to reduce death (mortality) and lost time from work and school, pneumonia, and other consequences of asthma (morbidity). The patient should be relatively free of side effects from treatment. To achieve this, a four-step approach has been recommended by the National Institutes of Health National Expert Panel.

40. Complete the chart below to show your understanding of the stepwise approach. Table 23-2 on page 516 of your text will help.

	SEVERITY	SYMPTOMS	LONG-TERM MEDICATIONS
A.	1: Intermittent		
B.	2: Mild persistent		
C.	3: Moderate persistent		
D.	4: Severe persistent		

41. Explain control of asthma in terms of the following criteria:

A. Symptoms: _____

_____

B. β_2-Agonists: _____

_____

C. Exercise: _____

_____

D. PEFR/FEV$_1$: _____

_____

E. Exacerbations: _____

_____

42. Give the criteria and actions for green, yellow, and red peak flow zones.

	ZONE	PEFR % PREDICTED	TREATMENT/ACTION
A.	Green		
B.	Yellow		
C.	Red		

43. Compare the use of inhaled corticosteroids and bronchodilators in asthma.

44. Name the two common side effects of inhaled steroids and two ways to control them.

   A. _____

   B. _____

   C. Control/reduce side effects:

      1. _____

      2. _____

45. Discuss the use of cromolyn/nedocromil sodium in asthma treatment.
   A. Indications

      1. Adults: _____

      2. Children: _____

   B. Acute attacks: _____

   C. What three problems could cromolyn protect against?

      1. _____

      2. _____

      3. _____

46. Leukotriene modifiers like Singulair are popular and useful for what specific type of asthmatic? Do these drugs replace steroids?

   _____

47. What type of drugs are the first-line treatment for all types of acute bronchospasm? _____

   _____

48. Name the two long-acting β-agonists, and explain the new FDA warnings.

Chapter **23** **Obstructive Lung Disease: COPD, Asthma, and Related Diseases**

49. Describe the use of methylxanthines such as theophylline in the treatment of asthma. What's a good dose, and how do you check?

50. What is the benefit of using anticholinergics like ipratroprium in the day-to-day management of asthma?

For a Good Time, Meet Me in the Emergency Department

The goal is to reduce death (mortality) and lost time from work and school, pneumonia, and other consequences of asthma (morbidity).

51. Name three factors you should monitor in a patient hospitalized with acute asthma.

A. _____

B. _____

C. _____

52. Give the criteria for hospital discharge for each of the following:

A. Pao_2: _____

B. PEFR: _____

C. Symptoms: _____

_____

D. Discharge medications: _____

_____

53. Management of asthma should be aggressive, including two specific types of medications along with oxygen. Discuss the use of β-agonists and steroids in this specific situation.

A. β-Agonists: _____

_____

B. Steroids: _____

_____

54. How can you prevent allergic reactions in asthmatic patients through immunotherapy?

55. Name some common outdoor and indoor allergens. Then give suggestions for control.

		ALLERGEN	CONTROL
A.	Outdoor		
B.	Indoor		

56. What is EIA? List three prophylactic drug treatments.

    A.   EIA = _____

    B.   Prophylaxis:

         1. _____

         2. _____

         3. _____

57. Define occupational asthma. What is the most common cause?

58. What is the only way to eliminate occupational asthma once an individual is sensitized? _____

_____

59. What drug is particularly helpful in the treatment of cough-variant asthma?

_____

60. List three medications that may be helpful in treating nocturnal asthma.

    A. _____

    B. _____

    C. _____

Chapter **23** **Obstructive Lung Disease: COPD, Asthma, and Related Diseases**

61. What recommendations would you make to a patient who has aspirin sensitivity?

62. What is the effect of pregnancy on asthmatics?

63. Discuss the use of asthma medications during pregnancy.

64. GER (Most of us call it GERD) can also play a role in asthma. Any ideas on how to help?

65. A surprising number of asthmatics have trouble with nose and sinus. No surprise to me, the nose and sinus are part of the respiratory system! What types of inhalers are needed here?

BRONCHIECTASIS

Bronchiectasis is a condition where airways are deformed and destroyed by chronic inflammation.

66. What is the clinical hallmark of bronchiectasis?

   _____

67. What test is now considered definitive for diagnosing bronchiectasis?

   _____

68. List the causes of local and diffuse bronchiectasis.
   A. Local

   1. _____

   2. _____

   B. Diffuse

   1. _____

   2. _____

   3. _____

69. Name the two primary treatments for bronchiectasis.

   A. _____

   B. _____

And if these don't work, the patient needs to have _____.

CASE STUDIES

Case 1

A 70-year-old man's chief complaint is dyspnea on exertion. He has a smoking history of two packs per day for the past 50 years. He has a barrel-shaped chest and much decreased breath sounds. His chest radiograph shows hyperinflation, especially in the apices; flattened diaphragms; and a small heart. He admits to a morning cough but denies significant sputum production.

70. What is the most likely diagnosis?

   _____

71. Calculate the patient's "pack-years." _____

72. What factor should you focus on to help the patient control his condition? _____

   _____

Case 2

A 60-year-old man has smoked a pack of cigarettes per day since he was a teenager. He complains of a chronic productive cough that is producing thick, yellow sputum. He is admitted to the medical

Chapter **23** **Obstructive Lung Disease: COPD, Asthma, and Related Diseases**

floor with a fever and shortness of breath. Blood gases reveal pH of 7.35, $PaCO_2$ of 50 mm Hg, and PaO_2 of 57 mm Hg. Physical exam shows pedal edema, distended neck veins, and use of accessory muscles of ventilation. He has scattered wheezing and rhonchi on auscultation.

73. What type of COPD is most likely in this case?

_____

74. What should you do with his sputum the next time he coughs productively?

75. What is the immediate respiratory treatment in this case?

76. What respiratory medications would you recommend?

Case 3

A 44-year-old man complains of dyspnea on exertion. He is a nonsmoker but drinks wine with his meals. He has a barrel-shaped chest and very decreased breath sounds. His chest radiograph shows hyperinflation, especially in the bases. History reveals that his father and uncle both died of "lung problems."

77. What is the most likely cause of the patient's COPD symptoms? Justify your answer based on the information presented.

78. What treatments are available for this condition?

A 15-year-old boy complains that he cannot catch his breath when he exercises. He states that he coughs a lot, especially in the winter. His breath sounds are clear, and his physical examination is unremarkable.

79. What do you suspect is the problem? _____

_____

80. How could a definitive diagnosis be made?

WHAT DOES THE NBRC SAY?

It will come as no surprise that the board exams place a special emphasis on COPD and asthma. The Clinical Simulation Examination Matrix states that you will see at least "two problems involving adult patients with COPD." You may also see a pediatric patient with asthma. *All* aspects of managing these patients may be included from pulmonary function testing to rehabilitation. Multiple choice exams, like the Written Registry and Entry-Level Examinations, do not specifically mention COPD or asthma in the matrices; however, diagnosis and management of these patients are heavily tested. Here are some sample questions. Circle the best answer.

Use the data presented below to answer questions 1 through 6.

A 20-year-old woman who has a history of asthma is brought to the emergency department in respiratory distress. Your assessment of the patient reveals the following:

pH	7.47
$Paco_2$	33 mm Hg
Pao_2	72 mm Hg
HCO_3^-	23 mEq/L
RR	28
HR	115
PEFR	200 L/min

81. Which of the following breath sounds would you expect to hear in this patient?
    A. inspiratory crackles
    B. expiratory wheezing
    C. inspiratory stridor
    D. expiratory rhonchi

82. The arterial blood gas results indicate the presence of _____.
    A. acute respiratory alkalosis
    B. acute metabolic alkalosis
    C. chronic respiratory acidosis
    D. acute respiratory acidosis

83. You are asked to initiate oxygen therapy. What would you recommend?
    A. simple mask at 10 L/min
    B. nonrebreathing mask at 15 L/min
    C. nasal cannula at 2 L/min
    D. air entrainment mask at 50% F_{IO_2}

84. What therapy would you recommend after the oxygen is in place?
    A. 2 puffs Atrovent (ipratropium) via MDI
    B. 0.5 ml Proventil (albuterol) via SVN
    C. intravenous aminophylline (theophylline) administration
    D. intravenous antibiotics

85. Blood gases are repeated 30 minutes after the oxygen therapy is initiated.
    pH   7.42
    $Paco_2$ 38 mm Hg
    Pao_2 86 mm Hg
    HCO_3^- 23 mEq/L
    RR   24
    HR   88
    PEFR   210 L/min

    Which of the following has shown significant improvement based on this information?
    A. compliance
    B. resistance
    C. oxygenation
    D. ventilation

86. Intravenous steroids and repeated bronchodilators have been given. The patient is now receiving 40% oxygen.
    pH   7.34
    $Paco_2$ 53 mm Hg
    Pao_2 74 mm Hg
    HCO_3^- 26 mEq/L
    RR   18
    HR   125
    PEFR   110 L/min

    What would you suggest at this point?
    A. increase of F_{IO_2} to 50%
    B. continuous nebulization of bronchodilators
    C. administration of intravenous bicarbonate
    D. intubation and mechanical ventilation

87. A patient with COPD and CO_2 retention is admitted for an acute exacerbation of her disease. The physician requests your suggestion for initiating oxygen therapy. Which of the following would you recommend?
    A. nasal cannula at 6 L/min
    B. air-entrainment mask at 28%
    C. simple mask at 2 L/min
    D. partial rebreathing mask at 8 L/min

88. A PFT on a 65-year-old woman indicates airflow obstruction with mild air-trapping. The patient is coughing up thick sputum. Which of the following diagnoses is most likely?
   A. cystic fibrosis
   B. pneumonia
   C. pulmonary fibrosis
   D. bronchiectasis

89. A PFT on a 56-year-old man with a history of smoking shows increased TLC and RV. The D$_{LCO}$ is reduced. What diagnosis is suggested by these findings?
   A. emphysema
   B. pneumonia
   C. sarcoidosis
   D. pneumoconiosis

90. Spirometry is performed before and after bronchodilator administration. Which of the following indicates a therapeutic response?
   I.   FEV$_1$ increased by 10%
   II. FVC increased by 300 ml
   III. PEFR increased by 5%
      A. I only
      B. II only
      C. I and II only
      D. I and III only

FOOD FOR THOUGHT

91. Because only 15% of smokers actually show big declines in airflow, why should we encourage all patients to quit smoking?

92. Patients with α_1-antitrypsin deficiency can now benefit from therapy. What is needed?

93. What is Xolair, and how does it work for asthma?

Chapter **23** **Obstructive Lung Disease: COPD, Asthma, and Related Diseases**

INFORMATION AGE

There are literally hundreds of thousands of references to this topic online, but I can tell you the best places to go and save you a lot of trouble.

- The American Lung Association (ALA) is a good place to start. Go to www.lungusa.org.
- But that is just a start. I think you must check out the Global initiative for Obstructive Lung Disease (GOLD) site: www.goldcopd.com. You can see that COPD and asthma are worldwide public health problems of epic proportion.
- Now try this: www.yourlunghealth.org. This site is all about COPD and includes a feature called "Ask Dr. Tom," where patients can e-mail renowned pulmonologist Dr. Tom Petty (see the NOTT trials). This site, along with ALA, is really good for patients and RTs.

Asthma

RTs can sit for the AE-C, or Certified Asthma Educator, exam to show their expertise in caring for asthma patients. So how do **YOU** become an expert? Start off at the ALA. Topics are nicely covered. There is lots of clear information, statistics, patient teaching materials, and more. After all, the ALA is the national expert on this subject.

RTs cannot know too much about asthma. The National Heart, Lung, and Blood Institute of the National Institutes of Health (NIH) is the definitive reference.

- You can find the latest version of this cornerstone of asthma therapy at www.nhlbi.nih.gov/guidelines/asthma/index.htm.
- And the asthma prevention plan: www.nhlbi.nih.gov/about/naepp/index.htm.
- Of course you wouldn't want to just look at that guideline because the Global Initiative for Asthma (GINA) has a wonderful guideline as well: www.ginasthma.com.
- At the National Asthma Educator Board (NAECB), we use both GINA and NIH guidelines to develop examination competencies. You really should not miss their site because this is how you will be able to become a certified educator after you graduate. Certified asthma educators are already in great demand with hospital and clinic employers, and they increasingly receive insurance reimbursement for their work: www.naecb.org.

24 Interstitial Lung Disease

> *There is a remedy for everything; it is called death.*
> Portuguese Proverb

There are an unbelievable number of interstitial lung diseases (ILDs). Individually, they are not common, but as a group, they represent a significant set of lung disorders. Sooner or later, you will encounter some of the members of this broad category of restrictive conditions. Fortunately, there are many common elements in the clinical signs, pulmonary function test (PFT) abnormalities, and treatment of most forms of ILD.

WORD WIZARD

Because there are so many new terms related to ILD in Chapter 24, a quick review will probably help you keep them straight. Match the correct definition with the correct term.

Terms	Definitions
1. _____ asbestosis	A. formation of scar tissue in the lung without known cause
2. _____ corticosteroids	B. respiratory disorder characterized by fibrotic infiltrates in the lower lobes
3. _____ cytotoxic agents	C. inflammatory reaction provoked by inhalation of organic dusts
4. _____ lymphangioleiomyomatosis	D. chemical that is lethal to living cells
5. _____ hypersensitivity pneumonitis	E. interstitial lung disease associated with inhalation of small inorganic particles
6. _____ idiopathic pulmonary fibrosis	F. restrictive disorder associated with pleural abnormalities and lung tumors
7. _____ interstitial lung disease	G. disorder of unknown origin that results in formation of epithelioid tubercles
8. _____ pulmonary Langerhans	H. hormones associated with control of body processes
9. _____ occupational lung disease	I. bone growth associated with numerous histiocytes and specific WBCs
10. _____ pneumoconiosis	J. abnormal airway smooth muscle growth
11. _____ pulmonary Langerhans histiocytosis	K. occupational disease most commonly seen in coal workers
12. _____ sarcoidosis	L. disorder caused by long-term exposure to sand and stone dust
13. _____ silicosis	M. star-shaped areas of disease associated with smoking

CLINICAL SIGNS AND SYMPTOMS OF ILD

14. Patients with ILD of many different etiologies will usually present with which two common complaints?

   A. _____

   B. _____

225

15. Describe the breath sounds usually heard in ILD. _____

_____

16. What two explanations does *Egan's* give for wheezing heard in patients with ILD?

A. _____

B. _____

17. Name at least two of the late signs of ILD.

A. _____

B. _____

18. Physical signs of underlying connective tissue disease include what three features?

A. _____

B. _____

C. _____

19. Describe the classic and late radiographic findings in idiopathic pulmonary fibrosis; use the colorful descriptive terms from *Egan's*. What are the late-stage findings?

A. Classic: _____

B. Late: _____

20. Discuss the effects of ILD on the following pulmonary function variables.

	VARIABLE	EFFECT OF ILD
A.	FEV_1	
B.	FVC	
C.	FEV_1/FVC	
D.	D_{LCO}	
E.	Lung volumes	
F.	Compliance	

SPECIFIC TYPES OF ILD

Because there are so many causes of ILD, it will help you to look at the primary groupings and some representative examples of each category.

21. What are the three most common types of occupational ILD?

    A. _____

    B. _____

    C. _____

22. What do these examples have in common?

23. Give at least one specific example for each of the following general categories of drugs that are associated with the development of ILD. (Hint: Box 24-1 on page 531 of your text is useful.)

	CATEGORY	EXAMPLE
A.	Antibiotic	
B.	Antiinflammatory	
C.	Cardiovascular	
D.	Chemotherapeutic	
E.	Illegal drugs	
F.	Miscellaneous agents	

24. Why is pulmonary involvement in connective tissue disorders often undetected until late in the course of the disease?

25. Name three common connective disorders associated with lung disease.

    A. _____

    B. _____

    C. _____

26. What is the name for chronic exposure to inhaled organic material that results in progressive scarring of the lung? _____

27. What factor is critical to identifying the cause of this condition? _____

_____

28. What is meant by the term "idiopathic?" _____

_____

29. Let's compare the two idiopathic lung diseases discussed in the text.

		Idiopathic Pulmonary Fibrosis (IPF)	Sarcoidosis
A.	Age		
B.	Symptoms		
C.	Treatment		
D.	Prognosis		

30. Discuss the common areas of treatment for hypersensitivity pneumonitis and occupational lung disease.

31. What is the primary drug (traditional) therapy for ILD? _____

_____

32. What is the most common respiratory therapy modality for ILD? _____

_____

33. What two vaccines are recommended to help avoid infections? What about pneumocystis?

A. Vaccines _____

_____

B. Pneumocystis: _____

_____

34. What is the only therapy shown to prolong life in end-stage ILD? _____

_____

CASE STUDIES

Case 1

A 48-year-old man is admitted for dyspnea on exertion and a dry cough of unknown origin. The chest radiograph shows bilateral reticulonodular infiltrates. Pulse oximetry indicates mild hypoxemia on room air. History reveals that the patient is a hay farmer.

35. What is the most likely diagnosis?

_____

36. What is the most likely cause of the lung disease? What are some other possible causes?

Case 2

A retired Pearl Harbor shipyard worker states that he has had a cough for some time but recently began expectorating some blood. He has bibasilar inspiratory crackles, with otherwise clear breath sounds. A chest radiograph shows reticulonodular infiltrates in both lower lobes. The radiologist also notes the presence of a small right-sided pleural effusion and the presence of pleural plaques and pleural fibrosis. PFTs reveal a normal FEV_1%, decreased TLC and RV, and a decreased D_{LCO}.

37. What is the most likely pulmonary diagnosis?

_____

38. What other information would be helpful in making a determination?

39. What type of disorder is suggested by the PFT results? _____

_____

WHAT DOES THE NBRC SAY?

The NBRC thinks you should know your PFT and physical examination findings pretty well! ILDs don't have a particular category on the boards, but they may be included as side issues to material like interpreting PFT results.

FOOD FOR THOUGHT

40. What is the general term for all lung diseases that cause a reduction in lung volumes without a reduction in flow

    rates? _____

INFORMATION AGE

- National Jewish Medical and Research Center has a good site at www.nationaljewish.org/disease-info/diseases/rheum/ild/.
- The American Lung Association is always a great Internet source for diseases. They have a section called "diseases from A-Z." Just check "I" for interstitial: www.lungusa.org.
- Check out this site if you are interested in finding out more about how medications may cause lung disease: http://pneumotox.com/. For example, antineoplastic agents are well known causes of interstitial disease. I use this site as a handy reference to check on drugs and how they may affect the lungs. Amiodarone is used to treat the heart but also can cause lung disease.

25 Pleural Diseases

Some men dream of doing great things. Others stay awake and accomplish them.
Author unknown

Imagine a piece of cake enclosed in Saran Wrap. Or, if you prefer collapsed lungs, a sandwich covered in that thin, tough clear stuff that we use to store food. Thinking about pleura always makes me think of plastic wrap. Like that clingy food protector, a breach in the pleura has important consequences. I hope you get a chance to play with some pig lungs while you're in training, but if you don't, you can always head for the kitchen!

WORD WIZARD

Chapter 25 introduces lots of important new terms. Match these pleural puzzlers to their definitions. You're going to need the glossary, but it will be worth it. Many of these words are commonly seen on board exams or in clinical practice.

Terms	Definitions
1. _____ bronchopleural fistula	A. pleural effusion high in protein
	B. air leak from the lung to the pleural space
2. _____ chylothorax	C. membrane covering the surface of the chest wall
	D. pleural fluid rich with triglycerides from a ruptured thoracic duct
3. _____ empyema	E. pleural pain
4. _____ exudative effusion	F. pus-filled pleural effusion
	G. blood in the pleural space
5. _____ hemothorax	H. abnormal collection of fluid in the pleural space
	I. pneumothorax without underlying lung disease
6. _____ parietal pleura	J. air under pressure in the pleural space
7. _____ pleural effusion	K. procedure that fuses the pleura to prevent pneumothorax
	L. air in the pleural space
8. _____ pleurisy	M. occurs when the lung is rapidly inflated after compression by pleural fluid
9. _____ Pleurodesis	N. pneumothorax that occurs with underlying lung disease
10. _____ Pneumothorax	O. low-protein effusion caused by CHF or cirrhosis
11. _____ primary spontaneous pneumothorax	P. chest wall puncture for diagnostic or therapeutic purposes
12. _____ reexpansion pulmonary edema	Q. membrane that lines the lung surface
13. _____ secondary spontaneous pneumothorax	
14. _____ tension pneumothorax	
15. _____ thoracentesis	
16. _____ transudative pleural effusion	
17. _____ visceral pleura	

18. How is the pleura of the American buffalo different from that of humans? What is the clinical significance for the buffalo, and when are humans in the same situation?

19. Describe the so-called "pleural space."

20. What is normal intrapleural pressure, and what effect does this have on fluid movement?

21. Explain why pleural pressures are different at the apex and lung bases.

PLEURAL EFFUSIONS

22. Give a brief explanation of how each of the following conditions can cause transudative pleural effusions. If you get lost, refer to Box 25-1 on page 541 of your text.
    A. CHF:

B.   Hypoalbuminemia:

C.   Liver disease:

D.   Lymph obstruction:

E.   CVP line:

23.   What is the most common cause of clinical pleural effusions?

24. What is the general cause of exudative pleural effusions?

_____

25. Give a brief explanation of the cause of these exudative pleural effusions.
A. Parapneumonic

B. Malignant

C. Chylothorax

D. Hemothorax

26. What change in pulmonary function is associated with pleural effusion?

_____

27. In what specific portion of the upright chest film is pleural effusion visualized?

_____

28. Describe the specific type of chest film used to improve visualization of pleural effusions.

29. What type of imaging is the most sensitive test for identification of pleural effusions?

_____

30. What are the three major risks of thoracentesis?

    A. _____

    B. _____

    C. _____

31. Identify the purpose of each of the chambers in the three-bottle chest tube drainage system shown here.

    A. _____

    B. _____

    C. _____

The standard three-bottle system is the basis for all commercial chest tube drainage systems.

32. What two symptoms are common to almost all cases of pneumothorax?

    A.   _____

    B.   _____

33. What is the most common type of traumatic pneumothorax and how is it treated? Give three examples.

34. Compare blunt and penetrating chest trauma as causes of pneumothorax. How does treatment differ in these two situations?

35. What special technique may be helpful to visual pneumothorax in a newborn?

    _____

36. Compare the two major types of spontaneous pneumothorax.

37. Tension pneumothorax can be a life-threatening medical emergency. It is a common board exam item. Please give short clear explanations for items A-D below.
    A.   Definition

    B.   Radiographic finding

C. Clinical signs

D. Treatment

38. Compare the outcomes of early clinical diagnosis and treatment of tension pneumo with delayed diagnosis.

39. How does oxygen administration assist in resolution of a pneumothorax?

40. What is BPF? How does mechanical ventilation perpetuate this problem? What special modes of ventilation may be indicated?

A. BPF = _____

B. Ventilators perpetuate BPF by: _____

C. Adjust ventilator for BPF patient by: _____

CASE STUDIES

Case 1

A mathematics instructor with a history of CHF is admitted with a complaint of pain on inspiration. Her respirations are rapid and shallow, and her heart rate is 104. The pulse oximeter shows a saturation of 93% on room air. Breath sounds are very decreased on the right side, with crackles in the left base. Chest wall movement is markedly less on the right. The chest radiograph shows opacification of the right lung, with shift of mediastinal structures to the left. Diagnostic percussion reveals a dull note on the right side.

Chapter **25 Pleural Diseases**

41. What do you think is wrong with this patient's right lung? Support your conclusion with at least five pieces of information from the case.

    A. "I think the patient has a _____ because

        1. _____

        2. _____

        3. _____

        4. _____

        5. _____

42. What would you recommend as the first respiratory intervention?

    _____

43. How could this disorder be resolved?

Case 2

A tall, thin, young male respiratory care instructor is admitted with a complaint of pain on inspiration. His respirations are rapid and shallow, and his heart rate is 104. The pulse oximeter shows a saturation of 93% on room air. Breath sounds are very decreased on the right side, and clear in the left base. Chest wall movement is markedly less on the right. The chest radiograph shows a dark area without lung markings on the right side, with shift of mediastinal structures to the left. Diagnostic percussion reveals increased resonance on the right side.

44. What do you think is wrong with this patient right lung? Support your conclusion with at least five pieces of information from the case.

    A. "I think this patient has a _____ because

        1. _____

        2. _____

        3. _____

        4. _____

        5. _____

45. What would you recommend as the first respiratory intervention?

46. How could this disorder be resolved?

WHAT DOES THE NBRC SAY?

Because pneumothorax can be caused iatrogenically and, may be life-threatening in mechanically ventilated patients, you will be expected to know how to recognize and treat this problem. While there is no special category called "pneumothorax," you can expect at least three questions related to this topic. You could almost say the NBRC is obsessed with tension pneumothorax.

In addition, you are expected to understand the causes of pleural effusion and how effusions are diagnosed and treated. Questions on assisting the physician in performing thoracentesis and equipment such as chest tubes and drainage systems are all on the boards because they are all connected to effusions and pneumothorax.

Circle the best answer.

47. Immediately after insertion of a central line via the subclavian vein, an intubated patient becomes dyspneic. The respiratory therapist should recommend which of the following diagnostic tests?
    A. 12-lead ECG
    B. chest radiograph
    C. ABG
    D. bedside spirometry

48. The middle bottle of a three-bottle chest drainage system is used as a _____.
    A. water seal
    B. fluid collection
    C. means of applying vacuum to the chest
    D. measurement of improvement of the pneumothorax

49. A chest tube is placed anteriorly between the second and third ribs. The tube is probably intended to treat a

    _____.
    A. chylothorax
    B. hemothorax
    C. transudative pleural effusion
    D. pneumothorax

50. A patient is suspected of having a pleural effusion. Which x-ray position is most appropriate to confirm this diagnosis?
    A. AP chest film
    B. lateral decubitus chest film
    C. apical lordotic chest film
    D. PA chest film

51. Thoracentesis is performed and 1500 ml of fluid is removed from the right chest. Which of the following is likely to occur as a result?
    A. pulmonary edema in the right lung
    B. stridor and respiratory distress
    C. pneumothorax in the right lung
    D. stelectasis in the right lung

52. All of the following would be useful in differentiating right mainstem intubation from left-sided pneumothorax *except* _____.
    A. chest radiograph
    B. diagnostic percussion
    C. auscultation
    D. lung compliance measurement

53. Following an IPPB treatment, a COPD patient complains of sudden severe chest pain. What is the respiratory therapist's first priority in this situation?
    A. Notify the physician of the problem.
    B. Initiate oxygen therapy.
    C. Recommend a chest radiograph.
    D. Perform an arterial blood gas.

54. A patient develops subcutaneous emphysema following a motor vehicle accident involving multiple rib fractures. What action should the respiratory therapist take in this situation?
    A. Perform bedside spirometry.
    B. Initiate oxygen therapy.
    C. Recommend a chest radiograph.
    D. Perform an arterial blood gas.

   There are *endless* variations on these themes. The subject material in Chapter 25 is limited and probably seems pretty straightforward. Be prepared to encounter this topic many times in both the clinical and board examination settings.

FOOD FOR THOUGHT

55. What is meant by the term "ascites?" Besides causing effusions, how could this affect respiratory function?

56. How is thoracentesis modified to prevent reexpansion pulmonary edema?

57. What is subcutaneous emphysema and what relationship does it have to pneumothorax?

INFORMATION AGE

Tension pneumothorax or any disorders of the pleural space are easy to check out on the Web. Google, a search engine, could show you radiographs, articles, and more. I got 322,000 hits on "tension pneumothorax" alone, and Google will assist you in refining your search. Try the following sites:
- www.emedicine.com
- www.nlm.nih.gov/medlineplus
- www.trauma.org

26 Pulmonary Vascular Disease

The person who moves a mountain begins by carrying away small stones.
Chinese Proverb

The invisible miles of delicate vessels in the lung remain hidden and ignored as they play their vital role in gas exchange and pressure regulation. Then a clot breaks loose and lodges in the pulmonary vascular highway, an accident that frequently has fatal consequences. Though rarely recognized, pulmonary embolism results in thousands of deaths each year in the United States. Chapter 26 reviews the incidence, pathophysiology, and treatment of pulmonary embolus and pulmonary hypertension, two conditions the respiratory therapist will encounter many times in the hospital setting.

WORD WIZARD

Complete the following paragraph by writing in the correct term(s) in the blank(s) provided.

When the pressure inside the lung vessels is elevated, a condition called pulmonary _____

exists. Prolonged bed rest could result in formation of a venous _____. Most clots form

in the _____ veins of the lower legs. The blood clot could travel to the lung where it is called

a pulmonary _____, or PE. If this process results in death of the lung tissue, it is called

pulmonary _____. Small particles of fat or air could also form an embolus. Chronic elevation

of pulmonary blood pressure will eventually cause a form of right heart failure known as cor _____.

MEET THE OBJECTIVES

1. How many people develop thromboembolic disease each year in the United States? _____

2. Is a PE likely to be fatal? _____

3. How often is the diagnosis missed? _____

4. Blood clots to the brain or heart often cause death of the tissue. Why is this uncommon in the lung?

5. Explain how pulmonary embolism (PE) increases alveolar deadspace?

6. Why does hypoxemia develop in some cases of PE?

7. What is the primary hemodynamic consequence of PE?

8. State the two most common symptoms of PE.

    A. _____

    B. _____

9. What are the three most frequent physical findings associated with PE?

    A. _____

    B. _____

    C. _____

10. What is the incidence of hemoptysis associated with PE? _____

11. What percentage of patients with PE have an abnormal ECG? _____

12. Name the two most common ECG abnormalities associated with PE.

    A. _____

    B. _____

13. How is the chest radiograph helpful in diagnosing pulmonary embolism?

14. How helpful are arterial blood gases (ABGs) in ruling out PE? What benefit does an ABG provide in these cases?

15. One rapid blood test has been developed to help rule out embolism. Why isn't D-dimer as good for some inpatients?

16. Which test is considered the "gold standard" for the diagnosis of DVT?

    _____

17. What tests might be useful in diagnosis of symptomatic proximal DVT?

18. Because of the high mortality rate, it is important to make a definitive diagnosis of pulmonary embolus. What two tests are reasonably sensitive and reliable in confirming this diagnosis?

    A. _____

    B. _____

19. What is the relationship of the ventilation ($\dot{V}$) and perfusion ($\dot{Q}$) portions of scans in making a high probability diagnosis of PE?

20. Discuss advantages and disadvantages of helical CT scans for PE.
    A. Advantages:

    B. Disadvantages:

ASSESS AND TEST

21. Prophylaxis for DVT is either pharmacologic or mechanical. Give three examples of each.
    A. Pharmacologic prophylaxis

       1. _____

       2. _____

       3. _____

B.   Mechanical prophylaxis

  1.   _____

  2.   _____

  3.   _____

22.   What is the standard pharmacologic therapy for existing DVT or PE? What is the mechanism of action? What are the risks?

  A.   Drug:

  _____

  B.   Action:

  _____

  C.   Risks:

  _____

23.   How are thrombolytics different than anticoagulants? Can they be given together?

24.   Give three examples of thrombolytic drugs.

  A.   _____

  B.   _____

  C.   _____

25.   List the mechanical options available for treatment of massive PE.

26.   When are vena cava filters indicated?

27. Define pulmonary hypertension.

28. Describe the epidemiology of IPH in terms of age, gender, symptoms, mortality, and genetic factors.

    A. Age: _____

    B. Gender: _____

    C. Genetics: _____

    D. Symptoms: _____

    E. Mortality: _____

29. How is IPH diagnosed?

30. Why is it so important to provide oxygen as needed to keep up the sats in this condition?

31. Which drug treatment is given via inhalation? _____

32. Pulmonary hypertension is a frequent complication of COPD. What percentage of elderly patients with COPD will

    develop significant pulmonary hypertension? _____

33. Explain the role of alveolar hypoxia in the development of pulmonary hypertension.

34. What other factors seen in COPD contribute to this condition?

35. What is the only treatment that improves survival in patients with COPD and pulmonary hypertension? What

    treatments might help? _____

CHAPTER HIGHLIGHTS

Identify the key points from Chapter 26. Complete the following questions by writing the correct
term(s) in the blank(s) provided.

36. Venous _____ is an important cause of morbidity and _____ in
    hospitalized patients.

37. One third of all deaths caused by pulmonary _____ occur within _____
    hour(s) of the symptoms.

38. The point of origin of pulmonary embolism is a deep venous thrombosis of the _____

    extremities or _____ in _____% of the cases.

39. Early recognition of PE and DVT is _____-_____.

40. _____ therapy reduces the risk of venous thromboembolism.

41. Treatment of venous thromboembolism includes anticoagulants such as _____ or

    _____.

42. Idiopathic pulmonary artery hypertension is a rare disease that affects _____ adult patients.

43. Drug treatment of IPAH includes _____ and vasodilators, but lung _____ is an option.

CASE STUDIES

Case 1

A 60-year-old man underwent total knee replacement. Two days after surgery, he complains of dyspnea and anxiety. Physical examination reveals a heart rate of 110, respiratory rate of 28, blood pressure of 115/80 mm Hg, and SpO_2 of 93% on room air. Breath sounds are clear except for faint inspiratory crackles in both bases.

44. Why is this patient at risk for PE?

45. What additional diagnostic tests would be helpful in ruling out other potential pulmonary

problems? _____

46. What treatment would you provide as a respiratory therapist?

_____

47. What medical treatment should be initiated if a diagnosis of PE is confirmed?

_____

WHAT DOES THE NBRC SAY?

Pulmonary embolism is so nonspecific in its clinical presentation that it does not have any separate category in the registry examination matrices. On the other hand, deadspace–to–tidal volume ratios (V_D/V_T) are definitely included. Evaluation of dyspnea, pulmonary hypertension, hypoxemia, and ventilation/perfusion scans are all mentioned. Cor pulmonale associated with COPD is a possible inclusion on the exam as well. Recommending anticoagulants is included in the pharmacology section.

You are expected to be able to make a differential diagnosis between heart attack, pneumothorax, and PE when a patient complains of sudden chest pain.

Circle the best answer.

48. A patient who is being mechanically ventilated shows an increased V_D/V_T ratio. Which of the following disorders could be responsible?
    A. atelectasis
    B. pneumonia
    C. pulmonary embolism
    D. pleural effusion

49. Which of the following is the most appropriate test to confirm the presence of a suspected PE?
    A. chest radiograph
    B. pulmonary angiography
    C. bronchogram
    D. arterial blood gas

50. A ventilation/perfusion scan reveals a defect in perfusion in the right lower lobe without a corresponding decrease in ventilation. Which of the following is the most probable diagnosis?
    A. right lower lobe atelectasis
    B. acute pulmonary embolus
    C. pneumothorax
    D. pneumonia

This topic will be covered more when we discuss hemodynamic monitoring!

FOOD FOR THOUGHT

51. What is the most common cause of pulmonary hypertension worldwide?

_____

52. Discuss the pros and cons of moving a critically ill ventilator patient to imaging for a $\dot{V}/\dot{Q}$ scan to confirm a suspected diagnosis of PE.

INFORMATION AGE

- The American Lung Association's site has some good, basic stuff: www.lungusa.org. Just click on "Diseases A-Z" and look under "P." You'll find several items.
- The Pulmonary Hypertension Association site is even better: www.phassociation.org. Of special interest to respiratory therapists on this site is information about inhaled prostacyclins for treatment of pulmonary hypertension!
- The Pulmonary Hypertension Central, which bills itself as the "definitive Internet resource for pulmonary hypertension": www.phcentral.org.
- National Institutes of Health (NIH) has information on PE: www.nlm.nih.gov/medlineplus/pulmonaryembolism.html.

> *To be good is noble, but to teach others to be good is nobler—and less trouble.*
> Mark Twain

Pulmonary edema is one mean clinical problem you will encounter frequently in the emergency department and intensive care units. While the symptoms and initial goals may be similar, cardiogenic (hydrostatic) and noncardiogenic (nonhydrostatic) pulmonary edema have very different etiologies and treatments. These are complex syndromes that will challenge you to use every skill and apply all you've learned. Despite all we have learned over the years, a fairly high mortality rate still exists, especially for acute respiratory distress syndrome (ARDS).

WORD WIZARD

My favorite acronym is "SNAFU": Situation Normal, All Fouled Up. Unfortunately, most medical acronyms aren't all that much fun, but you still need to learn them. Write out the definitions of Chapter 27's alphabet soup.

1. ALI: _____

2. APRV: _____

3. ARDS: _____

4. CHF: _____

5. ECMO: _____

6. ECCO2R: _____

7. GI tract: _____

8. HFV: _____

9. MODS: _____

10. PMNs: _____

11. PEEP: _____

I always hear people asking me to pass the AMBU (now a brand name) bag: the original AMBU meant Air Mask Bag Unit.

MEET THE OBJECTIVES

General Considerations

Let's talk about how to tell the various edemas apart. After all, the mortality from ARDS is 40%, so you really should try to figure this out! Start with a review of the normal physiology. When you're done, meet me at Box 27-3 on page 579 of your text.

12. Name two common conditions leading to hydrostatic pulmonary edema for each of the following general categories:

	CATEGORY	CONDITIONS
A.	Cardiac 1. 2.	
B.	Vascular 1. 2.	
C.	Volume overload 1. 2.	

Now let's go back to the beginning to look at the causes of ARDS. Check out Box 27-1 on page 573 of your text.

13. List four primary and four secondary risk factors for ALI/ARDS.
   A. Primary

   1. _____

   2. _____

   3. _____

   4. _____

   B. Secondary

   1. _____

   2. _____

   3. _____

   4. _____

The key thing in the ICU is to take this a step further and be able to compare. This is so important; the NBRC expects you to recognize the differences between these two wet, crackly, hypoxic lungs. Refer to Box 27-2 on page 577 of your text for a synopsis.

14. Compare CHF and ARDS in terms of the following criteria for diagnosis.

		CHF	ARDS
A.	Chest radiograph 1. Heart 2. Effusions 3. Infiltrates		
B.	Pulmonary capillary wedge pressure (PCWP)		
C.	Bronchoalveolar lavage fluid (BALF)		
D.	Four symptoms in common 1. 2. 3. 4.		

15. Briefly describe the pathophysiology of hydrostatic pulmonary edema.

16. Briefly describe the pathophysiology of nonhydrostatic pulmonary edema.

17. What five areas must be addressed to avoid secondary (iatrogenic) lung injury in ARDS?

    A. _____

    B. _____

    C. _____

    D. _____

    E. _____

Chapter **27** **Acute Lung Injury, Pulmonary Edema, and Multiple System Organ Failure**

18. What two general approaches are used to maintain adequate tissue oxygen delivery (D_{O_2}) in ARDS?

   A. _____

   B. _____

Ventilator Strategies

Most patients with ARDS will require artificial ventilatory support. Basically we're trying to avoid barotrauma, oxygen toxicity, volutrauma, sheering forces, etc. Good news for you—there are some fairly well-accepted criteria for tidal volume, peep, F_{IO_2}, and rate selection in ARDS. The following questions address the currently accepted methods for providing mechanical ventilation.

19. How does optimal PEEP differ from PEEP that delivers the best Pa_{O_2}? (The NBRC loves this one!)

20. In general, what level of PEEP is considered optimal?

   _____

21. We can avoid barotrauma by maintaining mean airway pressures at what value?

   _____

22. PEEP should be adjusted to maintain what F_{IO_2} and Pa_{O_2}?

   _____

23. Compare tidal volumes delivered in conventional mechanical ventilation versus volumes delivered to ARDS patients.

   A. Conventional volume range: _____

   B. ARDS volume range: _____

24. What is meant by "permissive hypercapnia?" What is the goal of this ventilator strategy?

25. In what two conditions is permissive hypercapnia contraindicated? Why?

A. _____

B. _____

Innovative Strategies

When the techniques previously described are not successful, we will have to try something different. Each of these methods has had some limited success. None are foolproof for every patient. In general, innovative strategies protect patients from developing lung injury and are especially useful for patients who need high levels of support like $F_{IO_2} > 60$.

26. The ARDS Net study showed that mortality is reduced when volumes are reduced to what levels? (This is so important I've asked you twice!) (Don't forget, it is ideal body weight, not actual body weight.)

_____

27. Describe high-frequency ventilation.

28. How does IRV differ from conventional ventilator modes?

29. What is the effect of IRV on survival of ARDS patients?

30. Pressure control ventilation (PCV) has a lot of potential since you can limit pressure trauma to the airway. Patients like the way it delivers lots of flow when they want it. What does the therapist need to monitor in PCV? What else that changes when the compliance or resistance changes?

Chapter **27** **Acute Lung Injury, Pulmonary Edema, and Multiple System Organ Failure**

31. Now that the new ventilator valves have solved the technical problems of airway pressure release ventilation (APRV) (and bilevel, as it may be called), why do you think this is a promising mode for ARDS?

32. How does APRV compare to IRV in terms of the patient?

33. How can patient positioning be radically altered to improve gas exchange?

34. Both ECMO and ECCO2R facilitate gas exchange via what type of device?

_____

35. What is the recommendation regarding ECMO and ECCO2R in routine management of ARDS?

_____

36. Exogenous surfactant is helpful in treating infant respiratory distress syndrome and when surfactant is washed out of the adult lung. What's the story on using this with ARDS in adults?

37. How is liquid ventilation accomplished?

38. What quality of perfluorocarbon compounds makes them attractive for use in ARDS? What are we waiting for?

Pharmacologic Treatments

A variety of drugs have been used to try to turn the tide in ARDS. A few have some limited success.

39. Surfactant is not currently recommended for ARDS. What patient group does respond to surfactant administration? _____

40. What was the potential role of nitric oxide (NO) in treating ARDS?

41. What type of abnormal hemoglobinemia is associated with the administration of NO?

_____

42. What is the consequence of sudden discontinuation of inhaled NO?

_____

43. Like surfactant, NO didn't work out for ARDS. What group of patients does receive NO?

_____

Chapter **27** **Acute Lung Injury, Pulmonary Edema, and Multiple System Organ Failure**

44. What specific advice is given in regard to steroids and ARDS?

_____

CHAPTER HIGHLIGHTS

Complete the following sentences by filling in the correct term(s) in the blank(s) provided.

45. CHF and ARDS are common causes of acute _____ failure that have similar initial

_____ presentations.

46. CHF-associated pulmonary edema is due to elevated _____ pressures in the pulmonary

_____.

47. ARDS-associated pulmonary edema results from _____ injury to the lungs.

48. It may be necessary to perform _____ or _____ in order to distinguish CHF from ARDS.

49. Recommendations regarding the treatment of ARDS have focused on supporting _____

_____ and systemic _____ function until the patient recovers from the underlying illness.

50. Ventilator strategies for patients with ARDS are designed to minimize ventilator _____

lung _____ by using _____, low _____

volumes, reduced airway _____, and nontoxic levels of inspired _____.

CASE STUDIES

Case 1

A 5 foot 6 inch, 143-lb (65-kg) teenager does not listen when his mom told him not to pop his pimples. Now he is in the ICU with a temperature of 103° F, blood pressure of 80/50 mm Hg, heart rate of 120, and an SpO_2 of 88% on 100% oxygen. His pulmonary capillary wedge pressure is 14 mm Hg, and cardiac output is 8 L/min. Breath sounds reveal coarse crackles throughout the lungs. The patient is intubated and currently is being ventilated with a tidal volume of 800 ml, rate of 14, and PEEP of 0.

51. What is the most likely diagnosis? Why?

_____

52. With regard to the oxygenation status, what changes would you recommend?

_____

53. With regard to the volume, what changes would you recommend?

_____

54. What is the maximum recommended mean airway pressure that should be delivered to this patient to prevent alveolar damage?

_____

Case 2

A 65-year-old, 143-lb (65-kg) woman was intubated after presenting in the emergency department with pulmonary edema and severe respiratory distress. Now she is in the ICU with a temperature of 97° F, blood pressure of 80/50 mm Hg, heart rate of 120, and an SpO_2 of 90% on 60% oxygen. Her pulmonary capillary wedge pressure is 24 mm Hg and cardiac output is 3 L/min. Breath sounds reveal coarse crackles throughout the lungs. The patient is intubated and currently being ventilated with a tidal volume of 700 ml, rate of 14, and PEEP of 10.

55. What is the most likely diagnosis? What's the underlying cause?

_____

56. With regard to the oxygenation status, what changes would you recommend?

WHAT DOES THE NBRC SAY?

Just like it says in Chapter 27, you need to be able to differentiate CHF and ARDS based on clinical presentation and diagnostic information. You should be able to maintain oxygenation and determine optimal PEEP. Management of these patients on the ventilator is a key part of ALL THREE EXAMINATIONS! Try the following questions.

Circle the best answer.

57. Which of the following would be useful in treating an elevated shunt in a patient with ARDS who is being mechanically ventilated?
    A. initiating SIMV mode
    B. initiating PEEP
    C. increasing the FiO_2
    D. adding expiratory retard

Chapter **27 Acute Lung Injury, Pulmonary Edema, and Multiple System Organ Failure**

58. Which of the following indicates the optimal PEEP setting?

PEEP	Pao$_2$	Cardiac Output
A.	5 cm H$_2$O	53 mm Hg	4.5 L/min
B.	10 cm H$_2$O	60 mm Hg	4.3 L/min
C.	15 cm H$_2$O	74 mm Hg	3.8 L/min
D.	20 cm H$_2$O	88 mm Hg	3.4 L/min

59. A patient is admitted to the ICU with a diagnosis of pulmonary edema. Which of the following breath sounds is consistent with this diagnosis?
    A. inspiratory stridor
    B. inspiratory crackles
    C. expiratory rhonchi
    D. pleural friction rub

60. A patient with ARDS being ventilated with the following settings:

Mode	Assist Control
F$_{IO_2}$	0.80
Rate	10
PEEP	5 cm H$_2$O
V$_T$	600 ml
Spo$_2$	82%

Which of the following would you recommend as possible ways to improve oxygenation?
    A. Increase the tidal volume.
    B. Increase the PEEP.
    C. Increase the F$_{IO_2}$.
    D. Increase the rate.

61. Which of the following would provide necessary information regarding fluid management in a critically ill patient with cardiogenic pulmonary edema?
    A. bedside pulmonary function testing
    B. intake and output measurements
    C. daily weights
    D. pulmonary artery catheter

62. Chest radiograph changes associated with noncardiogenic pulmonary edema include _____.
    I.   pleural effusion
    II. bilateral infiltrates
    III. enlarged left ventricle
        A. I and II only
        B. II only
        C. II and III only
        D. I and III only

63. Which of the following ventilator techniques have been suggested as useful in treating ARDS that does *not* respond to conventional therapy?
    I.   high-frequency ventilation
    II. airway pressure release ventilation
    III. supine positioning
    IV. pressure support ventilation
        A. I and II only
        B. II and III only
        C. III and IV only
        D. I and IV only

We'll come back to this subject again when we get to the chapter on hemodynamic monitoring!

Chapter **27** **Acute Lung Injury, Pulmonary Edema, and Multiple System Organ Failure**   Copyright © 2009, 2003, 1999 by Mosby, Inc., an affiliate of Elsevier Inc.

Shock lung, Da Nang lung, adult respiratory distress syndrome, wet lung, liver lung, and *noncardiogenic pulmonary edema* are all names for ARDS. This syndrome has been recognized ever since we began to save trauma victims during modern warfare.

64. What is the formula for ideal body weight? You can't get the right tidal volume without it.

65. Is ARDS a homogeneous or heterogeneous lung condition? Explain.

66. Lower inflection point (LIP or P_{flex}) is useful in setting appropriate PEEP and tidal volume levels. What is meant by the term LIP? How is it determined?

INFORMATION AGE

Petty and Ashbaugh first described ARDS and the use of PEEP to treat it in 1967! ALI is still a hot topic that requires you to be current in your clinical thinking. The Internet is an ideal way to stay on top of things.
- The American Thoracic Society has an important statement available in PDF format at www.thoracic.org, but you have to search the site for "ARDS position statement."
- When you are searching for information on this subject use the following terms:
  - Multiple organ dysfunction syndrome
  - ARDS
  - Acute lung injury
You will get lots of results that vary depending on the pathophysiology you want to research.
- One really good site on this subject for respiratory therapists is ARDSNet: www.ardsnet.org.
- For the patient and family perspective, try www.ards.org.
- Finally, try the American Lung Association: www.lungusa.org. Click on Diseases A-Z and you'll find ARDS at the top.

28 Lung Cancer

I kissed my first woman and smoked my first cigarette on the same day. I have never had time for tobacco since.

Arturo Toscanini

Respiratory cancer is a popular disease of the rich and famous—John Wayne, Humphrey Bogart, Sigmund Freud, Peter Jennings, Dana Reeves; the list goes on and on. Yet there is hardly a more dreaded word in our society than *cancer*. Lung cancer is the most frequently diagnosed cancer in the world and the most difficult to treat. There is no evidence that this cancer epidemic is slowing down.

WORD WIZARD

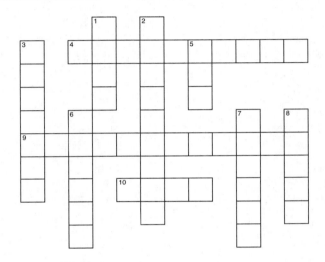

ACROSS

4. process by which tumor cells spread to distant parts of the body
9. drug treatment to cure cancer;
10. the "N" in the TNM

DOWN

1. small _____ cancer, also called oat _____ cancer
2. treatment of neoplastic growth using gamma rays
3. _____ genic carcinoma— cancer originating in the airway
5. staging system
6. opposite of malignant
7. malignant tissue growth
8. type of nodes where cancer spreads

MEET THE OBJECTIVES

1. How many cases of bronchogenic carcinoma were newly diagnosed in the United States in 2006? How many cases does the WHO estimate worldwide?

   A. _____

   B. _____

2. What percentage of cancer deaths are caused by smoking tobacco?

_____

3. Compare lung cancer deaths of men and women in the United States.

4. What percentage of the total population in the United States smoke? Which group of smokers is the largest? (Which group are you in?)

   A. Percent of population: Men _____ Women _____

   B. Most smokers: _____

   C. Are we winning the war against tobacco?

5. What is another name for passive exposure to smoke? _____

6. Describe the health risks of passive exposure to smoke.

7. Besides smoking, name four other major influences linked to an increase in lung cancer.

   A. _____

   B. _____

   C. _____

   D. _____

8. What is meant by the term *apoptosis?*

_____

9. List the four major histopathologic types of lung cancer along with the epidemiology they represent and a brief description of the cells. Try Table 28-1 for help.

TYPE OF CANCER	EPIDEMIOLOGY	DESCRIPTION
A.		
B.		
C.		
D.		

CLINICAL FEATURES

10. What are the four common sites of metastasis of cancer originating in the lungs?

A. _____

B. _____

C. _____

D. _____

11. What percentage of patients with lung cancer are asymptomatic at time of presentation?

_____

12. Local tumor growth in the central airways may cause many symptoms. Name four that a respiratory therapist could easily recognize.

A. _____

B. _____

C. _____

D. _____

13. Patients with pleural or chest wall involvement will typically have what two symptoms?

A. _____

B. _____

14. Explain what is meant by the term "paraneoplastic syndrome."

15. Give three examples of paraneoplastic syndromes commonly associated with lung cancers. Describe briefly, please.
A.

B.

C.

DIAGNOSIS

16. How do these imaging techniques fit into the diagnostic picture?
A. CT:

B.   CXR:

C.   PET:

17.   Two methods are used to obtain tissue for confirmation. Please describe
      A.   Flexible bronchosocopy (FB):

      B.   Transthoracic needle biopsy (TNB):

18.   Why is tumor staging so important?

19. Explain the meaning of the TNM staging system.

A. T = _____

   1 = _____

   2 = _____

   3 = _____

   4 = _____

B. N = _____

   O = _____

   1 = _____

   2 = _____

   3 = _____

C. M = _____

20. How is small cell cancer staged?

21. What's the consensus on mass screenings for people at high risk for lung cancer?

TREATMENT

22. Why is surgical resection the treatment of choice for all non–small cell lung cancers?

   _____

23. What patients are *not* candidates for surgery in terms of staging?

   _____

24. How are respiratory therapists involved in determining candidates for surgery?

_____

25. What test values for FEV_1 and D_{LCO} suggest a patient may safely (or may not!) undergo lobectomy or pneumonectomy?

26. Name the two nonsurgical therapy modalities.

A. _____

B. _____

27. What is the choice of therapy for small cell cancers?

_____

28. What is meant by *palliative* therapy? Give examples.

A. Medications:

B. Radiotherapy:

C. Bronchoscopy:

ROLE OF THE RESPIRATORY THERAPIST

We don't perform surgery or administer chemotherapy or radiation to patients. Still, lots of these people have preexisting lung disease or have airway problems.

29. Describe the role we play in
    A. Nicotine intervention:

    B. Diagnosis:

    C. Support:

CHAPTER HIGHLIGHTS

Complete the following sentences by writing the correct term(s) into the blank(s) provided.

30. _____ carcinoma is the leading cause of cancer deaths in the United States.

31. Approximately _____% of all lung cancers are linked to smoking.

32. _____ represents 40% of all lung cancers and currently is the most common type.

33. The _____ classification groups patients in stages or categories that correlate with

_____.

34. Patients with _____ cancer are classified in two stages: limited or extensive.

35. The most commonly used modalities of treatment for patients with non–small cell lung cancer are surgical resection, _____, and _____.

36. The most effective way to prevent lung cancer is to prevent _____.

Chapter 28 has five excellent case studies in the form of Mini Clinis, so I'm not going to reinvent the wheel. Four of these cases are particularly useful to the respiratory therapist.

Pancoast's Tumor

37. Will you be caring for patients with weakness and drooping eyelids? How is this different?

Paraneoplastic Syndrome

38. Confusion and generalized weakness are signs of what type of serious neurologic vascular accident?

Evaluating Surgical Risk

39. What therapy modalities might improve lung function prior to surgery for lung resection?

No Response to Antibiotics

40. What methods of diagnosis might be useful for the patient with copious amounts of clear, frothy sputum?

For once, the NBRC is relatively silent. Obviously you need to recognize that hemoptysis is an important sign of dysfunction that may relate to cancer or tuberculosis, among other diseases. You should be familiar with the imaging techniques (see Chapter 20 for more).

FOOD FOR THOUGHT

41. Besides lung cancer, what are the other significant health risks of smoking?

42. With the high incidence and known risk factors for lung cancer, you would expect to see screening techniques. Discuss this issue.

43. What is brachytherapy? _____

44. What is the *duty* of every respiratory therapist in regard to their patients who continue to smoke?

_____

INFORMATION AGE

- www.lungcancer.org is a peer-reviewed resource site.
- The government steps in with www.cancer.gov/cancertopics/types/lung.
- And don't forget the American Lung Association: www.lungusa.org. There are many pages on this excellent site.
- Finally, the grandma of them all: www.cancer.org.

29 Neuromuscular and Other Diseases of the Chest Wall

Expert: Someone who brings confusion to simplicity.
Gregory Nunn

Even if your lungs are normal, diseases that affect the brain, nerves, muscles, or bony thorax can lead to respiratory failure or hypoxemia. There are so many unusual conditions that produce muscular weakness that it can be difficult to keep them all straight. You will do fine if you focus on the general principles that apply to assessment and maintenance of the airway in these complex and often sad cases.

WORD WIZARD

I've always wondered if "neuromuscular" really meant you had a strong mind. Let's find out when you try matching these diseases to their definitions.

Diseases	Definitions
1. _____ ankylosing spondylitis	A. neuromuscular conduction disorder that particularly affects the face, throat, and respiratory muscles
2. _____ amyotrophic lateral sclerosis	B. chronic inflammatory disease that fuses the spine and affected joints
3. _____ flail chest	C. muscle wasting disease characterized by delayed relaxation of contracted groups
4. _____ Guillain-Barre syndrome	D. degenerative disease of motor neurons characterized by progressive atrophy
5. _____ Lambert-Eaton syndrome	E. inflammation of muscles caused by a rheumatologic disorder
6. _____ myasthenia gravis	F. unstable chest due to rib fractures exhibiting paradoxical movement on inspiration
7. _____ myotonic dystrophy	G. idiopathic polyneuritis characterized by ascending weakness
8. _____ polymyositis	H. abnormal curvature of the spine that may compromise ventilation
9. _____ kyphoscoliosis	I. neuromuscular conduction disorder associated with underlying malignancy

MEET THE OBJECTIVES

General Principles

10. Neuromuscular abnormalities affect four major groups of muscles that may result in respiratory problems. Name these four groups.

    A. _____

    B. _____

    C. _____

    D. _____

11. The three best recognized pulmonary dysfunctions of respiratory muscle weakness are

A. _____

B. _____

C. _____

12. What are the three common complaints of patients with respiratory muscle weakness due to neuromuscular disease?

A. _____

B. _____

C. _____

13. Give two representative diseases that affect each of the following locations in the respiratory system. (Hint: check out Table 29-1 on page 610 of your text.)

Location	Diseases
A. Cortex, upper motor	_____
B. Spinal cord	_____
C. Lower motor neurons	_____
D. Peripheral nerves	_____
E. Neuromuscular junction	_____
F. Muscle tissue	_____
G. Interstitial lung tissue	_____

14. Pulmonary function testing of patients with neuromuscular disease and otherwise normal lung tissue will demonstrate what type of ventilatory defect?

_____

15. What three specific tests are most useful in monitoring ventilatory function in patients with neuromuscular weakness?

A. Assess volumes with _____

B. Assess muscle strength via _____

C. Assess hypoxemia and hypercapnia with _____

16. How well does pulmonary function testing assess ability to protect the airway?

_____

17. What signs and symptoms suggest performing nocturnal oximetry or formal sleep testing?

_____

18. What is the primary treatment for severe respiratory muscle weakness? What is diaphragmatic pacing?

   A. Primary treatment: _____

   B. Diaphragmatic pacing: _____

19. What problem that may require respiratory therapy is often overlooked?

_____

Specific Neuromuscular Diseases

20. What is myopathic disease? Give two examples of common myopathies.

   A. What is it? _____

   B. Example 1 _____

   C. Example 2 _____

21. Discuss the role of nocturnal ventilation in patients with myopathic diseases.

22. Most cases of myasthenia gravis arise from what abnormality at the cellular level?

_____

23. What general category of drugs is used to treat myasthenia gravis?

_____

24. What surgical treatment may be effective in some cases of myasthenia gravis?

_____

Chapter **29** **Neuromuscular and Other Diseases of the Chest Wall**

25. List four predisposing factors to Guillain-Barre syndrome (GBS).

A. _____

B. _____

C. _____

D. _____

26. What percentage of patients with GBS will have respiratory muscle compromise?

_____

27. Bilateral interruption of the phrenic nerves that results in diaphragmatic paralysis is seen in what type of injury?

_____

28. Reversible unilateral diaphragmatic paralysis occurs frequently following what commonly performed surgery?

_____

29. Describe the chest radiographic presentation of unilateral diaphragmatic paralysis.

30. How is the paralyzed diaphragm visualized during fluoroscopy?

31. What is the percentage of new spinal cord injuries in the United States each year, and what percentage of these cases results in quadriplegia?

A. _____

B. _____

32. Define the high and middle/low classification of cervical cord lesions.
A. High:

_____

B. Middle/low:

_____

33. Describe the muscle groups affected by each of the following spine injuries. See the Mini-Clini on page 619 of your text!

   Level   **Muscle Groups**

   A. C1-2 _____

   B. C3-5 _____

   C. C4-8 _____

   D. T1-12 _____

   E. T7-L1 _____

34. What type of breathing is the hallmark sign of significant diaphragmatic weakness?

   _____

35. What percentage of patients with C3-5 injury will ultimately become liberated from mechanical ventilation?

   _____

36. Both stroke and traumatic brain injuries lead to disordered breathing. What is a stroke?

   _____

37. What are the two basic types of stroke?

   A. _____

   B. _____

38. Give examples of the effect on the respiratory system of strokes in the following locations in the brain (see Table 29-2 on page 620).

   Location   **Effect on Respiration**

   A. Cerebral cortex _____

   B. Bilateral hemispheric infarct _____

   C. Lateral medulla _____

   D. Mid pons _____

39. Aside from problems similar to stroke, brain trauma can cause what respiratory "fluid" problems?

   A. _____

   B. _____

Chapter **29** **Neuromuscular and Other Diseases of the Chest Wall**

40. Describe these two chest wall deformations that often occur together.

    A. Kyphosis:

    B. Scoliosis:

41. Describe the ventilatory defects and pulmonary function changes associated with severe kyphoscoliosis.

    A. Ventilation:

    B. Pulmonary function:

42. How is kyphoscoliosis treated in younger patients?

    _____

43. Describe the role of nocturnal ventilation in treating patients with kyphoscoliosis.

44. Describe the paradoxical chest motion that is the hallmark of flail chest.

45. Name three other pulmonary injuries frequently associated with flail chest.

    A. _____

    B. _____

    C. _____

46. Regardless of the physiologic mechanisms behind respiratory dysfunction, what are the mainstays of treatment for flail chest?

A. _____

B. _____

C. _____

CHAPTER HIGHLIGHTS

Complete the following sentences by writing in the correct term(s) in the blank(s) provided.

47. The key components of the respiratory neuromuscular system are the _____, the nerves,

the _____ junction, and the _____ of inspiration.

48. Weakness and _____ failure are the most important respiratory dysfunctions in many neuromuscular diseases.

49. Neuromuscular diseases can also cause _____ or hypoventilation, sleep

_____, aspiration, _____, and pulmonary hypertension.

50. Signs and symptoms of muscle weakness include exertional _____, orthopnea, soft

vocalizations, and a weak _____.

51. PFTs typically show a decreased _____ lung capacity, decreased _____

capacity, and decreased _____ inspiratory pressures.

CASE STUDIES

Case 1

A 27-year-old woman who was admitted from her physician's office following complaints of fatigue. Upon interview, the patient reports that she becomes weak after any exertion, especially in her arms. She also complains of difficulty swallowing. She denies any recent illness. Vital signs show a normal temperature and slightly increased heart rate and respiration. Inspection reveals that she has drooping eyelids and appears to have little tone in her facial muscles.

52. Based on this information, what is the most likely diagnosis?

_____

53. What drug therapy might help to confirm this diagnosis?

_____

54. Why is measurement of inspiratory and expiratory pressures a more sensitive test of muscle function that measurement of vital capacity?

Case 2

A 52-year-old man was admitted from his physician's office following complaints of fatigue. Upon interview, Mr. Brown reports that his feet felt numb yesterday and that his legs were weak when he got up this morning. He went to the physician because he thought he might be having a stroke. He states that he had the flu about 2 weeks earlier. Vital signs show a normal temperature and slightly increased heart rate and respiration.

55. Based on this information, what neuromuscular condition is likely?

_____

56. How would analysis of CSF be useful in making a diagnosis?

57. What two treatment strategies have improved outcome in this syndrome?

A. _____

B. _____

WHAT DOES THE NBRC SAY?

One or two cases on the Clinical Simulation Examination will be devoted to adult patients with neuromuscular or neurologic conditions. Myasthenia gravis, Guillain-Barre, tetanus, muscular dystrophy, and drug overdose are listed as examples in the matrix. You should be able to recommend or interpret the results of bedside tests such as vital capacity and maximum inspiratory pressure. So while there won't be too many multiple-choice questions on neuromuscular diseases, this is an important part of the testing process. Questions on the chest and spinal trauma are also included on your boards. In particular, you should pay attention to the subject of flail chest. Here are a few questions for practice.

58. A 23-year-old patient with flail chest is transferred to the ICU for observation following a motor vehicle accident. After 2 hours, the patient complains of increasing dyspnea and arterial blood gas analysis is performed.

    pH   7.27
    $Paco_2$ 55 mm Hg
    Pao_2 61 mm Hg

    What action should the respiratory therapist recommend at this time?
    A. Place the patient on oxygen therapy.
    B. Initiate mask CPAP.
    C. Administer a bronchodilator drug.
    D. Initiate mechanical ventilation.

59. A patient with Guillain-Barré syndrome has had serial vital capacity measurements.

    0900   3.1 L
    1100   2.6 L
    1300   2.1 L
    1500   1.6 L

    In regard to these data, what should the respiratory therapist recommend?
    A. Increase the monitoring to every hour.
    B. Administer Tensilon.
    C. Provide intubation and mechanical ventilation.
    D. Continue to monitor the patient every 2 hours.

60. A vital capacity below what value indicates the need for intubation and ventilation in a patient with acute neuromuscular disease?
    A. 30 ml/kg
    B. 20 ml/kg
    C. 15 ml/kg
    D. 10 ml/kg

61. A patient with myasthenia gravis presents in the emergency department with profound muscle weakness. Administration of which of the following will improve ventilation?
    A. pancuronium
    B. neostigmine
    C. epinephrine
    D. atropine

62. The presence of paradoxical chest motion on inspiration following a motor vehicle accident most likely indicates _____.
    A. flail chest
    B. pulmonary contusion
    C. pneumothorax
    D. hypoxemia

FOOD FOR THOUGHT

63. ALS is the disease that strikes down heroes in the prime of life. Prognosis is poor. Two new ideas for ALS include Riluzole and NSIF. Please discuss.
    A. Riluzole:

B. NSIF:

INFORMATION AGE

There are many different kinds of neuromuscular and chest wall diseases. The Internet is a fair resource for general information.

- For those who will work in pediatrics, the Muscular Dystrophy Association: www.mdausa.org.
- The ALS Foundation Web site: www.alsa.org.
- The Internet Handbook of Neurology is interesting: www.neuropat.dote.hu/nmd.htm.

Once you know the specific illness you want to look up, the Internet is an excellent way to get info. For specific diseases like myasthenia gravis, try www.nlm.nih.gov/medlineplus/myastheniagravis.html.

As a student working on a paper or a practitioner who works with specific patient populations, I highly recommend doing a Web search. Each condition will have good information on their association Web site.

30 Disorders of Sleep

Most people spend their lives going to bed when they're not sleepy and getting up when they are.

Cindy Adams

Does someone you love snore excessively? Whenever I ask that question, hands go up in the audience. Does that mean the snorer has sleep apnea? Have you ever wondered just exactly what you do while you're sleeping? The polysomnography lab is just the place to find out. Many respiratory therapists (RTs) have found rewarding careers in the sleep or neurodiagnostic lab setting.

Another reason RTs are interested in disorders of sleep are the cardiopulmonary consequences of sleep apnea. Finally, even in the acute care setting, you will be called on to deal with patients who utilize CPAP or bilevel airway pressure devices to control their apnea. Once again, you will find yourself in the position of being the expert on the assessment and equipment involved in treating this not-so-unusual condition.

WORD WIZARD

Acronyms can be fun if they sound cool, like SCUBA (Self-Contained Underwater Breathing Apparatus). Too bad most of the medical acronyms are dull. Give the full name of the following acronyms from Chapter 30. (You're probably already familiar with some of these by now.)

1. BiPAP: _____

2. CSA: _____

3. CPAP: _____

4. RDI: _____

5. EEG: _____

6. EPAP: _____

7. IPAP: _____

8. OSA: _____

9. PSG: _____

10. UVPPP: _____

11. AHI: _____

MEET THE OBJECTIVES

12. What is the definition of sleep apnea? What about hypopnea?

13. How does OSA differ from CSA?

14. What is the estimated incidence of OSA in the adult population?

    _____

15. Why does airway closure occur during sleep?

16. Name five adverse cardiopulmonary consequences of untreated OSA.

    A. _____

    B. _____

    C. _____

    D. _____

    E. _____

17. Name two neurobehavioral and two metabolic consequences of untreated OSA.
    Neurobehavioral

    A. _____

    B. _____

    Metabolic

    C. _____

    D. _____

18. List three factors that predispose a patient to OSA.

    A. _____

    B. _____

    C. _____

19. Describe the six common clinical features seen in many cases of OSA.

    A. _____

    B. _____

    C. _____

    D. _____

    E. _____

    F. _____

20. What is the current gold standard for making a diagnosis of OSA?

    _____

21. An apnea-hypopnea index of what value is consistent with moderate to severe sleep apnea? What is considered

    normal? _____

22. What are the three goals of treatment for OSA?

    A. _____

    B. _____

    C. _____

23. Discuss the behavioral options that should be pursued in all patients with sleep-disordered breathing.

24. Why do you think nocturnal CPAP has become the first-line medical therapy for OSA?

25. How does CPAP work to relieve OSA?

26. Discuss the issue of patient compliance with nasal CPAP therapy.

27. Explain how the titration of bilevel positive airway pressure therapy differs from that of CPAP.

28. Describe five of the common minor side effects of positive-pressure therapy. Identify what you can do to help the patient solve these annoying problems.

A. _____

B. _____

C. _____

D. _____

E. _____

29. What is the role of tracheostomy in treating sleep apnea?

30. What is the success rate of UPPP, and what is the current recommendation regarding this procedure as a treatment for OSA?

CHAPTER HIGHLIGHTS

Identify the key points from Chapter 30. Complete the following questions by writing the correct term(s) in the blank(s) provided.

31. The three types of sleep apnea are obstructive, _____, and _____.

32. The predominant risk factor for airway narrowing or closure during sleep is a _____ or _____ upper airway.

33. The long-term adverse consequences of OSA include poor _____ functioning as well as increased risk of _____ morbidity and mortality.

34. Risk factors for OSA include _____ gender, age greater than _____ years, upper body _____, and habitual _____.

35. The first-line medical therapy for OSA is _____.

36. _____ positive airway pressure therapy may be useful in salvaging patients who have difficulty complying with CPAP.

37. _____ therapy may be an option for a select group of patients who have undergone extensive upper airway analysis and do comply with medical therapy.

38. In mild to moderate OSA, _____ _____ can be an effective alternative therapy.

CASE STUDIES

KISS is another one of my favorite acronyms. *Keep it simple* . . . and this is simple. No way could I improve on the excellent cases in your textbook.

WHAT DOES THE NBRC SAY?

The NBRC usually considers CPAP to be a ventilator mode or freestanding strategy to improve oxygenation but that is changing. Nasal CPAP (and BiPAP, which by the way, is a trademark of a particular company, not a generic term) are included. To be specific, CPAP devices (mask, nasal, or bilevel) are mentioned, and you need to know about the equipment and the therapy. You may even see a simple tracing like you see on Figure 30-1, A on page 627 of your text.

39. An RT notes in the medical record that a patient is receiving BiPAP therapy with a machine he brought from home. Which of the following is the most likely diagnosis for the patient?
    A. pulmonary emphysema
    B. congestive heart failure
    C. obstructive sleep apnea
    D. atrial fibrillation

40. A sleep study shows simultaneous cessation of airflow and respiratory muscle effort. These findings are consistent with _____.
    A. pulmonary hypertension
    B. obstructive sleep apnea
    C. congestive heart failure
    D. central sleep apnea

41. Which of the following is *true* regarding BiPAP therapy?
    I.   Expiratory pressure is always set above inspiratory pressure.
    II. BiPAP units are pneumatically powered.
    III. IPAP should be increased until snoring ceases.
        A. I and III
        B. II only
        C. II and III
        D. III only

FOOD FOR THOUGHT

What is the Epworth Sleepiness Scale? The best way to screen people in a simple manner, that's all. I suggest you go to Stanford University Web site and find out. This will score you automatically: www.stanford.edu/~dement/epworth.html.

If you want to gain more professional expertise on this subject, look no further than the journal *Respiratory Care*, which has completely devoted editions to sleep-disordered breathing!

INFORMATION AGE

The trick here is to get the information you want. Searching for "sleep apnea" will give you a headache, believe me. "Obstructive sleep apnea" will yield better results, and so will "sleep disordered breathing" and "polysomnography." Some key words work better than others.
- The American Sleep Apnea Association is a nonprofit organization that maintains a good site: www.sleepapnea.org.
- The British site Sleep Study.org has lots of useful information including an excellent historical section: www.sleepstudy.org/Index.htm.

31 Neonatal and Pediatric Respiratory Disorders

Any man who hates dogs and babies can't be all bad.

Leo Rosten

There's hardly a more joyous event than bringing new life into the world—unless you look at it from the perspective of the respiratory therapist (RT). We don't see the healthy babies, just the sick ones! I am amazed that we RTs have children of our own . . .

WORD WIZARD

Try this matching exercise to test your ability to understand the new terms and acronyms found in Chapter 31.

Terms	Definitions
1. _____ RDS	A. poor clearance of lung fluids (type II RDS)
2. _____ croup	B. aspiration of fetal feces
3. _____ GERD	C. chronic problem from alveolar trauma and oxygen toxicity
4. _____ PPHN	D. life-threatening upper airway infection
5. _____ MAS	E. virus-induced subglottic swelling
6. _____ TTN	F. acute infection of the lower airways
7. _____ SIDS	G. leading cause of death in infants <1 year old
8. _____ epiglottitis	H. complex syndrome of newborn hypertension
9. _____ BPD	I. stomach problem association with asthma
10. _____ bronchiolitis	J. surfactant deficiency in preemies

BABY BLUES

11. How many babies in the United States have RDS?

_____

12. What is the primary pathophysiology in infants with RDS?

_____

_____

13. Describe the four clinical signs of RDS that are listed below.

A. Respiratory rate: _____

B. Breathing pattern: _____

C. Auscultation: _____

D. Audible sounds: _____

14. How is the definitive diagnosis usually made?

15. Discuss the four main therapies for treating RDS.
    A. CPAP: starting values? Device?

    B. Ventilator: when do you start? Goal of PEEP?

    C. Surfactant: when to give? Positioning?

    D.   HFV: what does it mean?

16. How does the chest radiograph of a baby with transient tachypnea of the newborn (TTN) (type II RDS) differ from that of primary RDS?

17. List two typical respiratory treatments for TTN.

    A. _____

    B. _____

18. Meconium aspiration is usually associated with what fetal event?

    _____

19. What age baby usually has MAS? _____

20. Name the three primary problems in MAS.

    A. _____

    B. _____

    C. _____

21. Immediate treatment of the MAS baby is vital! What should you do?

    A. Upon delivery: _____

    B. Repeat until: _____

    C. If the condition worsens: _____

22. In some ways, bronchopulmonary dysplasia is a result of our efforts to save preterm infants. What are the five events implicated in causing BPD?

A. _____

B. _____

C. _____

D. _____

E. _____

23. What is the "best management" of BPD, and how and where does this begin?

A. Best: _____

B. How: _____

C. Where: _____

24. Please define "periodic breathing," and compare that to "abnormal apneic spells."
A. Periodic breathing:

B. Abnormal apneic spells:

25. Describe how the following strategies work to alleviate infant apneic events.
A. Tactile stimulation:

B. CPAP:

C. Caffeine (xanthines):

D. Doxapram (Dopram):

E. Transfusion:

26. Persistent fetal circulation may result in hypertension in the newborn. Name the three types of PPHN and at least one factor that might have caused the problem.

	TYPES	FACTORS
A.		
B.		
C.		

27. What's the basic idea behind each of these treatments for PPHN?
    A. Oxygen

    B. Glucose

    C. Inotropes

    D. Sedation

    E. HFV

    F. Inhaled NO

    G. ECMO

28. An infant with profound cyanosis at birth most likely has one of two conditions. Name them.

    A. _____

    B. _____

29. What are the four defects seen in tetralogy of Fallot?

    A. _____

    B. _____

    C. _____

    D. _____

30. Acyanotic heart diseases are also seen in newborns. PDA is of special interest to RTs. Describe PDA. Name two treatments.
    A. Description:

B. Treatments:

NEONATAL RESUSCITATION

I just can't think of anything more exciting than neonatal resuscitation; except flying in the back of a small plane and doing neonatal resuscitation. RTs are always key members of the transport team. Refer to the American Academy of Pediatrics Neonatal Resuscitation Protocol. Go to www.aap.org/nrp/nrpmain.html, and you'll find out the scoop.

PEDIATRIC PROBLEMS

Kids get sick a lot and they have little airways. The combination of infection and airway problems like reactive airways and cystic fibrosis makes for a lot of visits to the emergency department (ED).

Sudden infant death syndrome (SIDS) is the leading cause of death in infants less than 1 year of age in the United States, with about 7000 deaths each year! Diagnosis isn't made until a previously healthy baby dies unexpectedly. That's pretty sad, don't you think?

31. What is the cause of SIDS? _____

_____

32. Describe the typical profile of a baby who dies of SIDS.

_____

_____

33. What sleeping position is strongly linked with SIDS?

_____

34. Identify the four infant characteristics often seen near the time of death.

A. _____

B. _____

C. _____

D. _____

35. Once an at-risk infant is identified, what can be done to try to prevent a SIDS death?

36. What is gastroesophageal reflux disease (GERD)? Name a few of the many respiratory problems this condition can trigger.

37. What group of kids usually gets bronchiolitis?

_____

38. RSV is one particularly nasty virus that's the culprit in many cases of bronchiolitis. Tell me about:

A. Immunization. Who gets it?

_____

B. What does RSV stand for?

_____

C. How is the diagnosis made?

_____

39. Dyspnea, tachypnea, wheezing, and cough are common in these kids. If they have to be hospitalized, what respiratory treatments are indicated? Name at least four.

A. Bronchodilators, what's the controversy?

_____

B. Why give antibiotics for a virus? _____

C. Hygiene? _____

D. What's Ribavirin? _____

For more information, go to www.rsvinfo.com.

CASE STUDIES

Bronchiolitis, croup, epiglottitis, and cystic fibrosis are all serious and relatively common pediatric respiratory disorders that you should be able to recognize and differentiate from each other.

Case 1

A mother brings her previously healthy 1-year-old to the ED. She states that her baby had a cold 2 days ago, but he still has a slight fever and has been coughing. Mom became concerned when she heard audible wheezing. A treatment with albuterol in the ED has had no effect. Vital signs are essentially normal, except for a slight elevation in respiratory rate. The chest radiograph shows mild hyperinflation with no signs of consolidation. Pulse oximetry shows a saturation of 94%.

40. What diagnosis is most likely?

    _____

41. How can a diagnosis of RSV be ruled out?

    _____

42. The physician decides to send mom and baby home. What treatment would you recommend?

Case 2

A 3-year-old is brought to the ED with respiratory distress and a barking cough (like a seal!). The child has been sick for several days with a low-grade fever and stuffy nose. Examination reveals moderate inspiratory stridor and retractions. The pulse oximeter shows a saturation of 88% on room air. A lateral neck film identifies subglottic narrowing with a "steeple sign."

43. What is the most likely diagnosis?

    _____

44. What aerosolized medication is traditionally delivered?

45. When should you add nebulized budesonide?

46. How would you deliver oxygen to this child?

_____

Case 3

A 5-year-old is brought to the ED with labored breathing and a high fever. Examination reveals marked inspiratory stridor. The child is listless, and dad says he has had a sore throat. When you talk to the boy, he responds very quietly with short answers. A lateral neck radiograph identifies a "thumb sign."

47. What is the most likely diagnosis?

_____

48. What organism is usually responsible for this condition? How could you confirm?

_____

49. What is the immediate treatment for this condition? Who should perform the intervention and

where? _____

50. What should not be done? _____

A grandmother brings her son's 2-year-old in to the clinic because "his breathing just isn't right." She states, "This boy is coughing all the time. Besides, he isn't growing very well, and when I kiss him his skin tastes salty!"

51. How would your diagnosis be confirmed?

   _____

52. What dietary modifications are needed in cystic fibrosis?

   _____

53. Name four respiratory treatments aimed at decreasing airway obstruction.

   A. _____

   B. _____

   C. _____

   D. _____

54. Nebulizing drugs here is one of the key treatments. Tell me more about:
   A. Mucolytic drugs:

   B. 7% solution:

   C. Who's this Tobi?

If you want to get serious about this disease, please go to the Cystic Fibrosis Foundation at www.cff.org.

WHAT DOES THE NBRC SAY?

The Entry-Level Examination may ask you a couple of questions related to pediatrics, usually recall questions, but this is not the primary proving ground for this area of knowledge. The Registry tests make detailed references to the material in Chapter 31. Neonates are pretty much on the Registry tests. The Examination Matrices (all of them!) contain these items (just a partial list!):

Perinatal data
- Maternal history
- Perinatal history
- Apgar scores
- Gestational age
- L/S ratio
- Preductal and postductal studies

Recommend procedures
- Umbilical line
- Transcutaneous monitoring

Inspect the patient
- Apgar score
- Gestational age
- Retractions
- Transillumination of the chest

Inspect lateral neck and chest radiographs

Equipment
- Oxygen hoods and tents
- Specialized ventilators-oscillators, high frequency

The Clinical Simulation Examination Matrix makes it clear that you will have one pediatric and one neonatal problem. Basically, you can't be an RT without specialized, in-depth neonatal and pediatric knowledge. That's why most schools have a separate course and text for this topic. BUT *Egan's* contains much of the information you need to pass your boards. These cases are typical examples from the clinical simulations:

Neonatal

Delivery room management, resuscitation, infant apnea, meconium aspiration, respiratory distress syndrome, congenital heart defect.

Pediatric

Epiglottitis, croup, bronchiolitis, asthma, cystic fibrosis, foreign body aspiration, toxic substance ingestion, bronchopulmonary dysplasia.

Try these multiple choice questions. Circle the best answer.

55. A premature infant is experiencing episodes of apnea and cyanosis. The respiratory therapist should recommend which of the following?
    A. albuterol
    B. Narcan
    C. Exosurf
    D. theophylline

302

56. A 5-year-old child presents in the ED with complaints of a severe sore throat. The child has inspiratory stridor and muffled phonation. He has a fever of 40°C. His mother states he will not drink anything, so she brought him in. The most likely diagnosis is _____.
   A. croup
   B. bronchiolitis
   C. foreign body aspiration
   D. epiglottitis

57. Which of the following tests is helpful in establishing a diagnosis of cystic fibrosis?
   A. sweat chloride
   B. L/S ratio
   C. Apgar score
   D. pneumogram

58. Which of the following is the most appropriate imaging technique to help confirm a diagnosis of croup?
   A. computed tomogram
   B. PA chest film
   C. lateral neck film
   D. bronchogram

59. A 4-year-old child with LTB presents in the ED with moderate stridor and harsh breath sounds. The RT should recommend which of the following?
   A. albuterol
   B. racemic epinephrine
   C. immediate intubation
   D. aminophylline

FOOD FOR THOUGHT

My students were just asking me "What's the difference between an infant, baby, child . . . ?" Here's some definitions for you that aren't in *Egan's:*

- **Fetus:** The unborn offspring from the end of the eighth week after conception (when the major structures have formed) until birth. Up until the eighth week, the developing offspring is called an embryo.
- **Premature baby:** A baby born before 37 weeks of gestation have passed. Historically, the definition of prematurity was 2500 grams (about $5^1/_2$ pounds) or less at birth. The current World Health Organization definition of prematurity is a baby born before 37 weeks of gestation.
- **Neonate:** This is a newborn baby. If the baby leaves the newborn nursery, goes home, and comes back to the hospital, he or she may be put into the pediatric unit.
- **Post-term baby:** A post-term baby is born 2 weeks (14 days) or more after the usual 9 months (280 days) of gestation.
- **Child:** This is a person 6 to 12 years of age. An individual 2 to 5 years old is a preschool-aged child. Sometimes we use the following criteria: Ages 1 to 8 for a child. Obviously size is important when you're talking about ET tubes and drug dosages, because some children are quite large.

P.S.: You might try a site like www.medterms.com if you need to look up words. I know I do.

INFORMATION AGE

- American Academy of Pediatrics: www.aap.org
- If you like resuscitation, you'll just love this heart site, which has all the pediatric advanced life support (PALS) stuff: www.heart.org/presenter.jhtml.
- Virtual Children's Hospital has been resurrected and you can find the files at www.vh.org/pediatric.

32 Airway Pharmacology

All things are poison and poison is in all things. Whether it is a medication or a poison . . . depends on the dose.
Paracelsus

When the first edition of *Egan's* came out in 1969, only a limited number of drugs were available by inhalation. Most of those medications are no longer used, due to the advent of newer, more specific agents with longer action and less side effects. New categories of inhaled medicines require the respiratory therapist (RT) to have a strong grasp of pharmacologic principles and the specific indications and actions for these newer tools for managing the airway. You'll need to stay on top of things; even as I write, a new nebulized drug has been approved for COPD (Brovana) and an inhaled drug has been approved for diabetes (Exubera). You will be the one who can advise physicians, nurses, and patients on methods and options for producing bronchodilation, reducing the inflammatory response, clearing secretions, and treating infection.

WORD WIZARD

Try this matching exercise to test your ability to understand the new terms found in Chapter 32.
(You may have to really dig for some of these—use the chapter, the glossary, and a medical dictionary if necessary!)

Terms	Definitions
1. _____ indication	A. time it takes to metabolize $1/2$ drug dosage
	B. drug may not be given for any reason
2. _____ tolerance	C. effect of acetylcholine on smooth muscle
	D. reason for giving a drug to a patient
3. _____ adrenergic	E. undesired effect of a drug
4. _____ vasopressor	F. drugs that mimic the effect of epinephrine
	G. has receptor affinity and exerts an effect
5. _____ pharmaceutical	H. mimics the effect of acetylcholine
6. _____ muscarinic	I. drug that exerts a constricting effect on blood vessels
7. _____ pharmacodynamic	J. phase related to route of administration
	K. dilation of the pupil of the eye
8. _____ side effect	L. phase related to mechanism of action
	M. maximum effect from a drug dosage
9. _____ absolute contraindication	N. time it takes a drug to start working
	O. how long the drug's effect lasts
10. _____ leukotriene	P. increasing dose needed for effect
11. _____ mydriasis	Q. has receptor affinity but produces no effect
	R. rapidly developing tolerance
12. _____ agonist	S. compounds that produce allergic or inflammatory responses
13. _____ pharmacokinetic	T. phase related to metabolism of a drug

Continued

14. _____ cholinergic

15. _____ antagonist

16. _____ tachyphylaxis

17. _____ onset

18. _____ peak effect

19. _____ duration

20. _____ half-life

JUST SAY YES

21. What is the most common route of administration that is used by RTs?

    _____

22. Name four advantages of this route.

    A. _____

    B. _____

    C. _____

    D. _____

23. Name two disadvantages of this route.

    A. _____

    B. _____

24. How do medications delivered by this route usually end up in the systemic circulation?

    _____

25. Describe the two primary divisions of the autonomic nervous system in terms of name, main neurotransmitter, and effect on bronchial smooth muscle.

	DIVISION	OTHER NAME	NEUROTRANSMITTER	AIRWAY MUSCLE EFFECT
A.	Sympathetic			
B.	Parasympathetic			

ADRENERGIC BRONCHODILATORS

26. State the three receptors of the sympathetic nervous system and their basic effects.

	RECEPTOR	PRIMARY EFFECT
A.		
B.		
C.		

27. Give the generic name, brand name, strength, and dose for the following commonly used beta-adrenergic bronchodilators.

	GENERIC NAME	BRAND NAME	STRENGTH	DOSE
A.	Racemic epinephrine SVN			
B.	Epinephrine SVN Epinephrine MDI			
C.	Albuterol SVN Albuterol MDI			
D.	Levalbuterol SVN Levalbuterol MDI			
E.	Pirbuterol MDI			
F.	Salmeterol DPI			
G.	Formoterol DPI			
H.	Arformoterol SVN			

28. Epinephrine and racemic epinephrine are bronchodilators, but these drugs are usually administered to:

A. Stimulate what receptor? _____

B. Produce what effect? _____

C. Accomplish what clinical goals? _____

29. What would you recommend if a patient experienced bronchospasm from a CFC inhaler?

_____

30. It is especially important that you know how long it takes for a drug to start working and reach its maximum effect and how long the drug will last. Fill in the information for the drugs listed below.

	DRUG	ONSET	PEAK EFFECT	DURATION
A.	Xopenex			
B.	Micronefrin			
C.	Proventil			
D.	Serevent			
E.	Formoterol			
F.	Arformoterol			

31. List the most common side effects of bronchodilator drugs. Which one is number 1?

A. _____

B. _____

C. _____

D. _____

32. Adverse reactions are more serious, but less frequently seen. List six potential adverse effects you must watch for in patients receiving adrenergic bronchodilators.

A. _____

B. _____

C. _____

D. _____

E. _____

F. _____

33. What should you monitor when administering any drugs via the aerosol route?

A. _____

B. _____

C. _____

D. _____

And the fifth vital sign?

E. _____

34. What specific tests or data can be obtained to monitor the effects of bronchodilator therapy?

A. _____

B. _____

C. _____

D. _____

35. How would you assess long-term bronchodilators?

A. _____

B. _____

C. _____

D. _____

E. _____

Excessive use of these medications might result in what undesirable outcome?

_____

_____

ANTICHOLINERGIC BRONCHODILATORS

36. Generally, ipratropium is indicated for use in what types of patients?

_____

37. Fill in the blanks to complete your knowledge of ipratropium.

NAME	BRAND NAME	STRENGTH	DOSE
Ipratropium bromide			
MDI (HFA)			
SVN			
Nasal			
Tiotropium			

38. Now try this one.

DRUG	ONSET	PEAK EFFECT	DURATION
Ipratropium			
Tiotropium			

39. What medication is available by MDI with both ipratropium and albuterol? What are the possible advantages and disadvantages of this medication?

40. Describe the side effects to watch for when administering this class of drugs.

Common side effects

A. _____

B. _____

MDI occasional side effects

A. _____

B. _____

SVN occasional side effects

A. _____

B. _____

41. Why does *Egan's* talk about the eyes of patients who get treatments? How do we protect them (and us!)?

_____

MUCUS CONTROLLING AGENTS

42. Describe the mucoactive agents available for nebulization?

	AGENT	BRAND NAME	DOSE	INDICATION
A.				
B.				
C.				
D.				

43. Bronchospasm is a common side effect of the administration of mucolytic agents. How would you recommend modifying the therapy to prevent or treat this problem?

44. What types of short- and long-term assessments should you make to monitor the effectiveness of these drugs?

45. When is mucoactive therapy a potential danger to a patient? Your book discusses three potential scenarios where you could make things worse.

INHALED GLUCOCORTICOIDS

Like bronchodilators, there are a lot of inhaled steroids out on the market. You can expect many of your patients to be receiving these medications. Physicians, patients, and family members have many misconceptions about steroids, including "steroid phobia." Again, it's up to you to be the expert and to be able to clearly explain the use of these very important tools in the fight against asthma.

46. How long will it take for inhaled steroids to have a noticeable effect on the symptoms of asthma?

47. What significance does this have in terms of patient education?

48. The most common side effects of inhaled steroids are local ones (as opposed to systemic). Name the four most common problems.

    A. _____

    B. _____

    C. _____

    D. _____

49. Besides a reservoir device, what two additional recommendations are made by GOLD and NAEPP in regard to corticosteroid inhalers?

50. What would you assess to determine if the steroids were working in the long run?

_____

The National Institutes of Health 1997 Asthma Education and Prevention Program guidelines contain definitive information on the use of drug therapy for the treatment of asthma. You can get a copy of these guidelines from the American Lung Association or your instructors or you can download the information from the NIH Web site (see "Information Age" at the end of this chapter for access to the NAEPP guidelines and the most current update EPR3, which was just released at the time of this writing).

NONSTEROIDAL ANTIASTHMA DRUGS

Drugs that prevent the release of histamine or block the release or effects of other mediators of inflammation are hot items right now. These drugs, whether oral, inhaled, or injected, hold tremendous promise for treating asthma and preventing the long-term pulmonary consequences of this increasingly serious condition. They fall into the category of "controllers" rather than "quick relief" drugs like albuterol.

51. What is believed to be the mode of action of cromolyn sodium?

_____

52. Which two mediator antagonists are recommended for use in young children? (Hint: Look at Table 32-6)

_____

53. Which of these mediator antagonists is available by inhalation?

_____

54. List the number 1 side effect for each of the following:

A. Cromolyn sodium (Intal): _____

B. Nedocromil (Tilade): _____

C. Zafirlukast(Accolate): _____

D.   Zileuton(Zyflo): _____

E.   Montelukast (Singulair): _____

55.   No one can pronounce it, but omalizumab, or Xolair (easier, 'zo-lair'), can make a dramatic difference for severe asthma that is caused by what type of response? Based on the time between shots, how long do you think this might take to start working? (The answer is not in *Egan's;* just check Table 32-6 and guess.)

TREATING INFECTION BY THE AEROSOL ROUTE

It should make sense to you that lung infections can be treated by aerosolizing medications. This technique for delivery is limited to very specific situations.

56.   What agent may be nebulized to treat PCP (pneumocystis pneumonia) seen in severely immunocompromised patients?

_____

57.   Why isn't the drug used much anymore?

_____

_____

58.   What are the common undesired respiratory side effects of administration? What modification of therapy would you recommend if they occur?

59.   While PCP is not a hazard to healthy people, patients with AIDS often have what other disease that is transmitted via the airborne route?

_____

60. Describe the use of Ribavirin in terms of indication, patient population, and special equipment need for administration.

    A.   Indication: _____

    B.   Type of patient: _____

    C.   Special equipment: _____

61. What about Tobi?

    A.   Drug: _____

    B.   Organism: _____

    C.   Nebulizer: _____

62. While not yet approved for inhalation in the United States, what other drug can be nebulized safely for gram-negative bugs?

_____

_____

INFLUENZA

Influenza can be fatal to the elderly and those with heart or lung problems. While vaccination is still the best protection, there is an inhaled drug that shortens the course and alleviates symptoms.

63. What's the drug? What's the problem with giving it to asthma and COPD patients?

    A.   Drug: _____

    B.   Problem: _____

No FDA-approved drugs are available specifically for inhalation right now. When I was a young therapist, I nebulized amphotericin B to administer to patients with fungus in their lungs on many occasions. A lot more science has been developed since then, but we still don't have good dosing schedules, any new classes of drugs, or adequate variety of delivery systems.

64. Invasive pulmonary fungal infections like aspergillosis love the lungs of the immunocompromised. Intravenous amphotericin B is the drug of choice. But when poor blood flow limits intravenous delivery to the lungs, you may consider aerosolizing amphotericin B. Describe a dosing and treatment plan.

65. What could go wrong with the lungs if you give this stuff, and what would you do about it?

INHALED VASODILATORS

People have been inhaling vasodilators for recreation for years, and now we have medications like nitric oxide for newborns. Iloprost can be nebulized to administer to adults with pulmonary hypertension.

66. What is the brand name of the iloprost, and what is the nebulized name?

A. _____

B. _____

67. What could go wrong?

INHALED INSULIN

Inhaled insulin is a great example of the wave of drug delivery for the future. Inhaled drugs don't hurt! I expect to see more large molecules being aerosolized now that Exubera has broken through.

68. Who should resist inhaling insulin until we know more?

_____

CASE STUDIES

Case 1

A patient who has asthma is admitted to the hospital for the second time in 2 months. She has not been able to get relief and is using her albuterol inhaler frequently.

69. In addition to inhaled beta agonists, steroids are commonly administered to *reduce* inflammation associated with asthma. Name one inhaled steroid and recommend a dose.

_____

70. What device is important to use along with MDIs to prevent deposition of these drugs in the mouth?

_____

71. Why should this patient rinse her mouth after use of her inhaled steroid?

_____

72. Recommend another drug that can be delivered by MDI as a long-term controller to prevent *release* of inflammatory mediators.

_____

73. What long-acting bronchodilator may help this patient sleep through the night without being awakened by dyspnea and wheezing?

_____

Case 2

Cystic fibrosis is diagnosed in a 7-year-old. This patient has extremely thick mucus (like glue!). Auscultation reveals scattered wheezing and rhonchi.

74. What drug would you recommend aerosolizing for treatment of the thick mucus?

75. What other drug should be given to treat the wheezing?

_____

76. Lee has *Pseudomonas* in his sputum. What could you nebulize to treat gram-negative bad boys in

CF? _____

Case 3

A 67-year-old man with long-standing COPD characterized by chronic bronchitis is coughing up copious amounts of very thick white sputum. He complains that his chest feels tight, and he cannot catch his breath. His albuterol inhaler is not providing relief.

77. What bronchodilator is appropriate to add to the therapeutic regimen?

_____

78. What mucolytic may be considered if other means of sputum clearance are ineffective? Why might this drug be counterproductive?

WHAT DOES THE NBRC SAY?

Sure enough, those scholastic scoundrels at the NBRC have scattered a number of drug questions strategically throughout the tests. In fact, pharmacology appears in at least six different parts of the matrix!

Try these exercises. Circle the best answer.

79. A patient with pneumocystis pneumonia is unable to tolerate oral antibiotics due to gastrointestinal side effects. Which of the following would you recommend?
    A. aerosolized acetylcysteine (Mucomyst)
    B. aerosolized albuterol (Proventil)
    C. aerosolized dornase alfa (Pulmozyme)
    D. aerosolized pentamidine iethionate (NebuPent)

80. An asthmatic patient presents in the emergency department with dyspnea, hypoxemia, and wheezing. All of the following are appropriate at this time *except* _____.
    A. administration of oxygen
    B. nebulized cromolyn sodium (Intal)
    C. nebulized albuterol (Ventolin)
    D. measurement of peak expiratory flow rates

81. Following extubation, a patient has mild stridor. Which of the following would you recommend at this time?
    A. administration of oxygen
    B. aerosolized albuterol (Proventil)
    C. aerosolized virazole (Ribavirin)
    D. aerosolized racemic epinephrine (Vaponefrin)

82. After administering a corticosteroid via MDI, the RT should ask the patient to perform which of the following actions?
    A. Rinse and gargle with water.
    B. Deep breathe and cough.
    C. Inhale an adrenergic bronchodilator.
    D. Inhale via a spacer device.

83. The heart rate of a patient receiving an adrenergic bronchodilator rises from 80 to 94 per minute during the treatment. Which of the following actions is most appropriate?
    A. The RT should discontinue the therapy.
    B. Let the patient rest for 5 minutes.
    C. Continue the treatment.
    D. Reduce the dosage of the bronchodilator.

84. A physician calls in an order for bronchodilator therapy for a patient with COPD. The order states "0.05 ml of albuterol in 3 ml of normal saline via SVN four times per day." The RT should _____.
    A. deliver the treatment as ordered
    B. recommend substituting Atrovent
    C. carefully monitor heart rate during the treatment
    D. call the physician to verify the order

FOOD FOR THOUGHT

You might be wondering how you can retain all this drug information. It's not easy! Especially when you might not use many of these medications on a regular basis. One suggestion I have for you is a time-honored technique. Make drug cards. All you need is some 3 × 5 or 4 × 6 index cards. Write out the following on each card (or type on the computer and glue or tape to the card):

- Generic and brand names of the drug
- Routes (like MDI, oral, SVN)
- Dose
- Strength
- Adverse reactions and side effects
- Contraindications
- Patient teaching points

Another trick is to make a memory matrix. You can use a spread sheet program to do this or any paper. Make rows down the left with the drug names and columns across the top with headings like indication, dose, etc. You can put most of this chapter on one page!

85. Besides treatment of excessively thick mucous, what can mucomyst be used for?

_____

86. Primatene Mist is a commonly used asthma inhaler that is available without a prescription. What drug is found in this MDI? What are potential problems with patients taking this drug?

INFORMATION AGE

Naturally you can look up any particular drug on the Internet, so that's easy enough.
   There are other things you can do with the Web.
- The FDA site is a great place to find out what's happening now. Is APIB approved? Is Advair safe? Go to www.fda.gov.
- Maybe you want the 2006 EPR3 asthma guidelines from the NIH! Go to www.nhlbi.nih.gov/guidelines/asthma/index.htm.
- Pharmacology is always changing, always new. No textbook can keep up to date with the latest information, so your journals and the Internet are your best source. I really appreciate this site: http://pneumotox.com. Pneumtotox.com tells you all about the effects of drugs on the lung! For example, amiodarone is used to treat various cardiac arrhythmias. What are the long-term pulmonary problems with this medication?
- For more information on some of the new drugs, go to www.brovana.com, www.exubera.com, and www.nektar.com. The latter is the site for Amphotericin B Inhalation Powder, which has been approved for orphan drug status and fast-track trials.

33 Airway Management

When you can't breathe, nothing else matters.
American Lung Association Motto

Airway management is one of my favorite subjects. It is very satisfying to help patients breathe better in such a dramatic fashion. While there is no substitute for experience, Chapter 33 will help you learn how to use equipment, tubes, and techniques to deal with airway emergencies. You will want to become an expert in every aspect of this subject so that you can become a skilled knowledgeable provider and a resource for other health care professionals. The chapter has a ton of material but it all falls into three basic areas:

- Airway clearance devices and techniques
- Insertion and maintenance of artificial airways
- Special airway management procedures

"THE HALLS ARE ALIVE WITH THE SOUND OF MUCUS..."

Patients who can't clear their own secretions are at risk for all kinds of problems like increased work of breathing, atelectasis, and lung infections. It's our job to get in there and clean out those airways. Respiratory therapists (RTs) suction both the upper and lower airways.

---

10 Commandments for Endotracheal Suctioning

I.   Thou shall assess thy patient.
II.   Thou shall use the correct vacuum setting.
III.   Thou shall use the right catheter size.
IV.   Thou shall preoxygenate and hyperinflate thy patient.
V.   Thou shall withdraw 1 to 2 cm prior to suctioning.
VI.   Thou shall suction on withdrawal only.
VII.   Thou shall limit the duration to 10 to 15 seconds.
VIII. Thou shall reoxygenate and hyperinflate after each attempt.
IX.   Thou shall only irrigate when indicated.
X.   Thou shall monitor thy patient.

---

1. Oral suctioning alone is usually accomplished with a rigid plastic tube called a tonsil tip. What's the other common name for this device?

   _____

2. Why do you need to be careful when you're putting a device in someone's mouth? (Hint: Did you ever stick your toothbrush too far into the back of your mouth?)

   _____

   _____

ENDOTRACHEAL SUCTIONING

Endotracheal suctioning is a vital, but potentially risky procedure. Closely following the rules will greatly reduce your chances of causing an adverse reaction. The AARC Clinical Practice Guidelines in your textbook give a good overview of this subject.

3. Describe the cause and how to prevent each of the following complications.

	COMPLICATION	CAUSE	PREVENTION
A.	Hypoxemia		
B.	Cardiac arrhythmia		
C.	Hypotension		
D.	Atelectasis		
E.	Mucosal trauma		
F.	Increased ICP		

4. Discuss the advantages and disadvantages of closed-system multiuse catheters.
    A. Advantages:

    B. Disadvantages

5. What special catheter is used to facilitate entry into the left mainstem bronchus?

    _____

6. How should you position a patient for nasotracheal suctioning?

    _____

7. How is the catheter prepared to prevent trauma during this procedure?

    _____

8. What specialized airway is used to facilitate repeated nasal suctioning?

_____

9. What device do you need to include when you want to collect a sputum specimen during suctioning?

_____

ESTABLISHING THE ARTIFICIAL AIRWAY

Start off by learning the parts of the two most important artificial airways used to maintain adequate ventilation.

WORD WIZARD

Establishing the Artificial Airway

Complete the following paragraph by writing in the correct term(s) in the blank(s) provided.

_____ tubes are long, semirigid tubes, usually made of _____ chloride or some other type of plastic. A typical ET tube has nine basic parts. The proximal end (sticking out of the mouth) has a standard _____-mm adaptor. The body of the tube has _____ markings in centimeters. The tube ends in a _____ tip. There is a port, or slot, cut in the side of the tip called a _____ eye. This slot helps ensure gas flow if the tip is obstructed. Just above the tip, a _____ is bonded to the tube, that can be inflated to seal the airway to prevent aspiration or provide for _____ pressure ventilation. A small filling tube leads to a _____ balloon. This small balloon has a spring-loaded _____ with a connector where a syringe can be attached to allow inflation or deflation. A _____ indicator, or line, is embedded in the wall of the tube body to make it easier to see the tube position on a chest x-ray.

Another commonly used tube, inserted through a surgical opening in the trachea, is called a _____ tube. These tubes are also made of plastic, or occasionally metal such as _____. The _____ cannula forms the primary structural unit of the tube. Like the ET tube, a _____ may be attached near the end to seal the airway. A _____ is attached to the proximal end to prevent slippage and provides a means to secure the tube to the neck. Many tubes have a removable _____ cannula with a standard _____-mm adaptor. This cannula can be removed for cleaning. A special device called an _____ has a rounded blunt end and is used to facilitate insertion.

ET TUBES

There are three specialized endotracheal tubes you should know about: double-lumen, jet ventilation tubes, and CASS tubes. Pay attention, this is board material!

321

10. What type of lung disease requires the use of a double-lumen ET tube?

_____

These are also called Carlen's, or endobronchial, tubes. What is the name of the special type of ventilation used

with this tube? _____

11. High-frequency jet ventilation tubes look like standard tubes with two additional lines. What are they?

A. _____

B. _____

12. Continuous aspiration of subglottic secretions is the generic name for the Hi-Lo Evac Tube. What is the reported

benefit of the CASS or Hi-Lo Evac Tube?

_____

INTUBATION PROCEDURES

13. What is the preferred route for establishing an emergency tracheal airway?

_____

14. Name the four types of practitioners who most commonly perform endotracheal intubation.

A. _____

B. _____

C. _____

D. _____

15. Why is suction equipment needed for intubation?

_____

16. Describe two common troubleshooting procedures used when the laryngoscope does not light up properly.

_____

17. How are tube sizes selected for infants?

_____

18. How are tube sizes selected for adults? How does size differ for men and women? Do you agree with the sizes for men and women in Table 33-2 on page 707 of your textbook?

_____

19. Prior to insertion, how should the RT test the tube?

_____

20. How is the head positioned to align the mouth, pharynx, and larynx?

_____

21. What other actions *must be taken* before making any attempt to intubate?

_____

22. How long may you attempt intubation? Why do you think we have a rule like this one?

_____

23. Name at least two anatomic landmarks *besides the glottis* to be visualized prior to intubation.

    A. _____

    B. _____

24. Compare the use of the Miller and Macintosh laryngoscope blades during the intubation procedure.

_____

25. Your textbook describes eight methods for bedside assessment of correct tube position. While none of these methods absolutely confirms position, they are essential assessments to make right after the tube is placed. Heart association says there should be three surveys of intubation. Fill in the information from Box 33-4 on page 709 of your textbook.

    Primary Survey = Physical Assessment

    A. _____

    B. _____

    C. _____

Secondary = Bedside Measurement Devices

A. _____

B. _____

C. _____

D. _____

E. _____

The third survey method is the gold standard; can you guess what it is?

_____

26. What is the disadvantage of using capnographic or colorimetric analysis of carbon dioxide to assess intubation in a cardiac arrest victim?

27. What is the final step of confirmation?

_____

28. Give two examples of clinical situations where nasotracheal intubation might be preferred over oral intubation.

A. _____

B. _____

29. Describe the two techniques used for nasal intubation.

A. _____

B. _____

30. Let's compare oral and nasal intubation. Each has advantages and disadvantages. Place a letter "O" by items that match oral intubation and a letter "N" by items that go with nasal intubation. Check out Table 33-1 on page 704 for help.

A. avoids epistaxis and sinusitis   _____

B. greater comfort for long-term use   _____

C. easier to suction   _____

D. larger tube   _____

E. greater risk of extubation   _____

F.   improved oral hygiene   _____

G.   bronchoscopy more difficult   _____

H.   increased salivation   _____

I.   reduced risk of kinking   _____

J.   decreased laryngeal ulceration   _____

K.   increased risk of sinusitis   _____

TRACHEOTOMY

31.   What is the primary indication for performing a tracheotomy?

_____

32.   When is tracheotomy the preferred primary route of airway management?

_____

33.   Describe the sequence for removing an ET during the tracheotomy procedure. You might want to remember this

procedure! _____

PERC ME UP!

The percutaneous, or bedside, tracheal tube insertion is by the most common method for ICU patients in our islands. I hope you get to watch or assist while you're in school.

34.   Compare the location of placement in percutaneous and traditional surgical tracheostomy.

35.   Name at least three advantages of the percutaneous technique compared with traditional surgical tracheotomy.

A.   _____

B.   _____

C.   _____

36. Compare the following laryngeal injuries associated with intubation in terms of symptoms and treatment.

	INJURY	SYMPTOMS	TREATMENT
A.	Glottic edema		
B.	Vocal cord inflammation		
C.	Laryngeal ulceration		
D.	Polyp/granuloma		
E.	Vocal cord paralysis		
F.	Laryngeal stenosis		

37. Name the three most common tracheal lesions.

A. _____

B. _____

C. _____

38. Compare tracheal malacia and tracheal stenosis in terms of cause, pathology, and treatment.

	INJURY	CAUSE	PATHOLOGY	TREATMENT
A.	Malacia			
B.	Stenosis			

39. Describe the tracheoesophageal fistula in terms of cause, complications, and treatment.

40. Tracheoinnominate fistula is a rare, but serious complication. What are the clues and what are the immediate and corrective actions taken? What is the survival rate?

CARE AND FEEDING OF YOUR NEW ARTIFICIAL AIRWAY

Once placement of an artificial airway is successfully completed the real fun begins. As an RT, you will be expected to secure the airway, maintain adequate humidification, manage secretions, care for that cuff, and troubleshoot problems that arise—some of which are life threatening.

41. What is the most common material used to secure endotracheal tubes? Tracheostomy tubes?

_____

What's the alternative? _____

42. How do flexion and extension of the neck affect tube motion? What is the average distance the tube will move (in cm)?

TALK TO ME

43. People with endotracheal tubes can't talk and they shouldn't try. What device is used to help with communication?

_____

44. What is a "talking" trach? What are some of the problems with these gadgets?

45. A trach can be temporarily closed with a finger (the patient's finger or yours, with a glove of course!). A more effective solution in the long run is the Passy Muir valve. What do you need to do with the cuff? How about the ventilator?

HUMIDIFICATION

46. What is the worst problem that results from inadequate humidification of the artificial airway?

_____

47. What temperature range must be maintained in a heated humidification system to provide adequate inspired

moisture? _____

48. What device can be used as an alternative to heated humidifiers for short-term humidification of the intubated

patient? _____

Look into Chapter 35 for more details on this subject.

49. State at least four reasons why tracheal airways always increase the risk of infection.

A. _____

B. _____

C. _____

D. _____

50. Describe three techniques that can be used to decrease the risk of infection.

A. _____

B. _____

C. _____

51. What is the most common cause of airway obstruction in the critically ill patient?

_____

CUFF CARE

52. Describe the shape of a modern tube cuff.

_____

53. What is the recommended safe cuff pressure? What is the consequence of elevated cuff pressures?

A pressure of 25 cm H₂O is considered the top number for the board exams!

54. Describe the two alternative cuff inflation techniques.
    A. MOV

    B. MLT

55. What happens to cuff pressures when the tube is too small for the patient's trachea?

_____

56. How is the methylene blue test performed?

TRACH CARE

RTs and nursing personnel may share some of the tracheostomy care duties. These tubes require daily care to keep the wound clean and the tube functioning properly.

Your textbook makes changing a trach tube sound simple. It can be a harrowing experience. The first change is often performed by the surgeon. Be especially careful when:
- The neck is thick.
- The site is inflamed or infected.
- The trach is fresh.

57. What protective gear do you need to use when performing trach care?

_____

58. Briefly describe the eight basic steps of tracheostomy care.

A. _____

B. _____

C. _____

D. _____

E. _____

F. _____

G. _____

H. _____

ALWAYS have intubation equipment ready.

AIRWAY EMERGENCIES

59. State three airway emergencies.

A. _____

B. _____

C. _____

60. Give four reasons why a tube may become obstructed.

A. _____

B. _____

C. _____

D. _____

61. What simple technique is used to assess tube obstructions that are not relieved by repositioning the head or deflating the cuff? _____

62. If you cannot clear the obstruction, what action should you be prepared to take?

_____

63. What additional troubleshooting step can often be performed on patients with tracheostomies?

_____

64. What effects will occur with a cuff leak when a patient is being mechanically ventilated?

_____

65. What action should you be prepared to take if the cuff is blown?

EXTUBATION AND DECANNULATION

Extubation is a procedure commonly performed by the RT. You will need to be familiar with the indications for extubation and techniques used to minimize risk during this procedure.

66. The decision to remove the airway and to remove the ventilator are NOT THE SAME! What kind of patients might need to remain intubated even after the ventilator is removed?

_____

67. Describe two methods for performing a "cuff-leak test."
    A.

    B.

By the way, we have NOT come up with a magic number for a leak that predicts success. No leak is bad, more leak is good. That's it.

68. List five types of equipment you will want to assemble *prior* to extubation.

   A. _____

   B. _____

   C. _____

   D. _____

   E. _____

69. You will need to suction which two places before extubating? Name them and describe the correct sequencing for

   this important step. _____

70. Describe the two different strategies for removing the tube itself.

   A. _____

   B. _____

71. What therapeutic modality is usually applied immediately after extubation?

   _____

72. List two or three of the most common problems that occur after extubation.

   _____

73. The worst complication of extubation is laryngospasm. What can you do if this persists for longer than a few seconds?

74. A common complication of extubation is glottic edema. How will you recognize *and* treat this problem?

75. Oral feeding should be withheld for how long following extubation? Why?

_____

76. State the three methods for weaning from a tracheostomy tube. Give one advantage and one disadvantage for each technique. This is national exam material.

	TECHNIQUE	ADVANTAGE	DISADVANTAGE
A.			
B.			
C.			

AIRWAY ALTERNATIVES

You might need to have a few more airway tricks up your sleeve. LMAs are increasingly popular devices, especially in the operating room and the EMS settings. Combitubes are also a part of the prehospital setting. Both of these tubes are now a part of Advanced Cardiac Life Support (ACLS) training. Emergency cricothyroidotomy may be needed if the upper airway is obstructed. Paramedics may put these in but RTs usually do not.

77. Give three advantages of the LMA.

A. _____

B. _____

C. _____

78. Give two disadvantages of the LMA.

A. _____

B. _____

79. Why is the Combitube so useful in the field?

_____

BRONCHOSCOPY

While rigid scopes are usually used in the operating room, flexible bronchoscopy is often done at the bedside with the RT playing a key role in patient preparation and monitoring during the procedure.

80. State one advantage and three disadvantages of the rigid bronchoscope.

81. Give an example of a specific drug and the general goal for each of the following classes of premedication used in bronchoscopy.

	DRUG CLASS	EXAMPLE	GOAL
A.	Tranquilizer		
B.	Drying agent		
C.	Narcotic-analgesic		
D.	Anesthetic		

82. What drugs would RTs nebulize prior to the procedure on a nonintubated patient? What about after the procedure?

A. Before: _____

B. After: _____

83. What three types of cardiopulmonary monitoring devices are considered essential for this procedure?

A. _____

B. _____

C. _____

84. What are some of the activities we might perform while assisting with the procedure?

A. _____

B. _____

C. _____

CASE STUDIES

Case 1

During your first day of clinical training in the ICU, a patient sustains a cardiac arrest. Your clinical instructor asks you to assist in preparing the equipment needed for endotracheal intubation. The patient is a small 56-year-old woman.

85. What size endotracheal tube should you select?

_____

86. How should you test the tube prior to insertion?

_____

87. How will you test the laryngoscope and blade for proper function?

_____

88. Once the tube is inserted, how can you quickly assess placement?

89. A colorimetric CO_2 detector is attached to the ET tube. The end-tidal CO_2 is 2% on exhalation and 0% on inhalation as the chest rises with bagging. What does this suggest regarding the effectiveness of the chest compressions?

_____

Case 2

After your heart-pounding initiation into resuscitation, it is time to check the other ventilator patients in the unit. A 19-year-old woman with a head injury is receiving mechanical ventilation via a cuffed No. 8 tracheostomy tube with an inner cannula. As you enter the room, the high-pressure alarm is sounding.

90. How will you determine the need for suctioning in this situation?

_____

91. What vacuum pressure should be set prior to suctioning?

_____

92. What size suction catheter is suggested using the Rule of Thumb found in *Egan's?*

_____

93. How long, and with what F_{IO_2}, should you preoxygenate this patient?

_____

94. After suctioning, you will need to check the cuff pressure. What is a safe cuff pressure?

_____

WHAT DOES THE NBRC SAY?

Chapter 33 is the longest one we've had so far! That must mean this is extremely important material. The NBRC agrees! The Examination Matrix says you must perform procedures to achieve maintenance of the airway including artificial airway care, adequate humidification, cuff monitoring, positioning, and removal of secretions. They go on to include modification of the management of artificial airways including changing the type of humidification, inflating or deflating the cuff, and initiating suctioning. You should be able to assemble and check the function of the airways and the intubation equipment. Finally, you need to assist the physician in performing bronchoscopy, tracheostomy, and, of course, intubation. The actual number of airway questions varies from exam to exam, but you should be prepared for at least six to eight questions on any given test.

Circle the best answer.

95. Which of the following will decrease the risk of damage to the trachea from the endotracheal tube cuff?
    I. minimal leak technique
    II. maintaining cuff pressures of 30 to 35 cm H_2O
    III. minimum occluding volume technique
    IV. inflating the cuff to 25 mm Hg
       A. I and II
       B. I and III
       C. II and III
       D. III and IV

96. The diameter of the suction catheter should be no larger than
    A. one-tenth the inner diameter of the ET tube
    B. one-third the inner diameter of the ET tube
    C. one-half the inner diameter of the ET tube
    D. three-fourths the inner diameter of the ET tube

97. A patient with a tracheostomy tube no longer requires mechanical ventilation. All of the following would facilitate weaning from the tracheostomy *except* a(n) _____.
    A. fenestrated tracheostomy tube
    B. cuffed tracheostomy tube
    C. tracheostomy button
    D. uncuffed tracheostomy tube

98. Extubation is performed on a patient with an endotracheal tube. Presence of which of the following suggests the presence of upper airway edema?
    A. rhonchi
    B. crackles
    C. wheezes
    D. stridor

99. All of the following are useful in nasotracheal intubation *except* a _____.
    A. laryngoscope handle
    B. stylette
    C. Miller blade
    D. Magill forceps

100. While performing endotracheal suctioning, an RT notes that flow through is minimal and secretion clearance is sluggish. Which of the following are possible causes of this problem?
    I. The vacuum setting is greater than 120 mm Hg.
    II. The suction canister is full of secretions.
    III. There is a leak in the system.
    IV. The tube cuff is overinflated.
       A. I and II
       B. I and IV
       C. II and III
       D. III and IV

101. Rapid, initial determination endotracheal tube placement can be achieved by _____.
    I.   auscultation
    II. arterial blood gas analysis
    III. measurement of end-tidal CO_2
    IV. measurement of S_{PO_2}
        A. I and II
        B. I and III
        C. II and IV
        D. III and IV

102. A patient with a tracheostomy tube shows signs of severe airway obstruction. A suction catheter will only pass a short distance into the tube. The RT should _____.
    A. remove the tracheostomy tube
    B. inflate the cuff of the tube
    C. ventilate the tube with positive pressure
    D. remove the inner cannula

103. Which of the following can be used to assess pulmonary circulation during closed-chest cardiac compressions?
    A. capnometry
    B. arterial blood gas analysis
    C. pulse oximetry
    D. blood pressure monitoring

104. Prior to performing bronchoscopy, an RT is asked to administer a nebulized anesthetic to the patient. What medication is most appropriate to place in the nebulizer?
    A. Versed
    B. atropine
    C. morphine
    D. lidocaine

FOOD FOR THOUGHT

Here's an idea that could help you learn a topic as huge, complex, and important as this one: digital flashcards. Take photographs of equipment, scan pictures from books, and download from the Internet to create a pile of pictures. Set up a slide show and you've got digital flashcards. My students find this a fun and effective way to learn, and they help each other out on the project.

INFORMATION AGE

When I searched Google for "endotracheal tube PowerPoint presentations," I got about 35,000 hits! You can do better than that!
    Try
- The Internet Journal of Airway Management: www.ijam.at. It has good stuff and a cool "virtual airway museum."
- E-medicine has a good area on tracheostomy at www.emedicine.com/ent/topic356.htm.

There is literally an astonishing amount of material on airway management on the Internet, so you need to have a pretty good idea of what you are looking for when you start to search. You'll want to narrow things down with "artificial airway emergencies," not "airway emergencies," if that's what you're hoping to find. If you do use Google, try switching to images or video mode; you might be pretty surprised at what you get!

34 Emergency Cardiovascular Life Support

We're in the resuscitation business, not the resurrection business.
Anonymous RT

Nothing is more satisfying than being a part of the team that helps save someone's life!

A successful resuscitation is an exciting event that you will remember forever. Of course, a poorly managed effort is completely frustrating, and attempting to save someone who should never have cardiopulmonary resuscitation (CPR) in the first place is about as depressing as it gets. Because respiratory therapists play an integral role in hospital resuscitations, you will want to know both the basic and advanced life support techniques. Chapter 34 summarizes the important concepts of these two activities and provides you with knowledge skills you will be expected to demonstrate on your boards. **There is no substitute for formal training and certification in basic and advanced life support!**

WORD WIZARD

Acres of Acronyms

You must have noticed by now that medicine loves acronyms. I found 15 in Chapter 34 that will enable you to talk the talk. (Walking the walk is another story altogether!)

Write out the full definition of each acronym below.

1. ABCD: _____

2. ACLS: _____

3. AED: _____

4. AHA: _____

5. ARC: _____

6. BLS: _____

7. BVM: _____

8. CDC: _____

9. CNS: _____

10. CPR: _____

11. FBAO: _____

12. EMS: _____

13. NRP: _____

14. PALS: _____

15. SCA: _____

CAUSES AND PREVENTION OF SUDDEN DEATH

16. What is the primary cause of sudden death among adults in the United States?

_____

17. What is the most common rhythm immediately after cardiac arrest? What are the two basic treatments?

A. Rhythm: _____

B. Treatments: _____

_____

BASIC LIFE SUPPORT

18. Compare adult, child, and infant resuscitation for the following categories (see Table 34-1 on page 745 of your text).

	CATEGORY	ADULT	CHILD	INFANT
A.	Obstructed 1. Mild 2. Severe 3. Unresponsive			
B.	Breath every:			
C.	Compression 1. Hands 2. Ratio 3. Cycles 4. Depth 5. Rate 6. Pulse			

19. You wouldn't want to do CPR on someone who is just sedated. Once you carefully assess unresponsiveness, you need HELP! What should you do in each of these situations?
    A. Collapsed outside hospital call:

    _____

    B. In the hospital call:

    _____

    C. How do you quickly check for "signs of life?"

    _____

    _____

20. When is the jaw-thrust maneuver indicated?

    _____

21. How can you determine if a victim is breathing?

    _____

22. Describe the technique for mouth-to-mouth breaths for adults and children. What is the hazard to the *victim* in this procedure?
    A. Adults:

    B. Children:

    C. Infants:

Chapter **34** **Emergency Cardiovascular Life Support**

D. Hazard:

23. When is mouth-to-nose indicated in adults?

_____

24. Mouth-to-tube or stoma? Seriously, folks, you might be able to bring yourself to do this on a loved one, but in the hospital, you will want to modify this technique. What would you do?

_____

25. How is assessment of pulselessness different in adults and infants?

_____

When can you just "go by the monitor" and not assess the patient's pulse?

26. How is hand positioning for chest compression different in adults, children, and infants?
A. Adults:

B. Children:

C.   Infants:
   1.   First method:

   2.   Second method:

27.   Describe the modifications to CPR that you need to consider under these special circumstances:
A.   Near drowning:

B.   Electrocution:

28.   Once CPR is begun, it is normally only stopped for what three reasons?

A.   _____

B.   _____

C.   _____

29.   Health care providers and lay providers might do CPR a little differently in terms of rates and ratios.

A.   One rescuer gives _____ compressions to _____ breaths in adults.

B.   Two rescuers give _____ compressions to _____ breaths in adults.

C.   Children and infants get _____ compressions to _____ breaths with two rescuers.

Chapter **34**   **Emergency Cardiovascular Life Support**

WHO PUT THE "D" IN DEFIBRILLATION?

The American Heart Association (AHA) added defibrillation (D) to the ABCs because it is lifesaving in many cases of sudden cardiac arrest.

30. A person with sudden cardiac arrest is probably in what rhythm?

    _____

31. What is the treatment for this rhythm?

    _____

32. Why is early defibrillation so important? What's the timeline?

33. How can you easily and quickly determine the effectiveness of ventilations and compressions delivered during CPR?

    A. Ventilation: _____

    B. Compression: _____

34. CPR can have complications. Give a way to avoid these classics?

    A. Neck injury: _____

    B. Gastric inflation: _____

    C. Vomiting: _____

    D. Internal trauma (liver laceration): _____

    E. FBAO removal: _____

35. CPR is contraindicated under what two circumstances?

    A. _____

    B. _____

36. What barriers does the CDC suggest to protect us during CPR?

    _____

344

37. What is the universal distress signal for foreign body obstruction of the airway?

_____

38. When should back blows be used on an adult victim?

_____

39. Give another name for the abdominal thrust maneuver.

_____

When should you avoid this maneuver in an adult?

_____

What should you do if you cannot or should not perform the abdominal thrust on a choking victim?

40. Describe four ways you can tell that you have effectively removed a foreign body from the airway.

A. _____

B. _____

C. _____

D. _____

ADVANCED CARDIAC LIFE SUPPORT

RTs are often called on to perform oxygenation, assessment, and airway management techniques during resuscitation. I recommend that you take the AHA course in ACLS. Besides making you a smarter member of the code team, it will enhance your marketability to employers. Many hospitals use rapid response or "precode" teams of an RT and RN to get the jump on emergencies. You'll need to follow protocols like ACLS to assess and treat.

41. What concentration of oxygen should be administered during a life-threatening emergency?

_____

42. Describe characteristics of the ideal mask.

43. What is the technique to select the best-sized oropharyngeal airway (OPA)?

44. Name and describe the two basic types of oral airways.

A. _____

B. _____

45. What could go wrong if you insert an oral airway in a conscious victim?

_____

46. What airway would you choose for the patient who cannot tolerate an oral airway?

_____

47. Describe two ways to insert an oral airway without pushing the tongue back.

A. _____

B. _____

48. How would you lubricate the following airways prior to insertion?

A. Oral: _____

B. Nasal: _____

49. Why is an endotracheal tube the preferred method for securing the airway during CPR?

50. Describe the proper way to ventilate during resuscitation to avoid hazards like auto-PEEP and increased intrathoracic pressures that might reduce effectiveness of the resuscitation effort.

51. When should the endotracheal route of drug administration be used? Hint: Check out the Mini Clini. . . .

52. What is the primary treatment for pulseless ventricular tachycardia and ventricular fibrillation?

_____

53. Give three examples of drugs that can be delivered via the ET route.

   A. _____

   B. _____

   C. _____

54. What modification to dosage and technique must be made for endotracheal instillation of emergency drugs?

_____

55. What initial energy level is recommended for electrical countershock during ventricular fibrillation? How about any subsequent shocks?

56. Explain the difference between cardioversion and defibrillation.

57. When is electrical pacing indicated?

_____

58. What are the two primary types of pacing?

A. _____

B. _____

DRUG THERAPY

59. Identify the drug indicated to treat each of the following. (Check out Table 34-2 on page 767 of your text.)

	EVENT	DRUG THERAPY
A.	Ventricular tachycardia	
B.	Pulseless electrical activity	
C.	Asystole	
D.	Poor cardiac contractility	
E.	Hypotension	
F.	Hypertension	
G.	Ventricular fibrillation	
H.	SVT	
I.	Coronary artery occlusion	
J.	CHF/pulmonary edema (fluid overload)	

CASE STUDIES

We're going to skip the cases and get straight to the board exam questions for once!

The Examination Matrix no longer makes it clear what you need to know in regard to resuscitation. They do tell you there are eight questions in the category between the Certified Respiratory Therapist (CRT) and Written Registry Examination (WRE). Be familiar with the following concepts for treating cardiopulmonary collapse:

A. BCLS

B. ACLS

C. PALS

D. NRP

Questions are mostly simple recall and application of facts. The matrix also mentions laryngoscopes, all the tubes, and CO_2 detectors. If you pay attention to this one chapter, you'll get those eight questions right! Admittedly, there is a lot to know. I don't think there is any substitute for an ACLS or PALS course to complete your knowledge in preparation for work in the ICU or the examinations. In fact, the examination matrices are clear that you must know ACLS, BLS, PALS, and NRP information even if you are not certified in these techniques! Finally, the Clinical Simulation Examination may present you a case on resuscitation as well.

Here are a few sample questions. Circle the correct answer.

60. When is the jaw-thrust technique indicated to help maintain an open airway?
    A. when foreign body obstruction is suspected
    B. following trauma to the head
    C. in cases of suspected neck injury
    D. during most CPR efforts

61. While attempting mask-to-mouth ventilation, an RT notes that the chest does not rise with each breath. The most appropriate action to take at this time is to _____.
    A. intubate the patient
    B. switch to bag-mask ventilation
    C. use an oxygen-powered breathing device
    D. give another breath after repositioning the head

62. Where should you check the pulse of an unresponsive infant?
    A. brachial artery
    B. carotid artery
    C. femoral artery
    D. radial artery

63. Upon entering a hospital room, you see a physical therapist administering CPR to a patient who is lying on the floor. Your first action would be to _____.
    A. move the patient onto the bed
    B. call for help
    C. take over chest compressions
    D. deliver two slow breaths to the airway

64. What is the correct number of rescue breaths to deliver during mouth-to-mouth ventilation of an adult victim?
    A. 6 breaths per minute
    B. 12 breaths per minute
    C. 16 breaths per minute
    D. 20 breaths per minute

65. An unconscious patient begins gagging during your attempt to insert an oropharyngeal airway. The correct action to take at this time would be to _____.
    A. insert a smaller oral airway
    B. intubate the patient
    C. perform the jaw-thrust maneuver
    D. insert a nasal airway

66. The correct ratio of compressions to ventilation during two-rescuer CPR of an adult is _____.
    A. 15:2
    B. 30:1
    C. 2:15
    D. 30:2

67. The ideal airway to use during a resuscitation effort is a(n) _____.
    A. oropharyngeal airway
    B. nasopharyngeal airway
    C. fenestrated tracheostomy tube
    D. oral endotracheal tube

68. A patient is coughing and wheezing after accidentally aspirating a piece of meat. At this time, the RT should _____.
    A. allow the patient to clear his airway
    B. perform the Heimlich maneuver
    C. deliver five back blows
    D. call for help

69. Upon entering an ICU room, a RT observes ventricular fibrillation on the cardiac monitor. The most appropriate treatment for this rhythm is _____.
    A. CPR
    B. administration of lidocaine
    C. administration of epinephrine
    D. defibrillation

70. During a resuscitation effort, no IV line can be established. The RT should recommend _____.
    A. intraosseous infusion of the medications
    B. endotracheal instillation of the medications
    C. insertion of a central line
    D. aerosol administration of the medications

71. The effectiveness of chest compressions in producing circulation can be measured by _____.
    I. pulse oximetry
    II. capnography
    III. transcutaneous monitoring
    IV. arterial blood gases
        A. I and II only
        B. II and III only
        C. II and IV only
        D. I and IV only

72. A patient has atrial fibrillation with serious signs and symptoms that do not respond to medications. The treatment of choice would be _____.
    A. vagal stimulation
    B. defibrillation
    C. oxygen administration
    D. cardioversion

Get the picture? Any question on the subject of resuscitation is fair game. Start by learning the basic rates, depths, and management techniques. Then move on to the advanced material.

FOOD FOR THOUGHT

73. How can we improve the quality of care given during codes?

74. Who provides emotional support to the family of a resuscitation victim? The health care providers?

INFORMATION AGE

You can get plenty of help online.
- There is a lot of helpful information on ACLS at www.acls.net.
- Information on NRP can be found at www.aap.org/nrp.
- Information on PALS at http://www.geocities.com/nyerrn/er/pals.htm

35 Humidity and Bland Aerosol Therapy

Water, taken in moderation, cannot hurt anyone.
Mark Twain

I recently traveled to Las Vegas to attend the AARC's International Respiratory Congress. After the first night in the hotel room, I woke up with a dry, sore nose. Have you ever traveled to a low-humidity environment and experienced a humidity deficit? Even your hair is unhappy in the dry air. Imagine what happens to patients when we give them dry gases to breathe. Or worse, when we bypass the upper airway's natural humidification system. Humidification is a simple thing, really, but then it's often the simple things in life that matter most.

WORD WIZARD

Complete the following paragraph by writing in the correct term(s) in the blank(s) provided.

The amount of relative humidity in gas can be measured by a device called a _____. When air does not have enough moisture to meet the normal _____ humidity of 44 mg/L, a humidity deficit is present. This problem may occur when the normal upper airway is bypassed by an endotracheal tube.

Secretions may become very thick or _____, resulting in airway obstruction. A _____ is a device that adds gaseous water to inspired air. When you heat a humidifier it can deliver more water to the lungs.

An artificial nose, or _____ and _____ exchanger, is a simple device that does not require a water-filled chamber. _____; devices that produce particles of water are also useful for adding moisture to inspired air. An electrically powered device called an _____ nebulizer, utilizes a _____ crystal, and produces a large output of small particles of water for deposition in the lung.

MEET THE OBJECTIVES

1. How are heat and moisture normally exchanged in your body?

   _____

2. List at least four consequences of prolonged inspiration of improperly conditioned gases.

   A. _____

   B. _____

   C. _____

   D. _____

3. Liter flows exceeding what value require humidification?

   _____

4. Give one other situation where you would **ALWAYS** provide humidification.

_____

5. List the two primary and two secondary indications for humidification (see Box 35-1).

   Primary   **Secondary**

   A. _____   A. _____

   B. _____   B. _____

6. What are the three variables that determine how well a humidifier works?

   A. _____

   B. _____

   C. _____

   Which is most important?

   _____

7. Bubble humidifiers are added to what type of oxygen delivery system?

   _____

8. What is the typical range for absolute humidity delivered by a bubble humidifier? What does this amount convert to in terms of relative body humidity?

   A. Output _____ to _____ mg/L

   B. Relative body humidity = _____ %

9. What safety device is incorporated into the design of a bubble humidifier?

   _____

10. Discuss the three primary advantages of passover humidifiers compared with bubble humidifiers.

    A. _____

    B. _____

    C. _____

11. Describe the principle of operation of each of the following artificial noses.
    A. Condenser humidifier:

B.   Hygroscopic condenser humidifier:

C.   Hydrophobic condenser humidifier:

12.   What are the five contraindications to using heat-moisture exchangers (HMEs), according to the AARC Clinical Practice Guideline on humidification during mechanical ventilation? (See page 786 of your text.)

A. _____

B. _____

C. _____

D. _____

E. _____

13.   Where does research suggest placing the HME in the breathing circuit?

14.   What is an "active HME?"

15. Both Pari Hydrate and Vapotherm offer unique humidification devices with wide-ranging clinical applications. Please briefly describe these popular new humidifiers.

A. Pari Hydrate _____

B. Vapotherm _____

16. Identify three possible risks of using heated humidifiers. (Hint: See Box 35-2 and the Clinical Practice Guideline!)

A. _____

B. _____

C. _____

17. Identify three hazards associated with water that "rains out," or condenses in humidified breathing circuits.

A. _____

B. _____

C. _____

18. How should you protect yourself from condensate?

19. What specialized breathing circuit circumvents (usually) the condensation problem?

20. The AARC recommends what range of alarm settings for electronically controlled heated humidifiers?

_____

21. What is the most reliable and scientific method used to determine the effectiveness of a humidification system? What do secretions tell you about effectiveness of humidification?

A. Scientific method

B. Secretions

22. Your textbook describes what really simple way to estimate the performance of an HME or heated-wire circuit without using a hygrometer?

_____

23. List the seven indications given in the AARC Clinical Practice Guideline for bland aerosol administration.

A. _____

B. _____

C. _____

D. _____

E. _____

F. _____

G. _____

24. Give three examples of solutions used to make bland aerosols.

A. _____

B. _____

C. _____

25. Identify the parts of the ultrasonic nebulizer (USN) shown here.

Functional schematic of a typical large-volume ultrasonic nebulizer. (Modified from Barnes TA: Core textbook of respiratory care practice, ed 2, St. Louis, 1994, Mosby.)

26. What preset variable determines the size of the aerosol particles generated by a USN?

_____

27. What adjustable control determines the actual amount of aerosol produced?

_____

28. USNs are primarily used to accomplish what specific clinical goal/procedure?

_____

29. When performing this procedure, what type of water is placed in the nebulizer cup?

_____

30. Identify the two primary clinical problems associated with tents and body enclosures?

    A. _____

    B. _____

31. Your text identifies six important problems associated with bland aerosol therapy. For each of these problems, give a possible solution or means of prevention.

Problem	Solution
A. Cross-contamination/infection	_____
B. Environmental safety	_____
C. Inadequate mist	_____
D. Overhydration	_____
E. Bronchospasm	_____
F. NOISE	_____

CHAPTER HIGHLIGHTS

Let's review some basic concepts from Chapter 35. Complete the following sentences by writing in the correct term(s) in the blank(s) provided.

32. Conditioning of _____ gases is done primarily by the _____.

33. Gases delivered to the trachea should be warmed to _____ to _____ °C

34. A _____ is a device that adds invisible molecular water to a gas.

35. A _____ generates and disperses particles into the gas stream.

36. _____ is the most important factor affecting humidifier output.

37. At high flows, some bubble humidifiers may produce _____, which can carry infectious bacteria.

38. Breathing circuit _____ must always be treated as _____ waste.

39. Bland aerosol therapy with sterile _____ is often used to treat _____ airway _____, overcome humidity _____ in patients with tracheal airways, and help obtain _____ specimens.

Use the algorithm on Figure 35-17 page 796 to choose the right humidity or bland aerosol system.

Case 1

A man is brought to the emergency department (ED) with a core temperature of 30°C after falling into a lake while ice-fishing. The patient is intubated with a No. 8 endotracheal tube. The patient is unconscious and requires mechanical ventilation.

40. Why can't you use an HME on this patient?

_____

41. What humidification system would you recommend?

_____

Case 2

A 32-year-old man is admitted to the medical floor with a diagnosis of *Mycoplasma pneumoniae*. He is receiving oxygen via nasal cannula at 5 L/min. He complains of a stuffy, dry nose a few hours after admission.

42. What humidification system would you recommend for this patient?

_____

43. Why is this patient unable to benefit from an HME?

_____

Case 3

A 57-year-old man who has undergone coronary artery bypass graft surgery (CABG) is being mechanically ventilated with a No. 8 ET tube pending recovery from the procedure. He has no secretion problems or history of lung problems. Body temperature is normal.

44. What humidification system would you recommend?

_____

WHAT DOES THE NBRC SAY?

You should be able to recommend and administer bland aerosol and humidity therapy. You should know when to change to another system. Selecting, assembling, cleaning, and troubleshooting are in there, too. Expect three to five questions, and especially expect something on HMEs and USNs.

Here are a few sample questions. Circle the best answer.

45. A respiratory therapist hears a loud whistling sound as she enters the room of a patient receiving oxygen via cannula at 6 L/min. In reference to the humidifier, what is the most likely cause of the problem?
    A. The top of the humidifier is cross-threaded.
    B. The humidifier has run out of water.
    C. The flow rate is set at less than the ordered amount.
    D. There is a kink in the oxygen supply tubing.

46. A USN is ordered for sputum induction. Which of the following solutions should be placed in the medication cup to accomplish this goal?
    A. sterile distilled water
    B. 0.45% NaCl solution
    C. 0.9% NaCl solution
    D. 3% NaCl solution

47. A large-volume all-purpose nebulizer is set at an F_{IO_2} of 40% and a flow rate of 10 L/min to deliver humidified oxygen to a patient with a tracheostomy. The nebulizer is producing very little mist. Which of the following could be done to improve the aerosol output?
    I.   Check the water level in the nebulizer.
    II. Increase the flow rate to the nebulizer.
    III. Drain condensate from the supply tubing.
    IV. Turn off the nebulizer's heating system.
        A. I only
        B. I and II only
        C. I and III only
        D. I, III, and IV only

48. While performing a ventilator check, the respiratory therapist observes a large amount of thin, white mucous in the tubing connected to the HME. Which of the following actions should be taken at this time?
    A. Rinse out the HME with sterile water.
    B. Suction the mucus from the tubing.
    C. Place the patient on a heated humidification system.
    D. Replace the HME.

49. Sputum induction via USN is ordered. The nebulizer will produce a 5 ml of water per minute output on the maximum amplitude setting. The treatment is to last for 15 minutes. How much solution should the RCP respiratory therapist place in the nebulizer?
    A. 5 ml
    B. 15 ml
    C. 50 ml
    D. 75 ml

FOOD FOR THOUGHT

50. The industry standard for adding simple humidification to an oxygen delivery system is a flow rate of greater than 4 L/min. Can you think of any situations where you might add humidification when the flow rate is lower than 4?

51. Why wouldn't you use Vapotherm or another similar system for every patient?

- Just for fun (respiratory fun), place yourself on a nasal cannula at 6 L/min (be sure to use a clean one!) or a simple mask at 10 L/min in the laboratory setting. Breathe through your nose for 10 or 15 minutes. How does it feel?
- Do you have access to Vapotherm or the other new high-flow devices? You may not be able to breathe on one, but we were able to comfortably breathe much higher flows than with a conventional bubble device.

INFORMATION AGE

I don't usually recommend corporate Web sites, but www.vtherm.com and http://pari.com/hydrate showcase exciting new devices.

The respiratory care program at University of Medicine and Dentistry of New Jersey (UMDNJ) has a great page, www.umdnj.edu/rspthweb/rstn2100/unit3.htm, that has lots of good resources and information!

36 Aerosol Drug Therapy

The pen is mightier than the sword! The case for prescriptions rather than surgery.
Marvin Kitman

Now that you have the drugs, what do you do with them? When I was a student, we gave almost all our medications via intermittent positive-pressure breathing (IPPB). It was expensive, complicated, and time and labor intensive and was not exactly customized to the customer! The good news was that we didn't have to know about so many delivery systems. You, of course, are expected to learn a wide variety of ways to deliver aerosolized drugs and find the most cost-effective and therapeutic method of delivery. Chapter 36 will get you off to a good start on this quest.

WORD WIZARD

Terminology Torture

By now you must have noticed that respiratory care has a language all its own. You won't go far without the passwords. Drug administration is no different, so you need to start by matching the following terms to their definitions.

Terms	Definitions
1. _____ aerosol	A. suspension of solid or liquid particles in a gas
2. _____ atomizer	B. difference between therapeutic and toxic drug concentrations
3. _____ baffle	C. device that produces uniformly sized aerosol particles
4. _____ deposition	D. device that removes large particles
5. _____ hygroscopic	E. device that produces non–uniformly sized aerosol particles
6. _____ inertial impaction	F. deposition of particles by collision
7. _____ MMAD	G. testimony of a witness (or, particles being retained in the respiratory tract!)
8. _____ nebulizer	H. absorbs moisture from the air
9. _____ propellant	I. measurement of average particle size
10. _____ therapeutic index	J. amount of drug left in the SVN
11. _____ residual drug volume	K. something that provides thrust

CHARACTERISTICS OF THERAPEUTIC AEROSOLS

12. Why is particle size so important in aerosol therapy?

13. What is the primary method of deposition for large, high-mass particles?

14. Particles of 10 microns or larger tend to deposit in what part of the respiratory tract? What about particles between 5 and 10 microns?

A. ≥10: _____

B. 5 to 10: _____

15. In what part of the lung would you like to deposit beta-adrenergic bronchodilator drugs? What particle size is needed to accomplish this goal?

A. Where: _____

B. Particle size: _____

16. It is extremely difficult to predict exactly what happens to particles once they enter the lung. What is the most practical way to determine how well you are delivering a drug?

_____

HAZARDS OF AEROSOL THERAPY

What is the number one hazard of aerosol drug therapy? Why, the drugs themselves, of course! (But you knew that . . .)

17. Nebulizers are a great source for nosocomial infections. Describe three of the CDC's recommendations for preventing this serious problem.

A. _____

B. _____

C. _____

18. List five aerosolized substances associated with increased airway resistance.

A. _____

B. _____

C. _____

D. _____

E. _____

19. What can you do to prevent bronchospasm from happening when you nebulize reactive substances?

_____

20. Aerosolizing drugs **always** has the potential for inducing bronchospasm. Describe at least four ways you can monitor this potential problem.

A. _____

B. _____

C. _____

D. _____

21. What group(s) of patients is most prone to harm from bland aerosols?

_____

22. What is meant by the term "drug concentration?" When is this most likely to occur?

AEROSOL DRUG DELIVERY SYSTEMS

I mentioned earlier that there are a lot of different delivery options available. Naturally, every company claims their system is the best. Let's see if we can figure out the best using the information in *Egan's*.

Metered-Dose Inhalers

Metered-dose inhalers (MDIs) are the most widely prescribed aerosol drug delivery system, even though they are not completely socially accepted. It's OK to pop your antacids in the boardroom, but most executives will hide their inhalers!

23. What is meant by priming the MDI?

24. What propellant was used in most MDIs, and why was this a problem? What new propellant is safer for patients

and the environment? _____

25. What other substances are found in MDIs that may produce clinical problems?

_____

365

26. What percentage of the drug in an MDI is actually deposited in the lung? Why is there so much variability?

_____

27. What is a "serious limitation" of pMDIs? How can you solve the problem?

_____

28. Put the following steps of optimal MDI delivery in order.

   A. Hold your breath   _____

   B. Breathe out normally   _____

   C. Wait 1 minute   _____

   D. Shake the canister   _____

   E. Hold the MDI two fingers from mouth   _____

   F. Slowly inhale as deep as you can   _____

   G. Warm the canister   _____

   H. Fire the canister   _____

29. What is the difference between a spacer and a holding chamber? Does it matter?

30. What class of inhaled drugs requires that you *always* use a spacer or chamber?

_____

31. How does the recommended breathing pattern differ with a holding chamber from that of a spacer or unassisted

   MDI? _____

32. Describe the Turbo or the Easihaler. How will these devices help patients get their medications?

_____

Dry Powder

Dry powder makes sense, because wet powder never did work. You'll want to get familiar with the four or five different types of devices in common use.

33.   What is a DPI? What's the big deal?

34.   How does DPI breathing technique differ from that recommended with an MDI?

_____

35.   What patients cannot use DPIs?

_____

36.   Name an example of an active DPI delivery system.

_____

37.   In general, what is the role of the DPI in management of acute bronchospasm?

Small Volume Nebulizers

Small volume nebulizers (SVNs) have been around a long time and are still widely used. They have an amazing number of aliases: mini-neb, acorn neb, hand-held neb, updraft neb, micro-neb, med neb . . . the list seems to go on forever. These devices are indicated when a patient is unable to physically use an MDI or cannot generate sufficient inspiratory flow rates for an MDI or DPI. Some drugs are only available for nebulization.

38.   List three potential power sources to drive the small medication nebulizer.

   A.   _____

   B.   _____

   C.   _____

39. How does an atomizer differ from an SVN? When would you want to use one?

40. What is the optimal flow rate and amount of solution to put in an SVN?

    A. Flow rate: _____

    B. Amount of solution: _____

41. Why is it so important to match nebulizer and compressor systems for home use?

    _____

42. Several nebulizers on the market are designed to reduce the amount of drug expelled into the atmosphere and wasted. Name two of these nebulizers.

    A. _____

    B. _____

43. What is meant by nebulizer "sputter," and why is it important to RTs?

44. What potential problem exists when you deliver an SVN via mask? How can you deal with this problem?

45. Explain what is meant by the "blow-by" technique used with infants, and discuss the effectiveness of this technique.

Large Volume Nebulizers

Large volume nebulizers are usually used to deliver bland aerosols (see Chapter 35). Special large volume nebulizers, like the HEART and HOPE nebulizers, are used to deliver continuous bronchodilator therapy. You may want to try one to deliver drugs when a severely obstructed patient does not respond to SVN treatments and needs a repeated series over time.

46. What potential clinical problem may exist with continuous bronchodilator therapy?

_____

47. Why is the SPAG generator unique? When is it indicated?

_____

Small Ultrasonic Nebulizers

Small ultrasonic nebulizers (USNs) have a lot of advantages: small uniform particles, and high output, and they can be used with ventilators.

48. List three advantages and three disadvantages of USNs to deliver medications (see Table 36-2 on page 826 of your text).

Advantages   Disadvantages

A. _____   _____

B. _____   _____

C. _____   _____

CASE STUDIES

Use the algorithms in Figures 36-28 (page 828) and 36-30 (page 830) in *Egan's* to answer the following questions about selection of aerosol drug delivery devices and doses.

Case 1

An alert cooperative 52-year-old man has recently been diagnosed with chronic bronchitis. He quit smoking (60 pack-year history) 6 months ago, but still has respiratory symptoms. He is in your pulmonary clinic today to receive his pulmonary function test (PFT) results and medications. The physician has ordered Atrovent and Flovent.

49. What method of delivery would you recommend for this patient?

_____

50. What other equipment is indicated?

_____

51. What general considerations for patient education would you stress for this patient?

_____

_____

52. How will you know that he is able to perform the therapy correctly?

_____

_____

Case 2

A 27-year-old man presents in the emergency department with acute respiratory distress. He is diagnosed with status asthmaticus. He has high-pitched diffuse wheezes, a respiratory rate of 24, heart rate of 106, and SpO_2 of 92%. His PEFR is 150 after 4 puffs of albuterol via MDI.

53. What are the possible options for treating this patient at this point?

_____

_____

54. What method of bronchodilator delivery would you recommend?

_____

_____

55. What is meant by "dose-response" assessment?

_____

_____

Case 3

You are asked to deliver a bronchodilator to a patient in the neurologic unit. When you arrive to assess the patient, you note that she is obtunded. Breath sounds reveal scattered rhonchi and wheezing in the upper lobes.

56. What method of bronchodilator delivery would you recommend in this situation?

_____

_____

57. What modification will you need to make?

_____

_____

58. Because peak flow is unlikely to be performed, how will you assess the effectiveness of therapy?

_____

_____

INTUBATED PATIENTS

Delivering bronchodilators to intubated patients has always been difficult. Much of the drug ends up in the circuit or the endotracheal tube. Assessment of effectiveness can be difficult as well. Both SVNs and MDIs can be used to achieve good results if you follow some guidelines and use the right equipment.

59. SVN dosages should be adjusted when delivered to an intubated patient by what amount?

   _____

60. What standard starting dosage is recommended for albuterol by MDI to a ventilator patient?

   _____

61. Where should you place the SVN in the ventilator circuit?

   _____

62. When should an MDI be activated for a ventilator patient?

   _____

63. What adjustments to dilution need to be made with the SVN for ventilator delivery?

   _____

64. What changes do you need to make to ensure delivery?

   A. HME: _____

   B. Flow-by: _____

   C. Alarms, limits: _____

WHAT DOES THE NBRC SAY?

It will come as no surprise that this information is on your boards. What is unusual is how little of this material is on the test considering the importance and frequency of aerosol drug administration in the clinical setting. One reason is that only recently have good studies been done to provide more scientific conclusions about how best to deliver medications. The matrix specifically mentions MDIs, spacers, DPIs, and pneumatic-powered nebulizers. Of course, peak flows and assessment are included. Continuous nebulization wasn't found in the matrix! Perhaps it will appear on the new exams that are coming soon.

Try the following questions. The following information pertains to questions 65 and 66. Circle the best answer.

Asthma has been recently diagnosed in a 16-year-old patient. The respiratory therapist is asked to teach the patient how to self-administer QVAR via MDI.

65. In addition to the inhaler, what other equipment would be needed to teach the patient?
   I.   spacer device
   II. pulse oximeter
   III. peak flowmeter
      A. I only
      B. I and II only
      C. I and III only
      D. II and III only

66. After performing the inhalation, the RT instructs the patient to perform a breath-holding maneuver. The purpose of this maneuver is to _____.
   A. promote a strong cough
   B. improve venous return
   C. improve inertial impaction
   D. increase medication delivery

67. While attempting to administer albuterol via SVN to a patient who has had a recent CVA, the RT notes that the patient is unable to hold the nebulizer or keep her lips sealed on the mouthpiece. The RT should recommend _____.
   A. switching to an MDI
   B. utilizing an aerosol mask for delivery
   C. discontinuing the medication
   D. subcutaneous administration of the medication

68. An MDI is ordered for a patient who is intubated and being mechanically ventilated and humidified with a heat-moisture exchanger (HME). Which of the following is the most appropriate way to administer the bronchodilator?
   A. Place the MDI in the expiratory limb of the ventilator circuit.
   B. Place the MDI between the HME and the endotracheal tube.
   C. Recommend changing the delivery method to a small volume nebulizer.
   D. Remove the HME during delivery of the drug.

69. An alert adult patient with asthma is receiving bronchodilator therapy via small volume nebulizer during a hospitalization. What recommendations should the RT make in regard to this therapy when the patient is ready for discharge?
   A. Recommend MDI instruction.
   B. Recommend oral administration of the medication.
   C. Recommend training in home use of the SVN.
   D. Recommend administration of the drug via IPPB.

70. Which of the following devices is most suitable for delivery of virazole (Ribavirin)?
   A. continuous large volume nebulizer
   B. small particle aerosol generator
   C. ultrasonic nebulizer
   D. atomizer

FOOD FOR THOUGHT

Chapter 36 ends with some important material on the subject of protecting the practitioner from continuous exposure to a wide variety of inhaled agents.

71. What two inhalational drugs have proved occupational risk for RTs?

   A. _____

   B. _____

72. Describe some of the physical ways to control environmental contamination when delivering medications that have potential side effects for the provider.

73. What do the terms HEPA and PAPR refer to?

_____

INFORMATION AGE

- A good place to start is the American Association for Respiratory Care (AARC) Web site (www.aarc.org), where you will find the Clinical Practice Guidelines for selection of an aerosol delivery device. (You can also find an excerpt of the guideline on page 827 of your text.)
- The online journal www.rcjournal.com is another good place to look.
- For more on Pari and Circulaire nebulizers, try www.pari.com and www.westmedinc.com.
- If you are interested in continuous bronchodilator therapy, all you need to do is type this subject into one of the search engines and you'll get an eyeful.

37 Storage and Delivery of Medical Gases

O Lord, help me to be pure, but not yet.
St. Augustine

One thing is for certain: every generation of respiratory care students since the dawn of time has had a good laugh at the engineers who thought up the name Pin Index Safety System (PISS). And what's up with that American Standard Safety System (ASSS)? Another thing I'm sure of is that we all have to learn more about medical gases than any other mortals on this planet! I have to admit this information has come in handy many times in the clinical setting, and it is good to be an expert when the delivery systems malfunction and no one else knows quite what to do but the respiratory therapist!

WORD WIZARD

Here's a little puzzle (see p. 376) to help you learn the new terms found in Chapter 37.

CHARACTERISTICS OF MEDICAL GASES

1. Name three gases categorized as nonflammable.

    A. _____

    B. _____

    C. _____

2. Most therapeutic gases will support combustion. Name three gases in this category.

    A. _____

    B. _____

    C. _____

3. Describe the four basic steps of the fractional distillation process.

    A. _____

    B. _____

    C. _____

    D. _____

4. What purity level is required for medical grade oxygen?

    _____

ACROSS

1. Valve that lowers gas pressure
3. _____ dioxide, used to treat hiccups
6. A device that controls both pressure and flow
7. Chemical named for this light gas
8. This meter controls the volume of gas per unit of volume
10. Type of "distillation" that produces oxygen
14. Gas used in treatment of severe asthma
16. Low pressure safety system
17. Pipe with many connections used to link gas cylinders together
19. Gas delivered in a yellow cylinder
20. _____ valves shut off the gas in case of a fire
22. Your mom told you not to say this, but it really is a safety system!
23. Gas delivered in a blue cylinder
26. The "P" in PISS
27. Gas that makes up 20.95% of air

DOWN

2. The "D" in DISS
4. Agency that classifies cylinders
5. Needle _____ adjust the flow in a Thorpe tube
7. Low density gas
9. Fixed orifice, variable pressure measuring or metering device
11. Rear end: also a safety system
12. Variable orifice, constant pressure flow metering device
13. Just say "NO"
15. Agency that sets standards for gas purity
18. Sets standards for design, construction, placement, and use of bulk oxygen systems
21. Gas with only one oxygen molecule
24. Slang term for cylinder
25. Second half of gas made by heating limestone in contact with water

5. Describe the two methods used to separate oxygen from air. What concentration is produced by each method?

A. _____

B. _____

6. Describe the devices used to produce medical grade air for hospital system and for home use.
   A. Hospital:

   B. Home:

7. Most medical grade carbon dioxide is used for what purpose?

   _____

8. What is heliox? What is it used for?

   _____

9. What is the primary medical use for nitrous oxide? What are some of the hazards of nitrous oxide administration?

10. How is nitric oxide being used in the neonatal setting?

_____

11. Describe two possible hazards of using nitric oxide.
   A.

   B.

12. Give the chemical symbol for each of the following medical gases.

   Gas   **Symbol**

   A. Oxygen   _____

   B. Air   _____

   C. Carbon dioxide   _____

   D. Helium   _____

   E. Nitrous oxide   _____

   F. Nitric oxide   _____

STORING MEDICAL GASES

High-pressure medical gas cylinders have been around for over 100 years. The modern cylinder is the subject of numerous regulations and rules that control manufacture, storage, and transportation of these potential dangerous steel bottles. Naturally, you will be expected to have considerable knowledge on this subject even if you don't use it on a daily basis!

13. Identify the cylinder markings on the diagram shown here.

Typical markings of cylinders containing medical gases. Front and back views are for illustration purposes only. Exact location and order of markings vary.

14. What do the symbols * and + mean when stamped on a cylinder?

A. * _____

B. + _____

15. Identify the proper color for these gas cylinders (in the United States).

A. Oxygen _____

B. Carbon dioxide _____

C. Nitrous oxide _____

D. Helium _____

E. Nitrogen _____

F. Air _____

16. Because cylinder color is only a guideline, how do you actually determine what gas is in a tank?

_____

17. What is the best way to determine the actual oxygen concentration in a cylinder?

_____

Chapter 37 **Storage and Delivery of Medical Gases**

Cylinders are either filled with gas or liquid. The liquid will either be at room temperature or in a cryogenic state.

18. Name two gases that can be stored in the liquid state at room temperature.

    A. _____

    B. _____

19. Explain why the pressure in a gas-filled cylinder is different than that of a liquid-filled cylinder.

20. Describe the methods for measuring the contents of a gas-filled cylinder and a liquid-filled cylinder.
    A.

    B.

21. Write the formula for calculating the cylinder factor for a gas-filled cylinder.

22. What are the factors for the "E" and "H" oxygen cylinders?

A. _____

B. _____

23. Now write the formula for calculating duration of flow in minutes.

_____

I promise we'll practice these calculations later in this chapter. They are important for clinical practice and for your board exams!

BULK OXYGEN

Try to imagine how much oxygen a large hospital needs every day. If you had 100 patients wearing oxygen at 6 L/min, you would need over 800,000 L for 1 day! Ventilators draw much more gas! You could do this with individual cylinders in each room, but think how much work that would involve. A bulk system, by definition, has at least 20,000 cubic feet of gas. Check out the cool picture on page 854, Figure 37-9. Better yet, go on a field trip and look at the bulk system with a hospital engineer.

24. Describe a gaseous bulk system. Be sure to discuss the manifold, the primary, and reserve banks.

25. Why do most hospitals use a liquid bulk oxygen system?

_____

26. Where are small liquid oxygen cylinders usually used?

_____

27. What is the critical temperature of oxygen? How is the bulk liquid oxygen maintained at this temperature?

28. What is the normal working pressure for a hospital oxygen piping system?

_____

29. What are zone valves? Give two reasons you might need to use these valves.

SAFETY SYSTEMS

Ah, the fabled safety systems. They come in two general types: those built into the cylinder valve stem to prevent rupture from high pressures, and indexed systems designed to keep you from giving the wrong gas to a patient.

30. Remember the gas laws? If a cylinder overheats, the pressure will rise. Describe the type of pressure release valve usually found in these cylinder stems.

A. Small cylinder: _____

B. Large cylinder: _____

31. Name the three basic indexed safety systems for medical gases. Both names!

Abbreviated Name   **Full Name**

A. _____   _____

B. _____   _____

C. _____   _____

32. A large cylinder of oxygen is described as follows: CGA-540 0.903-14NGO-RH-Ext. Explain what this means.

33. What type of cylinder uses pins and holes for the safety connection system?

_____

34. What system was established to prevent accidental interchange of low-pressure medical gas connectors? What do they mean by "low-pressure?"

_____

35. What is the purpose of the quick-connect system?

_____

REGULATION PRESSURE AND FLOW

Because a large cylinder of oxygen may have a pressure as high as 2400 psi, we need to have a way to lower this pressure and control it or our equipment (or the patient) could be harmed.

36. Describe the action of the following devices.

   A.   Reducing valve: _____

   B.   Flowmeter: _____

   C.   Regulator: _____

37. Describe the normal way each of the following is used in respiratory care.
   A.   Preset reducing valve:

   B.   Adjustable reducing valve:

   C.   Multiple-stage reducing valve:

38. What two hazards can be created when you open a cylinder attached to a high-pressure reducing valve?

Three categories of flowmeters are used in respiratory care. The next set of questions will test your knowledge of these commonly used devices.

39. What are two advantages and two disadvantages of flow restrictors?

	ADVANTAGES	DISADVANTAGES
A.		
B.		

40. Describe the Bourdon flowmeter.

_____

41. What is the chief advantage of the Bourdon-type flowmeter?

_____

42. How will indicated flow compare to actual flow when a Bourdon flowmeter meets up with downstream resistance? _____

43. What do Bourdon gauges actually measure? Thorpe tubes?

A. Bourdon: _____

B. Thorpe: _____

44. Compare indicated flow and actual flow in a compensated Thorpe flowmeter when downstream resistance occurs.

45. What happens to the float in a compensated Thorpe tube when you connect it to a 50 psi gas source?

_____

CASE STUDY

Case 1

A patient is to be transported from the ICU to the imaging department for a CT scan. The patient requires continuous supplemental oxygen at 10 L/min by mask. You will need to provide portable oxygen for the transport. An E cylinder is available.

46. What type of regulator is most appropriate for transport?

_____

47. How long will the cylinder last at the given flow rate if the pressure is 1000 psi?

Formula: _____

Calculation: _____

48. When you turn on the cylinder valve, a hissing noise is heard from the regulator. The flowmeter is off, so there must be a leak. What should you check to try to correct the leak?

A. _____

B. _____

MATHEMATICS

I told you we'd come back to the problem of cylinder duration calculations. Obviously, this is important—not just because it is on tests! Let's say you have to transport a patient by airplane, or send someone home with oxygen, or just go from the emergency department to the ICU. Will you have enough gas? Running out in the elevator is not really acceptable!

There are two ways to do this—the board-exam, precise way and the Rule of Thumb quick and dirty way.

Precise way first.

The two most common cylinders you will be using are the small E type and the larger H or K type. Factors are 0.28 and 3.14.

Example: You are sending a patient home by car. The E cylinder is full (2200 psi) and the patient is wearing a cannula at 2 L/min. How long will the O_2 last?

Start by writing out the formula. (You have to know this one.)

$$\text{Duration} = \text{psi} \times \text{Factor/Flow}$$

Now plug in the numbers.

Calculation: $2200 \times 0.28/2 = 616/2 = 308$ minutes

OK, how many hours is that?

$$308/60 = 5.1 \text{ hours}$$

49. Calculate duration of an E cylinder with 1500 psi running at 2 L/min.

Formula: _____

Calculation:

Answer: Minutes _____   Hours _____

50. Calculate the duration of an H cylinder with 1500 psi running at 2 L/min.

Formula: _____

Calculation:

Answer: Minutes _____   Hours _____

Now for the quick and dirty way.

0.28 is roughly ⅓. One third of 2200 is 700.

700 divided by 2 = 350 minutes, divided by 60 minutes in the hour = 5+ hours

You can see how you could get into trouble with this . . . ? Of course if the patient is taking a 30-minute trip home, it would hardly matter. Be sensible when you take shortcuts! A safer shortcut is to use ¼. One fourth of 2200 is about 550. Divided by 2, that is only 275 minutes, but you have a little cushion of extra gas.

P.S. If you use this on the boards, you could check your work pretty easily, or you might be able to skip the mathematics and just use the shortcut.

P.P.S. When I transport a patient who needs oxygen, I always start with a full cylinder if it is at all possible.

P.P.P.S. Remember that a full E cylinder will last 10 hours at 1 L or 1 hour at 10 L. This rule is easy to remember and can be useful.

WHAT DOES THE NBRC SAY?

You won't see too many questions on the material in Chapter 37. Cylinder duration is one common question, and usually involves duration of an E or H cylinder. Here are some typical questions for you to try.

Here are a few sample questions. Circle the best answer.

51. An H cylinder of oxygen is being used to deliver oxygen to a patient in a subacute care facility where no piped-in oxygen is available. The cylinder gauge shows a pressure of 1000 psi. The patient is receiving oxygen at 5 L/min by cannula. Approximately how long will the cylinder gas last at this flow rate?
    A. 1 hour
    B. 8 hours
    C. 10 hours
    D. 628 hours

52. A respiratory therapist notices that a flowmeter plugged into the wall outlet continues to read 1 L/min even though it is not turned on. What is the most appropriate action at this time?
    A. Replace the flowmeter.
    B. Include the extra liter in any calculations.
    C. Disassemble the flowmeter and replace the "O-rings."
    D. Do nothing; this is not an unusual situation.

53. A respiratory therapist has to transport a patient via air from the island of Maui to Honolulu. The patient is being manually ventilated with an oxygen flow set at 10 L/min. The cylinder gauge reads 2000 psi. How long will the cylinder last?
    A. 42 minutes
    B. 56 minutes
    C. 60 minutes
    D. 10 hours

54. When a respiratory therapist unplugs a Thorpe-type flowmeter, a huge leak occurs from the wall outlet. What action should the RT take at this time?
    A. Shut off the gas to the room with the zone valve.
    B. Shut off the bulk oxygen system.
    C. Plug the flowmeter back into the outlet.
    D. Call maintenance to fix the outlet.

FOOD FOR THOUGHT

55. What would happen if nitrous oxide leaked into the room in the emergency department or operating room setting?

56. What would you do if the bulk system at your hospital failed?

57. What protective gear is appropriate when opening a valve on a high-pressure cylinder?

_____

INFORMATION AGE

- Compressed Gas Association: www.cganet.com.
- Occupation Safety and Health Administration: www.osha.gov/SLTC/compressedgasequipment. This is OSHA's compressed gas site.
- Oklahoma State University has a site devoted to cylinder safety and has lots of useful information: www.pp.okstate.edu/ehs/links/gas.htm.

38 Medical Gas Therapy

Smile, breathe and go slowly.
Thich Nhat Hanh

My first job in respiratory therapy was that of oxygen technician. I was excited by the thought of being responsible for all those cannulas, masks, and humidifiers. The respiratory care profession has come a long way since then, but medical gas therapy is still a cornerstone of respiratory care. Of course we think of oxygen as a drug now, and things have changed a lot in our understanding of administering this powerful medication. The modern respiratory therapist (RT) must have a much firmer grasp of the goals and objectives of medical gas therapy than I did when I made my patient rounds 30 years ago.

WORD WIZARD

Let's try something different in the war of the words. My students always have a hard time with the spelling of medical terms. Check your ability by circling the correct spelling for this gas jargon.

1.	canulla	cannula
2.	reservore	reservoir
3.	lasitude	lassitude
4.	diaphramatic	diaphragmatic
5.	retanopathy	retinopathy
6.	hypoxemia	hypoxemea
7.	toxicity	toxisity
8.	infarction	infraction
9.	displasia	dysplasia
10.	pendent	pendant
11.	concentration	concintration
12.	entranement	entrainment
13.	wye	why

TANK JOCKEYS AND GAS PASSERS

We've been called some funny names in the past, but modern RTs don't just put masks on patient's faces. Any old knob twirler could figure out how to do that part of the procedure. Let's start by reviewing the reasons for giving oxygen and how to clinically recognize those needs.

14. What is acute hypoxemia? _____

15. What are the threshold criteria for defining hypoxemia in adults according to the AARC Clinical Practice Guideline?

    1. Pao_2 _____

    2. Sao_2 _____

16. Specifically, what beneficial effect does oxygen have on the symptoms of patients with COPD and chronic hypoxemia (besides treating hypoxemia!).

    A. COPD (and interstitial disease) _____

    B. Chronic hypoxemia _____

17. Describe the two compensatory mechanisms of the cardiopulmonary system when faced with hypoxemia.

 A. Lungs: _____

 B. Heart: _____

18. In what acute cardiac condition is oxygen therapy especially important?

 _____

19. What effect does hypoxemia have on the pulmonary blood vessels? What are the long-term consequences of this effect?

20. State the three basic ways to determine if a patient needs oxygen.

 A. _____

 B. _____

 C. _____

21. List six common acute clinical situations where hypoxemia is so common that oxygen therapy is usually provided.

 A. _____

 B. _____

 C. _____

 D. _____

 E. _____

 F. _____

22. Give two signs of mild and severe hypoxia for each of the following systems.

	SYSTEM	MILD	SEVERE
A.	Respiratory		
B.	Cardiovascular		
C.	Neurologic		

OXYGEN THERAPY RISKS

There are four great big problems associated with oxygen therapy (besides burning down the hospital!). Naturally, you need to know them.

Toxic Talk

23. Oxygen toxicity affects what two organ systems?

   A. _____

   B. _____

24. The harm caused by oxygen is influenced by what two factors?

   A. _____

   B. _____

25. Describe the effects of breathing excessive oxygen on the lung tissue.

26. What is meant by a "vicious circle" in reference to oxygen toxicity?

27. While every patient is unique, what general rule of thumb can be applied to prevent oxygen toxicity?

28. When should oxygen be withheld from a hypoxic patient to avoid the consequences of toxicity?

   _____

I Feel Depressed

29. What specific type of COPD patient is likely to experience depression of ventilatory drive while breathing

    oxygen? _____

30. Give two explanations for this effect.

    A. _____

    B. _____

31. When should oxygen be withheld from a hypoxic COPD patient to avoid depressing ventilation?

    _____

RLF or ROP? It's All the Same to Me!

32. Describe the pathophysiology of how excessive blood oxygen causes blindness in premature newborns.

33. During what time period after birth is a preemie likely to develop ROP?

    _____

34. How can you reduce the risk of ROP?

    _____

Absorbing Information

35. Describe how oxygen can cause atelectasis.

36. What groups of patients are at increased risk for absorption atelectasis?

    _____

37. How can you reduce the risk of absorption atelectasis?

_____

OXYGEN DELIVERY SYSTEMS

Now that you know why to give a patient oxygen and some of the hazards of administration, it's time to learn how to make tasty selections from the complex choices offered on the medical gas menu.

38. The three basic categories are low flow, high flow, and reservoir. Match the category to the description below.

Category	Description
A. Low flow _____	1. Always exceeds patient's inspiratory needs
B. Reservoir _____	2. Provides some of patient's inspiratory needs
C. High flow _____	3. May meet needs if no leaks occur

LOW FLOW

39. Why do you think the nasal cannula is the most commonly used low-flow system?

_____

40. When should you attach the cannula to a bubble humidifier?

_____

41. What maximum flow does the text suggest for newborns?

_____

Low-Flow Experiment

If you have access to a cannula, humidifier, and some medical oxygen, I think you should find out what it feels like to be a patient!
1. Attach the cannula to a flowmeter with the nipple adaptor (or "Christmas tree" if you like that term better).
2. Insert the prongs in your nose and set the flow to 1 L/min.
3. Try that for one minute.
4. Increase the flow by 1 L/min.
5. Continue this until you get to the 8 L/min maximum suggested by the text.
6. Try again with a humidifier.

Questions
- How well could you feel the gas at 1 L? What implication does this have for patient care?
- When did the flow start to become noticeable? Uncomfortable?
- What happened to the humidifier as the flow rates exceeded 5 L/min?

---

42. What is the primary advantage of using a transtracheal oxygen catheter?

_____

43. Why does the range of F_{IO_2} delivered by nasal cannulas vary so much?

44. Because you can't tell exactly how much oxygen the patient is receiving at any given moment from a cannula, how can you assess the effects of administering the drug?

_____

45. What are the advantages and disadvantages of reservoir cannulas?

A. Advantages _____

B. Disadvantages _____

46. In what setting are reservoir cannulas usually used?

_____

RESERVOIR

47. Use Table 38-3 on page 874 of your text to help you find the information about oxygen masks.

	MASK	F_{IO_2} RANGE	ADVANTAGE	DISADVANTAGE
A.	Simple			
B.	Partial rebreathing			
C.	Nonrebreathing			

48. What is the primary difference between the partial rebreathing and nonrebreathing masks?

_____

49. How can you tell if a nonrebreathing mask has an adequate flow rate?

_____

50. Give a solution for each of these common problems with reservoir masks.

Problem   **Solution**

A.   Confused patient removes mask   _____

B.   Humidifier pop-off activated   _____

C.   Mask causes claustrophobia   _____

D.   Bag collapses on inspiration   _____

E.   Bag fully inflated on inspiration   _____

Reservoir Experiment

Get a non-rebreather (NRB), a simple mask, a bubble humidifier, a nipple adaptor, and a flowmeter. Try to use a non-rebreather with two valves on the mask if you can find one.

1. **First,** try the simple mask without a humidifier. Set the flowmeter at 2 L/M and breathe from the simple mask for a few breaths. Now take deep breaths. Set the flowmeter at 10 L/M and try again.
2. **Next,** set up the NRB. Repeat the experiment. Breathe as deeply as you can and adjust the flowmeter until the bag doesn't collapse. **Try** the mask with one expiratory flap valve in place and with two (if possible).
3. **Finally,** attach the bubble humidifier, set the flow at 10, and put on the mask. Now increase the flowrate to 15, then flush.

Questions
- How did it feel to breathe on the simple mask at a low flowrate?
- What happened when you tried the NRB at a low flow?
- How did mask performance vary when you used 2 valves?
- What difference did the humidifier make?
- What happened to the humidifier when you increased the flow?

Remember, lab experiments should be done under lab conditions with appropriate supervision!

HIGH-FLOW

Air-entrainment systems are commonly used to provide high-flow oxygen because they are simple and inexpensive to operate. Oxygen is directed through a small tube, or jet, which creates a very high forward velocity. Air is entrained into the system, which dilutes the oxygen and increases the total flow rate.

51. Describe the effects of varying the jet size or entrainment port opening on F_{IO_2} and total flow rate.

	FACTOR	INCREASED SIZE	DECREASED SIZE
A.	Jet 1. F_{IO_2} 2. Flow		
B.	Port 1. F_{IO_2} 2. Flow		

Chapter **38** **Medical Gas Therapy**

52. Fill in the air-to-oxygen ratios for the following oxygen concentrations. (See Table 38-7 on page 883 of your text.)

A. 100% _____

B. 60% _____

C. 40% _____

D. 35% _____

E. 30% _____

F. 24% _____

53. What is the common name for an air entrainment mask (AEM)?

_____

54. Why does the AEM have larger openings on the side of the mask than a simple oxygen mask?

_____

55. What effect does raising the delivered flow from the flowmeter have on the F_{IO_2} delivered by an AEM?

_____

56. Air-entrainment devices are classified as high-flow. For what F_{IO_2} settings is this usually true?

_____

57. How do you boost the total flow when using an AEM?

_____

58. Why is this not possible with an air-entrainment nebulizer?

_____

59. There are four devices used to deliver gas from an air-entrainment nebulizer to the patient. Choose the device(s) that fits each of the following patients. (See Figure 38-16 on page 884.)

Patient	Aerosol Delivery Device
A. Tracheostomy tube	_____
B. Endotracheal tube	_____
C. Intact upper airway	_____
D. After nasal surgery	_____

60. Describe an easy way to tell if an air-entrainment nebulizer is providing sufficient gas to meet the patient's needs.

61. Give one example of a specialized flow generator that produces an aerosol, and one example that produces dry gas. These devices produce high flow and high FIO_2, thus solving the problem created with nebulizers and AEMs! (See Figures 38-18 and 38-19 on page 886-887 for an example.)

   A. Aerosol: _____

   B. Dry: _____

62. What effect does downstream resistance to flow have on FIO_2 and total flow delivered by a typical AEM or nebulizer entrainment system?

High-Flow Experiment

You will need an AEM, oxygen analyzer, and an air-entrainment jet nebulizer with a length of corrugated tubing.
   1. First, set the AEM at 40% with a flow of 5 L/M of oxygen. Analyze the FIO_2 (detach the mask and put the analyzer tee on). Increase the flow to 8 L/M. Analyze again.
   2. Next, set up the nebulizer. Use 40% and a flow of 10. Analyze the output. Increase the flow to 12 and analyze again.
   3. Now pour enough water into the corrugated tubing to partially occlude it. Analyze. **Add** enough water to completely occlude the tubing. Analyze.
   4. Finally, drain out the water. Try to increase the flowmeter setting past 15.

Concentration Questions
   ■ What is the effect of altering flowrate on the AEM?
   ■ What is the effect of water (resistance) in the tubing of a jet neb?
   ■ What happened when you tried to increase the flow with the neb? Why?

MATHEMATICS

Oxygen–to–air entrainment ratios and total flow from air-entrainment devices is another one of the universal clinical and board exam expectations that has driven countless students to the brink of insanity. Take a slow, deep breath; exhale. Straighten shoulders. Engage . . . The way I see it, you have three choices.
   ■ Memorize the ratios for each FIO_2.
   ■ Learn the algebraic formula.
   ■ Learn the magic box.

You must learn and master this information!

If you like the first method, you must memorize every detail Table 38-7 on page 883. READ the fine print.
Or
Look at the Mini Clini "Computing the Total Flow Output of an Air-Entrainment Device" on page 882 of your text. A three-step method is provided for calculating the ratio and the subsequent total flow. Let's try one.

A patient is receiving oxygen at 40% via a Venti-mask with the flowmeter set at 8 L/min. What is the ratio of oxygen to air? What is the total flow?

Step 1: Compute the ratio

$$\frac{\text{Liters of Air}}{\text{Liters of O}_2} \quad \frac{(100-40)}{(40-21)}$$

$$\frac{\text{Liters of Air}}{\text{Liters of O}_2} \quad \frac{(60)}{(19)}$$

$$\frac{\text{Liters of Air}}{\text{Liters of O}_2} \quad \frac{3}{1}$$

Step 2: Add the numerator and denominator parts

$$3 + 1 = 4$$

Step 3: Multiply the sum of the parts by the oxygen flow rate

$$4 \times 8 = 32 \text{ L/min total flow}$$

Now you try.

63. What is the oxygen–to–air entrainment ratio and total flow for a patient who is receiving 60% oxygen via an entrainment nebulizer with the flowmeter set at 10 L/min?

   A. Step 1: Compute the ratio

   Formula: _____

   Calculation: _____

   Reduce answer to get ratio: _____

   B. Step 2: Add the parts

   C. Step 3: Multiply the sum of the parts by the O$_2$ flow rate

The "magic box" is my personal favorite. (See page 883, Figure 38-14 for an example.) Retry the sample problem above for the patient on 40%. Pretty nifty! The only problem with this method is that you substitute 20 (instead of 21) to make the math easy. At percentages below 40, your answers will start to vary from the algebraic method. You can solve this by using "21" for low percentages and "20" for 40% or more.

   Practice with your chosen method until you can solve for every F$_{IO_2}$. There is no way out of this!

BLENDERS

Oxygen blenders are another kind of "magic box." The blender requires a 50 psi input of air and oxygen. When you twirl the knob to set the F$_{IO_2}$, you are actually adjusting a proportioning valve. Turning toward a high percentage of oxygen makes the opening for oxygen larger and the opening for air smaller. Use of 100% closes the air side and only

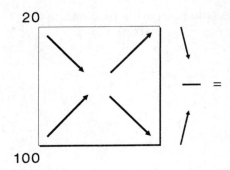

FIGURE 38-1 The magic box used to estimate air-to-oxygen ratio.

lets oxygen out. Vice versa for turning the knob toward 21%. The blender is a very handy device. It gives you high flow rates or 50 psi to power equipment at any F_{IO_2} you desire.

64. Describe the three-step process for confirming the proper operation of a blender (see Box 38-3).

A. _____

B. _____

C. _____

PUT THOSE KIDS IN A TENT!

The opening scene of the venerable "Marcus Welby, MD" television show depicted a man in an oxygen tent. You may see this being done on soap operas as well. Nowadays, enclosures are a simple way to deliver oxygen to infants and children.

65. What is the major problem with oxygen tents?

66. What is the highest F_{IO_2} you can expect to deliver with a tent?

67. Why is a hood the best method for delivering oxygen to an infant?

68. What minimum flow must be set for a hood? Why?

69. What harmful consequence occurs when flow rates into the hood are too high?

70. What effect will cold air flowing into the hood have on a premature infant?

_____

71. What is the best way to control oxygen delivery to an infant inside an incubator?

_____

72. What is the primary benefit of the infant incubator?

_____

HYPERBARIC OXYGEN

Life under pressure: that's hyperbaric oxygen, or HBO. We can administer oxygen to the patient at 2 or 3 atmospheres (ATA) to treat several acute and chronic problems. Originally designed for decompression sickness in divers, HBO operates according to Boyle's law. RTs often work with patients who require this mode of oxygen administration, and it is also common for RTs to work in hyperbaric units. So pick up your pencils and let's get on with the show!

73. Compare the monoplace and multiplace hyperbaric chambers.

	CHAMBER	O₂ DELIVERY	PATIENT	STAFF
A.	Monoplace			
B.	Multiplace			

74. List three acute and three chronic conditions where HBO is indicated. (Try Box 38-6 on page 894 of your text.)

Acute   Chronic

A. _____   _____

B. _____   _____

C. _____   _____

75. Under what circumstances is HBO indicated in cases of carbon monoxide poisoning? (See Box 38-7 on page 894 of your text.)

OTHER GASES

76. Two other therapeutic gases are administered by RTs. Give indications for each.

Gas   Indications

A. NO   _____

               _____

B. Helium   _____

               _____

77. What other gas is always mixed with helium? What is the most common combination?

_____

78. What physical property of helium results in decreased work of breathing?

_____

79. Helium is so diffusible that special balloons are used to hold it! What type of gas delivery device is used to administer helium to patients who are not intubated?

_____

Case 1

A 52-year-old college professor is admitted for chest pain and possible myocardial infarction (MI). Electrocardiogram (ECG) monitoring reveals sinus tachycardia. The chest pain has been decreased by the administration of nitroglycerin. Respirations are 20 per minute, and SpO_2 on room air is 92%.

80. What is your assessment of this patient's oxygenation status?

81. What is your recommendation in regard to administration of supplemental oxygen?

Case 2

A man has been admitted for exacerbation of his COPD. The patient is wearing oxygen at 2 L/min via nasal cannula. The pulse oximeter shows a saturation of 94% while at rest. The nurse calls you to ask for your assistance in evaluation of the patient's dyspnea during ambulation.

82. What changes occur in breathing pattern during exercise?

_____

83. How are low-flow oxygen devices affected by changes in breathing pattern?

_____

84. How would you assess dyspnea on ambulation for a patient wearing oxygen?

A patient is recovering from surgery following a head injury. The patient is trached and requires supplemental oxygen at 60% via T-piece. The flowmeter is set at 12 L/min. Each time the patient inhales, the mist exiting the T-piece disappears.

85. Air-entrainment nebulizers are considered high-flow delivery systems. Discuss this in terms of the

    disappearing mist. _____

86. What should be added to the T-piece to help deal with this problem?

    _____

87. Describe a common method of increasing the delivered flow when administering high F_{IO_2} via

    air-entrainment nebulizers. _____

88. What is the oxygen–to–air entrainment ratio for 60%?

    _____

89. What is the total flow in the system described in this case?

    _____

_____

WHAT DOES THE NBRC SAY?

There must be some reason why this chapter is so long. The NBRC will expect you to know about all types of delivery systems and when to use them. You should know when oxygen is indicated and recognize and minimize potential hazards and complications. The Entry-Level Exam will have at least 10 questions based on the topic of "conducting therapeutic procedures to achieve adequate arterial and tissue oxygenation." Heliox administration is covered on the Registry Exams, and you should be prepared for any of these gases. Answer the following questions. Circle the best answer.

90. During a suctioning procedure a patient experiences tachycardia with PVCs. Which of the following could be responsible for this response?
    A. inadequate vacuum pressure
    B. lack of sterile technique during the procedure
    C. fear of the suctioning procedure
    D. inadequate preoxygenation

91. A patient with a history of carbon dioxide retention is receiving oxygen at 6 L/min via nasal cannula. He is becoming lethargic and difficult to arouse. In regard to the oxygen delivery, what change would you recommend?
    A. Change to a 40% Venturi mask.
    B. Maintain the present therapy.
    C. Change to a partial rebreathing mask.
    D. Reduce the flow to 2 L/min and obtain an ABG.

92. A newborn requires oxygen therapy. Which of the following methods of delivery would you select?
    A. partial rebreathing mask
    B. oxygen hood
    C. Venturi mask
    D. oxygen tent

93. A patient is receiving oxygen therapy from a nonrebreathing mask with a flow rate of 10 L/min. The respiratory therapist observes the bag deflating with each inspiration. What action is indicated in this situation?
    A. Replace the mask with a cannula.
    B. Immediately perform pulse oximetry.
    C. Increase the flow to the mask.
    D. Change to a Venturi mask.

94. A patient is to receive a mixture of helium and oxygen. Which of the following delivery devices would be appropriate?
    A. nasal cannula
    B. oxygen tent
    C. Venturi mask
    D. nonrebreathing mask

95. An 80/20 mixture of helium and oxygen is administered. The oxygen flowmeter is set at 10 L/min. What is the actual flow delivered to the patient?
    A. 10 L
    B. 14 L
    C. 16 L
    D. 18 L

96. A patient is receiving 40% oxygen via an air entrainment mask with the flowmeter set at 8 L/min. What is the total flow delivered to the patient?
    A. 24 L/min
    B. 32 L/min
    C. 40 L/min
    D. 48 L/min

97. Water has accumulated in the delivery tubing of an aerosol system. This will result in all of the following *except*
    _____.
    A. increased F_{IO_2}
    B. decreased aerosol output
    C. increased total flow
    D. increased back-pressure in the system

98. A patient requires a flow rate of 40 L/min to meet his inspiratory demand for gas. He is to receive oxygen via a Venturi mask set at 24%. What is the minimum setting on the flowmeter to produce the appropriate flow?
    A. 1 L/min
    B. 2 L/min
    C. 3 L/min
    D. 4 L/min

FOOD FOR THOUGHT

99. Why does common use of the term "100% nonrebreather" create a clinical problem?

100. Why would an AEM be preferred over an air-entrainment nebulizer for a patient who has asthma or COPD?

INFORMATION AGE

- The respiratory program of the University of Medicine and Dentistry of New Jersey: www.umdnj.edu/rspthweb/rstn2100/unit2.htm.
- The University of Kansas Medical Center's respiratory care program has a good page on nitric oxide therapy: http://classes.kumc.edu/cahe/respcared/cybercas/nitricoxide/nother.html.
- You could put a phrase like "heliox therapy for asthma" or "nonrebreathing mask" into the search engine and get good sites.
- One more idea for you that's cool. A hot item in home care is the oxygen-conserving regulator. These devices work by sensing inspiration and pulsing a dose of O_2 to the patient. No flow occurs during exhalation, which saves a lot of gas! Sure beats a reservoir cannula!
  - You can see one of these at the Salter Web site: www.salterlabs.com/products. While Salter is a commercial site, if you click on "Resource Links," you can get a lot of neat resources and links.
  - But, the hottest of the hot is www.inogen.net/products. The portable oxygen concentrator is a breakthrough for many of our patients who want to travel or be free of cylinders!

I really could go on and on about oxygen, but you look like you need a break.

39 Lung Expansion Therapy

Cheer the patient up by having someone tell him jokes.
(Postoperative instruction to surgical residents in medieval text.)
A. De Mondeville, 1260-1320

Postoperative complications are dreaded by everyone involved: surgeons, nurses, third-party payers, and, yes, even patients. Postoperative pulmonary complications have been recognized as a problem for as long as surgery has been around, and respiratory therapists (RTs) have been at the forefront of the battle against atelectasis (incomplete expansion) and retained secretions for many years. Anesthesia, pain, medications, and preexisting lung disease are the enemy. Fortunately, we have a powerful arsenal of lung expansion devices and treatments on our side. (In addition to telling the patient jokes.)

WORD WIZARD

One of the problems associated with lung expansion therapy is to explain the goals, procedures, and equipment so the patient can understand. For each of the following terms or treatments, give a simple, short explanation in lay terms that even your kid brother could understand. (I'll help you get started, but you don't have to use my words if you don't need to.)

1. Atelectasis: "When you don't take deep breaths . . ."

   _____

2. Incentive spirometer (IS):

   A. "The purpose of this treatment is to . . ."

   _____

   B. "This device will . . ." _____

3. Sustained maximal inspiration (SMI): "I want you to take . . ."

   _____

4. Intermittent positive-pressure breathing (IPPB)

   A. "Your doctor has ordered a breathing treatment that will help you . . ."

   _____

   B. "This machine will . . ." _____

5. Continuous positive airway pressure (CPAP)

   A. "This treatment will . . ." _____

   B. "I am going to put a mask on your face . . ."

   _____

In fact, maybe you should try out your explanations on friends or family members to see if they make sense! Think of it as a play and act your part.

MEET THE OBJECTIVES

Answer the following questions to test your understanding of this chapter's objectives.

6. What is the definition of atelectasis?

   _____

7. What is resorption atelectasis, and when is it likely to occur?

8. What causes passive atelectasis?

9. Why are postoperative patients at highest risk for development of atelectasis?

10. What specific group of postoperative patients are at highest risk?

   _____

408

11. Name two other types of patients who have increased likelihood of developing atelectasis. Explain why.

A. _____

B. _____

12. Explain how each of the following may help provide clues that atelectasis is present or likely. (I use the exact same indicators to tell if the atelectasis is improving after lung expansion therapy, except for the history, of course.)

A. History

B. Breath sounds

C. Respiratory rate

D. Heart rate

E. Chest film

13. All modes of lung expansion therapy increase lung volume by increasing the transpulmonary pressure gradient. What are the two methods for increasing the gradient?

A. _____

B. _____

INCENTIVE SPIROMETRY

14. List three indications, two contraindications, and two hazards of incentive spirometry. (See Boxes 39-1, 39-2, and 39-3 on p. 906.)
    A. Indications

    1. _____

    2. _____

    3. _____

    B. Contraindications

    1. _____

    2. _____

    3. _____

    C. Hazards

    1. _____

    2. _____

15. Consider the top two complications. What are your ideas about dealing with these problems?
    A.

    B.

IPPY-BIPPY

I am not kidding—we called it ippy-bippy. Intermittent positive-pressure breathing (IPPB) is a time-honored way to pump someone up. That means ancient. Still, for the right patient this machine works well. It is also expensive, complicated, and intimidating to students. The first IPPB treatment I ever gave was to an RT who was in a motor vehicle accident! IPPB was first described by Motley in 1947 following its use in aviation medicine during the war.

16. Please give a brief general idea of how it works to inflate the lung when the patient cannot take a deep breath.

_____

17. Like IS, IPPB is used to treat atelectasis. Specifically, when would IPPB be indicated compared with IS?

18. What is the one absolute contraindication to IPPB?

19. List at least five additional partial contraindications.

A. _____

B. _____

C. _____

D. _____

E. _____

20. Name two common complications of IPPB administration.

A. _____

B. _____

21. What outcomes will tell you that your IPPB therapy has been effective? Name at least four. Try Box 39-8 on page 913 of your text if you get lost.

A. _____

B. _____

C. _____

D. _____

22. Name the three current PAP therapies. Which one is the best?

A. _____

B. _____

C. _____

D. The best one is . . . _____

23. Physiologic effects of CPAP are poorly understood but probably include:

A. _____

B. _____

C. _____

D. _____

24. Name two contraindications to CPAP therapy.

A. _____

B. _____

25. The text suggests the major complications of this therapy. Discuss each of the following problems.
    A. Hypoventilation:

    B. Barotrauma:

C. Gastric distention:

26. What alarm system is essential for monitoring patients receiving continuous mask CPAP?

27. Adequate flow is important to maintain CPAP levels. How does the author suggest you determine the initial setting?

Look at Figure 37-9 on page 916 in *Egan's*. I have assembled and used this type of system in the past. Currently, in my clinical sites, I see a device called EZ-PAP.

The company Web site is www.smiths-medical.com. To operate this simple PAP generator, you use flows of 5 to 15 L/min and the patient breathes as coached. Whether you use commercial CPAP/flow generators or your institution makes a continuous flow system, the methodology is sound and the patients breathe *spontaneously*.

CHAPTER HIGHLIGHTS

Complete the following sentences by writing in the correct term(s) in the blank(s) provided.

28. Atelectasis is caused by persistent _____ with _____ tidal volumes.

29. Patients who have undergone upper _____ or _____ surgery are at the greatest risk for atelectasis.

30. A history of _____ disease or _____ are additional risk factors.

31. The chest _____ is often used to confirm the presence of atelectasis.

413

32. Patients with atelectasis usually demonstrate _____ _____ breathing.

33. The most common problem associated with lung expansion therapy is the onset of respiratory _____,

which occurs when the patient breathes _____.

CASE STUDIES

Use the protocol found in Figure 39-8, page 918 of your text, and the section on "selecting an approach" to help answer the following questions.

Case 1

An alert, 34-year-old man is admitted for a hernia repair. He smokes 2 packs of cigarettes per day. Following surgery, the physician asks for your recommendation for therapy to prevent lung complications. The patient's vital capacity is 1.4 L and he weighs 80 kg with ideal body weight. He complains of cough but produces no sputum.

34. Discuss potential risk factors for atelectasis in this case.

_____

35. What therapy would you recommend for prevention of atelectasis for this patient?

_____

Case 2

A 70-year-old 5 foot 2 inch female patient is immobilized following hip replacement. Her predicted inspiratory capacity is 1.8 L. She is performing incentive spirometry at 500 ml per breath. Breath sounds reveal bilateral basilar crackles, and she is coughing up lots of thick mucus.

36. What is the minimum acceptable volume for incentive spirometry for this patient according to her predicted IC and her measured volume?

_____

37. What treatment would you recommend adding to the therapeutic regimen at this time?

_____

Case 3

An obese, mildly confused 59-year-old woman is recovering from CABG (open-heart surgery). The patient has persistent atelectasis with mild hypoxemia. Her radiograph shows an elevated left hemidiaphragm with air bronchograms in the left base. Vital capacity is 10 ml/kg ideal body weight. She has no prior lung disease, and is not coughing up any mucus.

38. What is the significance of the elevated diaphragm and air bronchograms seen on the chest film?

39. What treatment would you recommend? Why? What's the minimum goal for this therapy?

WHAT DOES THE NBRC SAY?

Lung expansion techniques like IS, IPPB, and CPAP are important parts of your board examinations. PEP is usually discussed under secretion management. The main difference between the CRT and RRT exams is the difficulty level of the questions. For example, the CRT exam is more likely to ask you to recall facts or apply them. The RRT exam asks more difficult questions that ask you to analyze information. Lung inflation is a very RICH topic for the boards:

- Assessment items: crackles, air bronchograms, elevated diaphragm
- Diagnostic studies: chest radiographs, oxygenation
- Equipment: spirometer, IPPB, circuit, disinfection
- Mathematics, communication, instructing the patient, and more!

Here are a few practice questions. Circle the best answer.

40. A patient complains of a "tingling" feeling in her lips during an incentive spirometry treatment. The RT should instruct the patient to _____.
    A. breathe more slowly
    B. take smaller breaths
    C. continue with the treatment as ordered
    D. exhale through pursed lips after each breath

41. Which of the following alarms are a vital part of the system when setting up CPAP therapy for treatment of atelectasis?
    A. exhaled volume
    B. high respiratory rate
    C. pulse oximetry
    D. low pressure

42. During administration of IPPB therapy, the practitioner observes the system pressure rise up suddenly at the end of inspiration. The RT should instruct the patient to _____.
    A. "Help the machine give you a deep breath."
    B. "Inhale slowly along with the machine."
    C. "Exhale gently and normally."
    D. "Exhale through pursed lips after each breath."

43. A patient is having difficulty initiating each breath with an IPPB machine. The practitioner should adjust the
_____.
   A. pressure limit
   B. peak flow
   C. F_{IO_2}
   D. sensitivity

44. Which control is used to increase the volume delivered by an IPPB machine?
   A. pressure limit
   B. peak flow
   C. F_{IO_2}
   D. sensitivity

45. Continuous positive airway pressure is used to increase which of the following?
   A. functional residual capacity
   B. peak expiratory flow rate
   C. FEV_1
   D. arterial carbon dioxide levels

46. An IPPB machine cycles on with the patient effort but does not shut off. The most likely cause of this problem is
_____.
   A. The pressure is set too low.
   B. The sensitivity is set incorrectly.
   C. There is a leak in the system.
   D. The patient is not blowing out hard enough.

47. How should you instruct a patient to breathe during incentive spirometry?
   A. "Exhale gently, then inhale rapidly through the spirometer."
   B. "Inhale deeply and rapidly through the spirometer."
   C. "Exhale until your lungs are empty, then inhale and hold your breath."
   D. "Exhale normally, then inhale slowly and deeply and hold your breath."

48. How often should a patient be instructed to use their incentive spirometer after they are taught to perform the procedure correctly?
   A. 10 breaths, four times per day
   B. 6 to 10 breaths every hour
   C. 10 to 20 breaths every 2 hours
   D. 6 to 8 breaths three times daily

49. A patient who has had surgery for an abdominal aortic aneurysm suffers from arrhythmias and hypotension after surgery. The physician asks for your recommendation for lung expansion therapy. The best choice in this situation would be _____.
   A. IS
   B. IPPB
   C. PEP
   D. CPAP

50. When adjusting the flow rate control on an IPPB machine, the RT would be altering the _____.
   A. maximum pressure delivered by the device
   B. effort required to initiate a breath
   C. volume delivered by the machine
   D. inspiratory time for a given breath

   I'll stop torturing you now, but I could go on and on. To get good at lung expansion therapy you will need to get out the equipment and practice in the lab. All of these treatments can be delivered to classmates in practice sessions until you are skilled with the devices, the coaching, and the breathing circuits. My students say the hardest part is learning to explain and coach therapy, not the equipment!

416

51. A really interesting topic in critical care is how best to reinflate the acutely restricted or atelectatic lung. "Lung recruitment maneuvers" is the correct name. Why don't you search out that one and explain BRIEFLY, IN YOUR OWN TERMS, how a lung recruitment maneuver is done.

INFORMATION AGE

- For an interesting treatise on trends in lung inflation therapy try: www.anaesthetist.com/icu/organs/lung/recruit/Findex.htm. Just search for lung recruitment.
- Your best bet on the subject of LI is the AARC Clinical Practice Guidelines: www.rcjournal.com/cpgs/index.cfm.

40 Bronchial Hygiene Therapy

Sputum is our bread and butter.
Anonymous Respiratory Therapist

Bronchial hygiene—well, it sounds better than "pulmonary toilet," which was the catch phrase when I was a student. After medical gas administration, playing with sputum is what makes our profession famous (or infamous). I distinctly remember my early clinical experience of asking a man to "cough it up" while I turned my head away to gag. That was before I got used to that lovely rattling sound. Join me now, for the halls are alive with the sound of mucus, and secretion management awaits!

WORD WIZARD

Acronyms Again?

After you've read Chapter 40 (You have read it, right?), you will have noticed an awful lot of acronyms (Check out Table 40-3 on page 942 if you don't believe me). Let's get those out of the way before we dive into bronchial hygiene. Write the definition for each of these mystic medical markings.

1. ACB _____

2. ARDS _____

3. AD _____

4. PDPV _____

5. CPT _____

6. CPAP _____

7. EPAP _____

8. FET _____

9. HFCWC _____

10. HZ _____

11. ICP _____

12. IPV _____

13. MI-E _____

14. PEP _____

AIRWAY CLEARANCE

Normal lungs generate a modest amount of mucus from the goblet cells, glands, and Clara cells. The mucociliary escalator whips that stuff up and out in no time. You hardly even notice. Of course, things go wrong. That's where we come in.

15. Name the four phases of the normal cough. Give examples of impairments for each (Table 40-1 on page 923).

Phase | Impairments

A. _____   _____

B. _____   _____

C. _____   _____

D. _____   _____

16. Compare the effects of full and partial airway obstruction caused by retained secretions.

A. Full obstruction, or _____ plugging, results in _____.

B. Partial obstruction increases _____ of breathing and leads to air _____.

17. Just for fun, state the airflow velocities and rise in lung pressures created by a good strong cough.

A. Expiratory velocity: _____ miles per hour!

B. Pleural/alveolar pressure: _____ mm Hg

DISEASE AND BAD CLEARANCE

18. Name at least three conditions that may cause internal obstruction or external compression of the airway lumen (opening).

A. _____

B. _____

C. _____

19. Name two obstructive lung diseases that result in excessive secretion of mucus and impairment of normal clearance.

    A. _____

    B. _____

20. List four neurologic or musculoskeletal conditions that impair cough.

    A. _____

    B. _____

    C. _____

    D. _____

SECRETION MANAGEMENT: GOALS AND INDICATIONS

Obviously getting the gunk out of the lungs is the main idea, but there's more to it, of course! The big picture is made up of acute conditions, chronic disorders, prevention, and assessment.

21. Name four acute conditions where bronchial hygiene is indicated.

    A. _____

    B. _____

    C. _____

    D. _____

22. Explain why you think bronchial hygiene is not useful in treating most cases of pneumonia or uncomplicated asthma.

Chronic

23. Discuss bronchial hygiene therapy for chronic lung conditions. How much sputum needs to be produced daily for the therapy to be useful? What are three typical diseases that we treat?

24. Describe the two well-documented preventive, or prophylactic, uses of this type of therapy.

A.

B.

25. In order to determine the need for bronchial hygiene therapy, you would assess the patient and the medical record. Give a brief explanation of the significance of each factors listed below (see Box 40-3 on page 925).

Factor	Significance
A. History	
B. Airway	
C. Chest radiograph	
D. Breath sounds	
E. Vital signs	

BRONCHIAL HYGIENE METHODS

There are five general noninvasive approaches to managing secretion problems. Within each general approach are several choices. You will need to customize therapy for each patient based on cost, effectiveness, clinical condition, and ability to participate in therapy.

Postural Drainage

26. Kinetic therapy has many pulmonary benefits. Name two *non*pulmonary benefits.

A.

B.

27. Postural drainage therapy includes up to four components, not counting cough. What are they?

A.

B.

C.

D.

28. List two absolute and two relative contraindications to turning.
    A. Absolute

       1. _____

       2. _____

    B. Relative

       1. _____

       2. _____

29. What does your book mean by "plumbing problems?"

30. Describe prone positioning.

    - What is it used for?

- What is the benefit?

- Prone positioning does not appear to increase _____ (yet!).

31. How long should you wait to schedule postural drainage after a patient eats? Why?

    _____

32. What is the minimum <u>range</u> of time for effective application of postural drainage therapy?

    _____

33. Give two recommended interventions for each of the complications of postural drainage listed below (check out Table 40-2 on page 930).

    Complication   **Interventions**

    A. Hypoxemia   _____

    B. Increased ICP   _____

    C. Acute hypotension   _____

    D. Pulmonary bleeding   _____

    E. Vomiting   _____

    F. Bronchospasm   _____

    G. Cardiac dysrhythmias   _____

34. Discuss vigorous cough efforts in relationship to position and postural drainage.

35. How long does it take to determine the effectiveness of postural drainage? If therapy is effective, how often should you reevaluate in the hospital? In the home?

A. How long? _____

B. Reevaluate hospital patients?

_____

C. Reevaluate home patients? _____

36. Describe at least five factors that must be documented after each postural drainage treatment:

A. _____

B. _____

C. _____

D. _____

E. _____

37. Describe percussion and vibration as techniques to loosen secretions. Are they really effective?

38. Compare manual and machine methods of percussion and vibration.

Cough It Up, Baby

Bronchial hygiene therapy is frustrating and sometimes useless if you can't get the patient to make an effective cough. Directed cough, cough staging, huff coughing, autogenic drainage, and active cycle of breathing are all really good tools you'll want to have in your bag of tricks. Each patient may require a combination of hygiene and coughing techniques. The latest research coming out as this text goes to press strongly suggests that cough and other clearance techniques are the most important part of bronchial hygiene.

39. How would you position a patient (ideally) for an effective cough? (Don't forget the part about the legs—try it!)

40. Standard directed cough must frequently be modified. Give three examples of types of patients who may need modified cough techniques.

   A. _____

   B. _____

   C. _____

41. What is splinting? _____

42. What special form of cough assistance is used with patients who have neuromuscular conditions?

   _____

43. Describe the forced expiratory technique (FET).

44. Describe the three repeated cycles of the ACB technique.

   A. _____

   B. _____

   C. _____

45. What is the primary problem with autogenic drainage?

   _____

46. Describe the two cycles of MI-E in terms of time and pressure.
   A. Inspiratory:

B. Expiratory:

Positive Airway Pressure

47. Positive airway pressure is a popular way to help mobilize secretions. What are the four indications for PAP adjuncts according to the AARC Clinical Practice Guideline?

A. _____

B. _____

C. _____

D. _____

48. What type of monitoring is essential regardless of the equipment used to deliver positive airway pressure to help mobilize secretions?

High-Frequency Compression/Oscillation of the Chest Wall

49. Describe the two general approaches to oscillation.

A. _____

B. _____

50. What do you think are the primary problems with vests and shells? What group of patients most commonly uses

the vest? _____

51. Describe the way IPV delivers gas to the airway.

52. Describe at least four of the benefits or advantages of the flutter valve as a secretion management tool.

A. _____

B. _____

C. _____

D. _____

Mobilization and Exercise

Early mobilization and frequent position changes are standards of care in preventing pulmonary complications after surgery or trauma.

53. Describe the benefits of adding exercise as a mobilization technique.

54. What should you specifically monitor when exercising patients with lung problems?

Case 1

Refer to Figure 40-13 on page 942 for some clues.

A 60-year-old professor who has had a colon resection for an intestinal tumor is receiving incentive spirometry to help expand his lungs. You are asked to assess the patient for retained secretions. Auscultation reveals coarse rhonchi bilaterally in the upper lobes. A few scattered crackles are heard in the bases. SpO_2 on room air is 94%. The patient states he is unable to cough up anything "because it hurts too much."

55. What technique could you use to decrease the pain associated with cough in a postoperative

patient? _____

56. What type of cough would you teach him?

_____

A 75-year-old woman with bronchiectasis states she coughs up "cups of awful mucus every day." She is admitted with a diagnosis of pneumonia.

57. What therapy is indicated while this patient is in the hospital?

_____

As you provide the therapy, you find out that the patient is a widow who lives alone. She takes albuterol treatments via SVN when she has difficulty breathing.

58. What therapy alternatives could you recommend for home use?

_____

WHAT DOES THE NBRC SAY?

They say, "Study hard and listen to Uncle Steve so you can pass your boards!" Well, OK, what they really say is this:

Remove Bronchopulmonary Secretions (Sounds like the RT commandment to me.)
- Conduct therapeutic procedures to remove bronchopulmonary secretions.
- Instruct and encourage proper coughing, AD, PEP, IPV, HFCWO, flutter.
- Perform postural drainage, percussion and/or vibration (use vibrators, percussors).

The only real difference between CRT and RRT is the difficulty level of the questions, not the actual content.

Here's a sample of what you can expect. Circle the best answer.

59. During the initial treatment, a PEP device is set to deliver a pressure of 15 cm H_2O. The patient complains of dyspnea and can only maintain exhalation for a short period of time. Which of the following should the RT recommend?
    A. Decrease the PEP level to 10 cm H_2O.
    B. Increase the PEP level to 20 cm H_2O.
    C. Discontinue the PEP therapy.
    D. Add a bronchodilator to the PEP therapy.

60. A patient is lying on her left side, one-quarter turn toward her back, with the head of the bed down. What division of the lung is being drained?
    A. lateral segments of the right lower lobe
    B. right middle lobe
    C. left upper lobe, lingular segments
    D. posterior segment of the right upper lobe

61. A patient is receiving postural drainage in the Trendelenburg position. The patient begins to cough uncontrollably. What action should the RT take at this time?
    A. Encourage the patient to use a huff cough.
    B. Administer oxygen therapy.
    C. Administer a bronchodilator.
    D. Raise the head of the bed.

62. In explaining the therapeutic goal of PEP therapy to a patient, it would be most appropriate to say _____.
    A. "This will help prevent pneumonia."
    B. "This will increase your intrathoracic pressure."
    C. "This will help you cough more effectively."
    D. "This will prevent atelectasis."

63. A COPD patient with left lower lobe infiltrates is unable to tolerate a head-down position for postural drainage. What action would you recommend?
    A. Perform the drainage with the head of the bed raised.
    B. Do not perform the therapy until 2 hours after the last meal.
    C. Administer a bronchodilator prior to the postural drainage.
    D. Notify the physician and suggest a different secretion management technique.

64. Active patient participation is an important part of which of the following procedures?
    I.   postural drainage
    II.   directed cough techniques
    III. airway suctioning
    IV.   positive expiratory pressure (PEP)
        A. I and II
        B. II and IV
        C. I and III
        D. III and IV

65. An RT is preparing a patient with bronchiectasis for discharge. Which of the following techniques would be most appropriate for self-administered therapy in the home?
    A. IPPB
    B. flutter
    C. suctioning
    D. percussion and postural drainage

FOOD FOR THOUGHT

66. How does hydration affect secretion clearance? What respiratory therapy modality can augment hydration of the airway?

67. Your text mentions never clapping directly over the spine or clavicles. Can you think of other places you should not clap? Use your imagination! (Could you get fired for clapping on certain parts of the anatomy?) So where *exactly* should you clap?

One more thing! When a patient has lung disease in only one lung, or "unilateral lung disease," positioning is very important. The rule of thumb is **down with the good lung.** When you put the good lung down, gravity takes the blood flow to the best ventilation. IF you put the bad lung down, perfusion goes to the bad lung and oxygenation can significantly worsen. There are some exceptions: lung abscess, PIE, and internal bleeding may require you to put the bad lung down. Otherwise, watch your patients for signs of distress if you turn them so the diseased lung is down!

- High-frequency oscillation delivered via a vest is a hot therapy being used for about 300 more conditions than just cystic fibrosis. In fact, there are hundreds of possible uses! Like ALS, MD, and transplants. Check it out at www.thevest.com.
- Another innovation is "vibratory PEP." Check out "Acapella" at www.smiths-medical.com. They make TheraPEP as well.
- If you're looking for a wide selection of information, I suggest you go to your search engine and type in "bronchial hygiene" or "secretion management." You'll get a lot of useful sites with these key words.

41 Respiratory Failure and the Need for Ventilatory Support

There's no success like failure, and failure's no success at all.
Bob Dylan

Chapter 41 is short, sweet, and essential to your understanding of why patients need mechanical ventilation. Remember, 44% of all the patients diagnosed with acute respiratory failure die in the hospital! Life seems to get worse before it gets better—only 36% died in the previous edition of this book. When you understand the material in this chapter, you will be ready to tackle the very complex and difficult subject of mechanical ventilation and critical care. Chapter 41 is really the gateway to becoming a registered respiratory therapist (RRT). The National Board for Respiratory Care (NBRC) places a special emphasis on the material in Section VI. Work hard on this chapter and it will help you pass your boards and . . . perhaps that 44% will have a better chance at survival.

WORD WIZARD

Here's a really short, sweet crossword puzzle to help you get over your fear of small words.

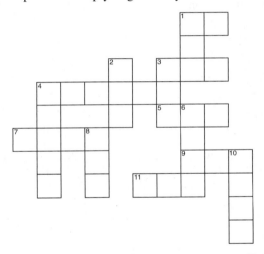

ACROSS

1. Preset minimum rate, patient can trigger breaths with set volumes
3. Maximum voluntary ventilation
4. Inability to maintain normal oxygen delivery to the tissues
5. Mode of ventilatory support designed to augment spontaneous breathing
7. Ventilatory support which patient breathes spontaneously at an elevated baseline
9. Measure of the output of respiratory muscles in cm H_2O pressure
11. Ventilator mode that uses high respiratory rates

DOWN

1. Another name for AC
2. Opposite of MIP
3. Also called NIF and MIF
4. Respirarory failure indicated by CO_2 greater than 50 in an otherwise healthy individual
6. Mode of support where spontaneous breaths are allowed between patient-triggered machine breaths
8. Mode of support in which breaths are delivered at a preset inspiratory pressure
10. Pressure above atmospheric during exhalation of a mechanical ventilator breath

SO, WHAT COULD GO WRONG?

1. Complete this sentence: "Put simply, respiratory failure is the _____.

2. What is the blood gas criteria for respiratory failure?

   A. Pa_{O_2}: _____

   B. Pa_{CO_2}: _____

3. What are the two general types of respiratory failure based on the type of physiologic impairment?

   A. Type I: _____

   B. Type II: _____

LET'S REVIEW

Egan's lists seven causes of hypoxemia. Of these, decreased F_{IO_2}, diffusion defect, and perfusion/diffusion impairment are not commonly seen in the acute care setting. $\dot{V}/\dot{Q}$ mismatch, shunt, venous admixture, and hypoventilation are common.

- $\dot{V}/\dot{Q}$ mismatch is usually a result of poorly ventilated areas that still get blood flow. A typical example would be bronchospasm.
- Shunt occurs when there is no ventilation at all. A typical example would be pneumonia or ARDS.
- Venous admixture is a low oxygen level in the blood returning to vena cava/lungs. A typical example would be CHF with low cardiac output or a low hemoglobin.
- Hypoventilation occurs in an essentially normal lung when CO_2 displaces O_2. A typical example would be a drug overdose.

It's not too hard to tell these conditions apart.

- $\dot{V}/\dot{Q}$ mismatch responds to oxygen therapy.
- Shunt does not respond to oxygen therapy.
- Hypoventilation present with a normal A-a gradient and responds to . . . ventilation!
- Venous admixture needs more cardiac output/more hemoglobin to deliver the Os.

4. What is the classic blood gas presentation of acute hypoxemic respiratory failure due to $\dot{V}/\dot{Q}$ mismatch or shunt? (Remember this one; it will show up to haunt you on the boards! Check out the Mini Clini "Differentiating Causes of Hypoxemia" on page 954 of your text for some help.)

   _____

TELL ME MORE, TELL ME MORE

5. What is the relationship between Pa_{CO_2} and alveolar ventilation?

6. *Egan's* states that there are three major groups of disorders responsible for acute hypercapnic respiratory failure (Type II). Give two examples of specific disorders representative of each category. Table 41-2 on page 956 provides a complete list.

    A. Decreased ventilatory drive

        1. _____

        2. _____

    B. Respiratory muscle fatigue/failure

        1. _____

        2. _____

    C. Increased work of breathing

        1. _____

        2. _____

7. Give an example of a condition that could cause greatly increased CO_2 production.

    _____

ACUTE-ON-CHRONIC RESPIRATORY FAILURE

8. How does the body compensate for chronically elevated carbon dioxide levels associated with COPD or obesity hypoventilation syndrome? _____

9. What happens to the normal blood gas classification of respiratory failure in patients with chronic respiratory failure?

10. Identify the five most common factors that lead to acute-on-chronic failure.

    A. _____

    B. _____

    C. _____

    D. _____

    E. _____

11. Name four treatment goals for this group of patients.

A. _____

B. _____

C. _____

D. _____

12. The complications from treating acute respiratory failure are as life threatening as the failure itself! Identify the likely causes of these pulmonary complications.

A. Emboli _____

B. Barotrauma _____

C. Infection _____

13. Give one example of each of these nonpulmonary complications of life in the ICU.

A. Cardiac _____

B. Gastrointestinal _____

C. Renal _____

14. Oh, go ahead; tell me three more complications associated with prolonged visits to the unit.

A. _____

B. _____

C. _____

TUBE 'EM

15. What is the primary goal of mechanical ventilation?

_____

16. Your board exams will expect you to identify these classic criteria for mechanical ventilation. Remember that no one criterion mandates ventilation (except apnea). See Table 41-3.

Mechanism	Critical Value
A. $Paco_2$	_____
B. pH	_____
C. VC (ml/kg)	_____
D. MIP	_____

E.   MVV   _____

F. V_E _____

G. V_D/V_T _____

H. $P(A - a)O_2$ on 100%   _____

I.   P/F ratio   _____

You need to learn these values! I am not kidding. Make flash cards. Make a memory matrix. Just do it.

17. Oxygenation indices like P/F ratio and A-a gradient are useful in determining the severity of failure. What P/F ratio is considered an indicator of profoundly impaired oxygenation?

18. Why is it useful to consider pH when evaluating carbon dioxide levels to determine the need to intubate and ventilate a patient? _____

ASSESSMENT OF FATIGUE

19. Define "MIP" and give the minimal value for most patients.

   A.   _____

   B.   _____

20. State the three types of muscle fatigue and give the cause.

   A.   _____

   B.   _____

   C.   _____

21. Respiratory *muscle weakness* is most likely to occur in what patient group?

   _____

22. Name three conditions that frequently lead to respiratory *muscle fatigue*.

   A.   _____

   B.   _____

   C.   _____

Chapter **41** **Respiratory Failure and the Need for Ventilatory Support**

Noninvasive ventilation is our best new strategy for supporting patients in failure. Chapter 45 will go in-depth. Here's an overview.

23. Define noninvasive ventilation.

24. NPPV can blow off the CO_2 and improve the Os via several mechanisms. List at least three.

    A. _____

    B. _____

    C. _____

25. When is NPPV useful for COPD?

26. What cardiac condition is also treated by NPPV?

27. What about NPPV for patients who have progressive neuromuscular disorders like ALS? Please discuss.

28. What is the main strategy for reducing lung injury in ARDS according to Chapter 41?

29. How does hyperventilation result in reduced ICP in head injury?

30. What is the target Pa_{CO_2} in these cases?

_____

31. What is the chief concern regarding use of PEEP to increase oxygenation in patients with acute head injuries?

32. Air-trapping, or hyperinflation, as a result of obstructive lung disease (COPD, asthma) causes what two complications in mechanically ventilated patients?

    A. _____

    B. _____

33. How are tidal volume and flow rate manipulated to reduce complications in mechanically ventilated COPD patients?

    A. Tidal volume _____

    B. Flow rate _____

34. What surprising technique was found to reduce auto-PEEP?

_____

CHAPTER HIGHLIGHTS

Complete the following sentences by writing in the correct term(s) in the blank(s) provided.

35. Acute respiratory failure is identified by a Pa_{CO_2} > _____ mm Hg and/or a Pa_{O_2} < _____ mm Hg in an otherwise healthy individual (at sea level, of course).

36. _____ respiratory failure is usually due to $\dot{V}/\dot{Q}$ mismatch or intrapulmonary _____, or _____.

37. _____ respiratory failure results from inadequate drive, respiratory muscle _____, or excessive work of _____.

38. Chronic respiratory failure may be represented by ABGs demonstrating _____ with evidence of metabolic compensation or _____ reflecting chronic hypoxemia.

39. The _____ status of the patient is the most important factor determining the need for ventilator support.

40. Excessive _____ is the most common cause of respiratory muscle fatigue.

41. Only patients with rapidly reversible conditions should undergo _____ ventilation in the acute setting.

42. The goal of therapy in acute hypercapnic respiratory failure is to guarantee a set _____ ventilation.

CASE STUDIES

Case 1

An alert, anxious 25-year-old woman presents in the emergency department (ED) complaining of chills, fever, and shortness of breath. An arterial blood gas is drawn on room air with these results:

pH	7.45
Pa_{CO_2}	32 mm Hg
Pa_{O_2}	50 mm Hg
HCO_3^-	23 mEq/L

43. Interpret this blood gas.

44. What is the A-a gradient?

45. What type of respiratory failure is present?

46. What do you recommend for initial respiratory treatment?

A 27-year-old is brought to the ED by paramedics following a drug overdose. The patient is obtunded. Blood gases are drawn on room air:

pH	7.24
$Paco_2$	60 mm Hg
Pao_2	65 mm Hg
HCO_3^-	26 mEq/L

47. Interpret this blood gas. _____

48. What is the A-a gradient? _____

49. What type of respiratory failure is present?

50. What is the appropriate initial respiratory treatment in this case?

Case 3

An alert 56-year-old man with a history of COPD presents in the ED complaining of dyspnea, which has worsened over the last few days. A blood gas is drawn on room air:

pH	7.26
$Paco_2$	70 mm Hg
Pao_2	50 mm Hg
HCO_3^-	32 mEq/L

51. Interpret this blood gas.

52. What is the A-a gradient?

53. What type of respiratory failure is present?

54. What initial respiratory treatments are indicated? What are we trying to avoid?

WHAT DOES THE NBRC SAY?

Stop. Do not pass Go. Do not collect $200! The information presented in Chapter 41 forms a fundamental basis for our understanding of respiratory failure. It is highly complex, combining blood gases, pathophysiology, and more. The NBRC is passionate about your understanding of this material and will present you with many similar situations. Assess. Interpret. Recommend. Treat. Modify. Wow! When you are working on these problems, always start by interpreting the ABG. Do this in the context of the patient's history. COPD should raise a red flag that suggests you think hard before you interpret or act. Here are some examples. Circle the best answer.

55. An RT is asked to evaluate a lethargic 50-year-old woman who is in respiratory distress following abdominal surgery. She is breathing spontaneously, on a 50% air-entrainment mask, at 32 breaths per minute. ABG results show

pH	7.28
$Paco_2$	55 mm Hg
Pao_2	60 mm Hg
HCO_3^-	26 mEq/L

Based on this information, what would you recommend?
A. Provide intubation and mechanical ventilation.
B. Increase the Fio_2 to 1.
C. Administer IPPB.
D. Administer bronchodilator therapy via SVN.

56. An alert, anxious 60-year-old man with a history of CHF presents in the ED with respiratory distress. Auscultation reveals bilateral inspiratory crackles. He has peripheral edema. ABG results drawn on a partial rebreathing mask show

pH	7.45
$Paco_2$	35 mm Hg
Pao_2	40 mm Hg
HCO_3^-	23 mEq/L

The most appropriate therapy for improving oxygenation would be
A. Provide intubation and mechanical ventilation.
B. Administer oxygen therapy via nonrebreathing mask.
C. Administer oxygen therapy via CPAP.
D. Administer bronchodilator therapy via SVN.

57. A man is being mechanically ventilated immediately after surgery for a closed head injury. Settings are:

Tidal volume	700 ml
Rate	10
Mode	AC
Fio_2	0.40
PEEP	0

ABGs show:

pH	7.37
$Paco_2$	44 mm Hg
Pao_2	86 mm Hg
HCO_3^-	24 mEq/L

Which of the following ventilator changes would you recommend at this time?
A. Increase the FIO_2.
B. Decrease the volume.
C. Increase the rate.
D. Increase the PEEP.

58. An adult patient is being mechanically ventilated following respiratory failure. Settings are

Tidal volume	800 ml
Rate	12
Mode	AC
FIO_2	0.60
PEEP	3 cm H_2O

ABGs show

pH	7.37
$Paco_2$	41 mm Hg
Pao_2	43 mm Hg
HCO_3^-	22 mEq/L

Which of the following ventilator changes would you recommend at this time?
A. Increase the FIO_2.
B. Decrease the volume.
C. Increase the rate.
D. Increase the PEEP.

59. A patient with a history of hypercapnia and COPD is intubated and placed on the ventilator following respiratory failure. 24 hours later, the patient is alert and breathing spontaneously.
Settings are

Tidal volume	800 ml
Rate	12
Mode	CMV (AC)
FIO_2	0.30
PEEP	0 cm H_2O

ABGs show:

pH	7.48
$Paco_2$	41 mm Hg
Pao_2	60 mm Hg
HCO_3^-	30 mEq/L

Which of the following ventilator changes would you recommend at this time?
A. Decrease the FIO_2.
B. Decrease the volume.
C. Change to pressure-controlled ventilation (PCV).
D. Change to synchronized intermittent mandatory ventilation (SIMV).

60. A 77-year-old man with COPD is admitted with acute bronchitis. Room air blood gas results show

pH	7.52
$Paco_2$	45 mm Hg
Pao_2	50 mm Hg
HCO_3^-	36 mEq/L

444

What intervention would be appropriate at this time?
A. CPAP with 24% oxygen
B. 28% Air entrainment mask
C. nasal cannula at 5 L/min
D. simple mask at 8 L/min

61. CPAP is indicated for treatment of patients with _____.
A. respiratory failure secondary to shunting
B. apnea
C. ventilatory failure with hypercapnia
D. hypoxemia secondary to V̇/Q̇ mismatch

Between the cases, the chapter, and these questions you should be getting the general idea!

FOOD FOR THOUGHT

Remember Table 41-3 (page 958), the one about measurable indications for ventilatory support?
    I didn't forget about that one. Your boards expect you to know this information, as part of the decision to intubate and ventilate, or as part of the decision to wean.

62. What clinical situations or condition suggests using ABGs to evaluate the need to intubate and ventilate? Compare this with situations better assessed by measures like VC and MIP.

We'll come back to this again in Chapter 47 when we talk about weaning.

INFORMATION AGE

- A good overview of CPAP and BiPAP in the treatment of failure: www.theberries.ns.ca/archives/CPAP.html.
- Another good overview at e-medicine: www.emedicine.com/MED/topic2011.htm.
- Here's a little juicy site: www.virtualrespiratorycentre.com.
- And, of course, MEDLINE: www.nlm.nih.gov/medlineplus/ency/article/000092.htm.
- You can use "respiratory acidosis" as another good search word.

42 Mechanical Ventilators

Just bag 'em till I get there.
Florida Society for RC T-Shirt

CMV, PSV, PCV, IMV, MMV, VAPS, ZEEP, NEEP, PEEP . . . bleep . . . brain reeling, neuronal meltdown. . . . Must try to understand Chapter 42 . . . must remain conscious. . . .

Once upon a time there were only three modes of ventilation: control, assist-control, and IMV. Ventilators were driven by pistons or bellows and an occasional light bulb glowed or buzzer sounded when there was a problem. Volume cycled, pressure limited was, well—just exactly what it sounded like. Times have changed. Ventilators cost more than new cars. Whether or not the explosion of technology in ventilator design has improved health care has yet to be determined, but you will have to try to make sense of it anyway.

WORD WIZARD

Ventilator Verbiage

Match these definitions to the key terms in the beginning of the chapter.

Definitions	Terms
1. _____ breath initiated by the ventilator	A. spontaneous breath
	B. control variable
2. _____ causes a breath to end	C. limit variable
	D. cycle variable
3. _____ manipulated by machine to cause inspiration	E. intermittent mandatory ventilation
	F. trigger variable
4. _____ controls the magnitude of inspiration	G. CMV
	H. CSV
5. _____ combination of machine and spontaneous breaths	I. mandatory breath
6. _____ machine breaths only—no spontaneous	
7. _____ spontaneous breaths only and no machine breaths	
8. _____ causes a breath to begin	
9. _____ breath initiated and ended by the patient	

HOW VENTILATORS WORK

10. What is a ventilator?

11. Describe the desired output of the ventilator in terms of the patient.

    _____

12. Identify three settings where ventilators use DC back-up power sources.

    A. _____

    B. _____

    C. _____

13. How are most modern intensive care ventilators powered?

    _____

14. Identify one setting where electrical power is undesirable.

    _____

15. What other mechanisms are used to drive a ventilator besides compressed gas?

    _____

I'M IN CONTROL

16. What does the output control valve do?

    A. Regulates: _____

    B. Shapes: _____

17. Setting an appropriate expiratory time (at least three time constants) is clinically important to avoid what

    dangerous condition? _____

18. What are the three variables that ventilators control?

    A. _____

    B. _____

    C. _____

19. Identify the five types of control circuits used in ventilators.

   A. _____

   B. _____

   C. _____

   D. _____

   E. _____

20. State two advantages of fluidic control circuits.

   A. _____

   B. _____

21. Control variables are how a ventilator manipulates inspiration. Fill in the blanks below to show what is constant and what changes for each control variable.

Control Variable	Constant	Varies With Changes in Lungs
A. Pressure	_____	_____
B. Volume	_____	_____
C. Flow	_____	_____

PHASE

22. Describe the basic purpose of the following phase variables in terms of the breathing cycle.

Phase Variable	Portion of Breathing Cycle Controlled
A. Trigger variable	_____
B. Limit variable	_____
C. Cycle variable	_____
D. Baseline variable	_____

23. Name the three ways to trigger the ventilator.

   A. _____

   B. _____

   C. _____

24. Time triggering divides each minute into segments allotted for each breath. This is the total cycle time. If the rate is 12 breaths per minute, what is the total cycle time? (Hint: Divide the minute into 12 equal parts!)

25. What is the normal setting range for pressure triggering? Flow triggering?

    A. Pressure _____ to _____ cm H_2O

    B. Flow _____ to _____ below the baseline flow

26. Which ventilator uses volume triggering? _____

27. Pressure support ventilation (PSV) is an example of a mode that has a limit (pressure) but is cycled off by another variable (flow). Define the term "limit variable."

    _____

28. Define the term "cycle variable."

    _____

29. What is the most common application of pressure cycling?

    _____

30. What lung inflation therapy uses a pressure-cycled machine?

    _____

31. Try to explain the difference between pressure limiting and pressure cycling.

    _____

32. What is the usual cycling parameter for pressure support ventilation?

    _____

33. Define the term "baseline variable."

    _____

34. What baseline variable is used on all modern ventilators?

    _____

35. Explain what is meant by these acronyms. Which is the default value for ventilators?

A. ZEEP: _____

B. NEEP: _____

C. PEEP: _____

A LA MODE

36. Define the phrase "mode of ventilation."

_____

37. You need to decide on a control variable to end inspiration. What are the two primary ways to end inspiration? (Hint: Look under "breathing pattern.")

A. _____

B. _____

38. What does "dual control" mean?

_____

39. Define spontaneous and mandatory breaths. Give another term for each.

A. Spontaneous: _____

B. Mandatory: _____

40. Explain the basic sequence of ventilation represented by each of these terms.

A. CMV _____

B. CSV _____

C. IMV _____

Recap
- All ventilators offer a mode that intermixes spontaneous breaths with ventilator breaths. This is called synchronized intermittent mandatory ventilation (SIMV).
- All adult ventilators offer a mode that is machine breaths only. Common names are continuous mandatory ventilation (CMV) and assist-control.
- All adult ventilators offer the choice of volume-controlled ventilator breaths (VC) and pressure-controlled ventilator breaths (PC) for any mode that offers a machine breath.
- All adult ventilators have a mode that is spontaneous breathing without machine breaths. This is called spontaneous or continuous positive airway pressure (CPAP) mode, or continuous spontaneous ventilation (CSV).
- All adult ventilators offer a way to augment spontaneous breaths with a pressure boost. This is called pressure support (PS or PSV).
- Some ventilators offer specialized modes like APRV, but this is really pressure-controlled (PC) IMV.

You may enjoy reading about the different controls. Ventilators actually have things like cruise control. Adaptive controls are truly new because the ventilator is capable of operating independently from the therapist. Expect fuzzy logic next, like in a fancy rice cooker!

SURF THE WAVEFORMS

Ventilator waveforms have been around for a long time, but when I was a student we couldn't really see them in action. Most modern ventilators are capable of displaying waveforms graphically so you can apply them clinically. For example, if you see that expiratory flow does not return to baseline before the next breath starts, you know that the patient is not able to exhale completely. You can then adjust the ventilator to allow complete exhalation, or try to treat the problem (by giving a bronchodilator, for example).

I only know two ways to help you learn waveforms.
- One method of learning this difficult subject is to practice drawing the waveforms.
- The other way is to go to a ventilator in the classroom or lab setting. Attach the ventilator to a test lung, turn on the graphics, and adjust the ventilator to deliver different settings and look at the waveforms that are produced. It will help you if an instructor is handy to guide you through this procedure!

Once you learn to identify the various waveforms, you can move on to the next step, which is to learn the problem pictures, what they mean clinically, and how to fix the problem. *Egan's* covers this area in Chapter 42.

41. Draw the following flow patterns. Look at Figure 42-12 on page 986 for **help.**

    A.   Rectangular   _____

    B.   Ascending ramp   _____

    C.   Descending ramp   _____

    D.   Sinusoidal   _____

Most ventilators allow the therapist to select the flow waveform from at least three of these four patterns. The pressure waveform will be determined by the mode you select.

CLINICAL APPLICATION OF VENTILATOR MODES

Continuous Mandatory Ventilation (CMV)

This mode allows the operator to greatly reduce patient work of breathing and control the minute volume. This is pretty good if the patient is apneic or exhausted or you want a specific Pa_{CO_2} level.

42. Pressure or volume may be used as the control variable for machine breaths. What happens to volume and airway pressure when compliance drops?

Control Variable	Volume	Airway Pressure
A. Pressure	_____	_____
B. Volume	_____	_____

43. Why is manipulation of mean airway pressure clinically important?

44. What is the primary goal of CMV? _____

_____

45. What are three potential harmful effects of excess triggering in CMV?

    A. _____

    B. _____

    C. _____

46. Use of VC-CMV allows the clinician fairly precise control over what values?

_____

47. When is PC-CMV indicated? _____

48. Why does PC improve patient comfort and ventilator synchrony?

_____

49. What parameter has to be closely monitored in PC to avoid volutrauma or ventilator-induced hypoventilation?

_____

50. Dual-control CMV may be useful when a patient has unstable or changing pulmonary mechanics. The ventilator makes small adjustments in pressure to maintain a good tidal volume. PRVC is one example of dual-control CMV. Give an example of a clinical situation where DC-CMV could be useful.

_____

Synchronized Intermittent Mandatory Ventilation (SIMV)

Once the most popular modes in the country! It's often used for weaning (although it can be a bit slow). SIMV also provides some work for the respiratory muscles and other benefits of spontaneous breathing. You set the level of support by determining how many machine breaths you want to give each minute.

51. What is the potential cardiac benefit of the spontaneous breaths seen in SIMV?

_____

52. What's the difference between IMV and SIMV?

_____

Chapter **42** **Mechanical Ventilators**

53. Guillain-Barré patients usually have normal lungs and a drive to breathe. What mode would you select?

54. PC-IMV or DC-IMV (if you have it) could be useful with what clinical situation involving COPD or asthma?

Why? _____

55. If you want to wean VC-IMV, you need to drop the rate. How do you wean PC-IMV?

_____

Spontaneous Ventilation (CSV)

In this mode, the patient begins and ends each breath. You can set the level of support the ventilator gives during the spontaneous breath, and you can set the baseline. There are lots of spontaneous breathing modes around, but TC, SPONT, CPAP, and PSV are terms used throughout our industry. CPAP and PSV are the most common in my area.

56. Give an example of initial pressure levels for CPAP mode.

_____

57. What does this accomplish physiologically?

_____

58. Pressure support is popular because of its many attributes. List at least four:

A. _____

B. _____

C. _____

D. _____

CASE STUDIES

Case 1

A 21-year-old patient is placed on a ventilator following a closed head injury. The physician desires to control this patient's ventilation to achieve a specific CO_2 level in the arterial blood.

59. What mode of ventilation would best achieve this goal?

_____

454

60. What would you recommend if the patient's breathing pattern is out of synch with the ventilator?

_____

Case 2

A 35-year-old woman with a neuromuscular disease is placed on a Puritan-Bennett 840 ventilator in CMV mode. The ventilator is set for A/C volume-cycled ventilation at a rate of 10, but the machine is triggering at a rate of 28. The patient looks pretty scared.

61. What is the most likely cause of the excess ventilator triggering?

_____

62. What mode of ventilation does *Egan's* suggest you use to solve this problem?

WHAT DOES THE NBRC SAY?

The following modes of ventilation are listed in the examination matrices.
- PCV
- SIMV
- PS or PSV
- CPAP
- PCV

For the more common traditional modes, you are expected to be able to recommend, initiate, adjust, etc.—in other words, everything! We'll get into this more in Chapter 44, so don't worry. The less common modes, like APRV, are not specifically mentioned, but you still need to know a little general information like when to recommend.

Here are a few practice questions. Circle the best answer.

63. A patient with ARDS is being ventilated with the following settings.

Mode	AC
V_T	800
Rate	14
FIO_2	80%
PEEP	15 cm H_2O

Peak pressures are unacceptably high while oxygenation remains poor. Which of the following changes may be beneficial in this situation?
A. Change the PEEP to 20 cm H_2O.
B. Increase the FIO_2 to 100%.
C. Initiate pressure control ventilation.
D. Place the patient on BiPAP by mask.

455

64. A patient is being ventilated in SIMV mode. The patient is making spontaneous efforts with tidal volumes of 150 ml. What modification would you recommend?
   A. Initiate PEEP.
   B. Initiate PSV.
   C. Change to CPAP mode.
   D. Change to CMV mode.

65. A patient with COPD and CO_2 retention is intubated following respiratory failure. The physician states that she wants to avoid overventilation and air-trapping. Which of the following modes would you recommend?
   A. SIMV
   B. AC
   C. CPAP
   D. APRV

66. A patient in the early stages of ARDS is intubated. The physician states that he wishes to minimize the possibility of volutrauma or barotrauma. Which of the following modes would you recommend?
   A. volume-controlled ventilation
   B. manual ventilation
   C. CPAP
   D. pressure-controlled ventilation

67. An 80-kg (176-lb) patient is being ventilated in pressure control mode. During a ventilator check, the therapist notes that the compliance has decreased from 40 ml/cm H_2O to 35 ml/cm H_2O. What effect will this change in compliance have on the patient–ventilator system?
   A. no effect
   B. increased peak airway pressure
   C. decreased mean airway pressure
   D. decreased tidal volume

FOOD FOR THOUGHT

Not all modes are used in all parts of the country. What are your hospitals using? Does practice vary between community hospitals and the trauma center? A good starting point for the new therapist is to learn a lot about the modes that are most commonly used in current practice where you live and where you do your clinical training. For example, if you are being assigned to do clinical in a small hospital where CMV and AC are the main modes, don't go in with the idea that you will implement bilevel mode on the 840 or APRV. Instead, learn as much as you can about the art of using CMV. The best RTs can make the best of whatever mode is used in their institution while acting as resources for the nurses and physicians. They pull the other modes out of their bag of tricks when the opportunity arises, *but only after making themselves experts.* Introducing a new ventilator or new mode of ventilation is fraught with hazards if in-service training doesn't come along with the changes.

INFORMATION AGE

- A nice tutorial on the differences between APRV, bilevel, and other advanced modes using pressure control is found at www.ccmtutorials.com/rs/mv/page13.htm.
- A short and fairly clear explanation of some of the newer modes of ventilation is found on "ISPUB", the Internet journal of anesthesia at www.ispub.com/ostia/index.php?xmlFilePath=journals/ija/vol4n4/ventilation.xml.
- Here's another thought for you—go online to www.medscape.com and register. It's free. This will give you access to over 100 online journals and other resources. I found lots of articles on mechanical ventilation.

43 Physiology of Ventilatory Support

Life is like riding a bicycle. You don't fall off unless you stop pedaling.
Claude Pepper (attributed)

Mechanical ventilation can be a life-sustaining procedure, but it is not natural. There are physiologic consequences to applying positive pressure to the lungs and chest. For better or for worse, we're currently married to this technology and you will need to understand what happens when you connect the patient to the machine.

WORD WIZARD

There aren't too many new words to learn in Chapter 43. Look up the definitions in the your glossary and write them out next to the words I've listed below.

1. barotrauma _____

2. time constant _____

3. biotrauma _____

4. transrespiratory pressure _____

5. patient–ventilator asynchrony _____

6. atelectrauma _____

7. mean airway pressure _____

8. transpulmonary pressure _____

LIFE UNDER PRESSURE

9. Which pressure is responsible for maintaining normal alveolar inflation?

_____

10. Which pressure gradient is required to expand the lungs and chest wall together?

_____

457

11. Which pressure causes airflow in the airways?

_____

12. What happens to transpulmonary pressure during normal inspiration? Exhalation?

A. Inspiration _____

B. Exhalation _____

13. What happens to transpulmonary pressure during inspiration with a negative pressure ventilator? Exhalation?

A. Inspiration _____

B. Exhalation _____

14. What is "tank shock?" _____

15. What happens to the airway and pleural pressures during inspiration with a positive-pressure ventilator?

_____

WHAT ABOUT OXYGENATION?

Remember type I failure? The mechanical ventilator can be used to improve oxygenation through a variety of methods.

16. Explain how mechanical ventilation improves oxygenation for each of the following causes of hypoxemia:

A. Hypoventilation _____

B. $\dot{V}/\dot{Q}$ mismatch _____

C. Shunt _____

17. What range of F_{IO_2} can a modern ICU ventilator deliver?

_____

18. State the formula for each of the following

A. D_{O_2} _____

B. Alveolar air _____

C. Arterial oxygen content _____

D. Minute ventilation _____

19. How is optimal PEEP determined in terms of F_{IO_2} and Pa_{O_2}?

_____

EFFECTS OF MECHANICAL VENTILATION

There are so many effects of mechanical ventilation that we need to break them down into little pieces to understand what happens when you attach that circuit to the ET tube!

Ventilation

20. What is the normal range of tidal volume during spontaneous breathing?

_____

21. It's important to set a tidal volume on the ventilator based on pathophysiology. What volume would you set for a patient with:

A. ARDS _____

B. COPD _____

C. Normal lungs _____

22. Besides increasing the volume, how can you increase minute ventilation with the ventilator?

_____

23. What effect does minute ventilation have on Pa_{CO_2}?

_____

24. Where is gas distributed by a normal spontaneous breath? What about a positive-pressure breath?

A. Spontaneous _____

B. PPV _____

25. How does perfusion, or blood flow, in the lung change during PPV?

_____

26. What's the net effect of all this redistribution on the $\dot{V}/\dot{Q}$ ratio?

_____

27. How would poor ventilator management result in respiratory acidosis?

_____

28. There are several ways you could assess this problem. Explain the importance of each the following:

    A.   Draw arterial blood _____

    B.   Check electrolytes _____

    C.   Check ECG _____

29. How would poor ventilator management result in respiratory alkalosis?

_____

30. There are several ways you could assess this problem. Discuss each of the following:

    A.   Draw arterial blood _____

    B.   Check electrolytes _____

    C.   Check ECG _____

31. Discuss the two methods for treating metabolic acidosis in mechanically ventilated patients. Each can be *a lifesaving* maneuver, so think carefully on this one!
    A.   Bicarbonate administration

    B.   Minute ventilation

LUNG MECHANICS

32. How long does it take for 95% of the alveoli in a normal lung to fill with air?

    A.   Time constants _____

    B.   Real time _____

    What about 98% of alveoli? _____ 99%? _____

33. What are the two major factors that affect alveolar time constants?

A. _____

B. _____

34. Compare a restrictive disorder like ARDS and an obstructive problem like COPD in terms of the time it takes for alveolar filling and emptying. Mark the blanks with a ↑ or ↓ to indicate how you would adjust the ventilator for these two groups of patients.

A. ARDS needs _____ inspiratory time and _____ expiratory time.

B. COPD needs _____ inspiratory time and _____ expiratory time.

35. You could help prolong the inspiratory phase for your restricted patient by making adjustments:

A. Inspiratory time setting should be _____.

B. Inspiratory flow setting should be _____.

36. You could help prolong the expiratory phase for your obstructed patient by making adjustments:

A. Inspiratory flow should be _____.

B. Mandatory ventilator rate should be _____.

C. Tidal volume should be _____.

37. What is meant by the term "peak inspiratory pressure?" What's the abbreviation?

_____

38. What is meant by the term "plateau pressure?" What's the symbol?

_____

39. We can protect patient lungs from damage caused by pressure by maintaining plateau pressures at less than

_____ cm H_2O.

40. See if you know how to adjust mean airway pressure. It's a little complicated! Circle "T" for "true" if the choice is one that would *raise the mean airway pressure*.

A. Increase peak pressure   T   F
B. Decrease inspiratory time   T   F
C. Synchronized IMV   T   F
D. Increase PEEP levels   T   F
E. Constant pressure pattern (PC mode, ↓ ramp flow)   T   F

41. OK, now tell me how increasing airway pressure affects the FRC and oxygenation.

A. FRC _____

B. Oxygenation _____

42. Does inspiratory positive pressure ventilation by itself increase the FRC? What can you add to maintain this capacity? _____

43. What will happen to compliance when too much PEEP is applied? Could you adjust the PEEP based on the changes in compliance? _____

44. Your vent patient has atelectasis and needs lung recruitment. You'll want to apply up to _____ cm H$_2$O PEEP for up to _____ to _____ minutes.

45. The pressure-volume curve is useful for establishing the point where the lung begins to open up. Give three names for this "lower" point.

   A. _____

   B. _____

   C. _____

46. Why does deadspace increase during mechanical ventilation?

   _____

WHAT ABOUT WORK OF BREATHING?

Ventilators are intended to decrease the work of breathing. Many patients who are in respiratory failure are exhausted and their breathing muscles need a break to recover.

47. What happens to the diaphragm if the ventilator does the work for too long?

   _____

48. What type of triggering reduces WOB in older ventilators? What about newer vents?

   _____

49. What inspiratory maneuver can be added to SIMV to reduce the work of breathing through the ET tube and ventilator circuit? _____

50. Since you can't really measure WOB at the bedside, what three variables does the experienced therapist use to determine whether WOB is excessive?

   A. _____

   B. _____

   C. _____

PHYSIOLOGIC EFFECTS OF VENTILATORY MODES

Mechanical ventilation is lifesaving. Unfortunately, it can also damage the lung. The RT is the advocate for the patient's lung tissue!

51. Look at Table 43-2 and give two negative pulmonary effects of too much PEEP.

    A. _____

    B. _____

52. Why is PEEP a problem with severe unilateral lung disease?

53. Identify two potential harmful effects of controlled CMV.

    A. _____

    B. _____

54. Name two advantages of IMV.

    A. _____

    B. _____

55. How can you identify a leak in the VC-CMV mode using ventilator graphics? What will you see?

    _____

56. What is the primary reason for using PC-CMV?

    _____

57. What is meant by "permissive hypercapnia"?

    _____

58. What are some of the possible benefits of APRV?

    _____

59. PSV overcomes airway _____ and improves tidal _____.

60. *Egan's* says that PSV will result in four beneficial effects. Name them.

A. _____

B. _____

C. _____

D. _____

61. In BiPAP, IPAP is the same as _____ and EPAP is the same as _____.

62. Bilevel CPAP was originally developed for treatment of obstructive sleep apnea. It has also been shown to be useful in acute care settings. Explain.

A. COPD _____

B. ARDS _____

63. What is the effect of CPAP on ventilation?

_____

64. Identify the important physiologic effect of CPAP.

_____

65. Explain ASV in terms of

A. Therapist inputs _____

B. Microprocessor controlled _____

What about weaning? _____

66. PAV is designed to improve what important relationship?

_____

67. Automatic tube compensation is not a mode of ventilation. What is it really? _____

_____

DOWN WITH THE GOOD LUNG!

68. Patients with unilateral lung disease greatly benefit from what type of positioning?

_____

69. What unique position improves oxygenation in ARDS?

_____

NOT JUST THE LUNGS!

Amazingly enough, positive pressure ventilation affects almost every important organ system in the body including the heart, kidney, liver, brain, and the gut. You thought you would just put the patient on the ventilator!

70. Briefly explain the negative effects of PPV on the heart.

_____

71. Why can patients with stiff lungs such as ARDS tolerate higher levels of PEEP in terms of the effect on heart and

blood vessels? _____

72. Normal patients can easily compensate for moderate increases in airway pressure. What patients are especially sensitive to the cardiovascular effects of PPV?

_____

73. Fluids can help a patient tolerate ventilation and so can drugs. Which drug would you use to treat

A. Low cardiac index _____

B. Low blood pressure _____

74. How can you use the ventilator to temporarily manage increased ICP?

_____

75. Explain the mechanism behind the drop in urine output in ventilated patients.

A. Direct _____

B. Indirect _____

76. There is a high incidence in GI bleeding in ventilator patients usually due to stress ulceration of the gastric mucosa. Name the two pharmacologic agents used to protect the GI tract.

A. Cytoprotective _____

B. Acid suppression _____

77. ICP is not the only CNS problem associated with mechanical ventilation. The ICU experience results in fear, anxiety, and pain. Name one sedative and one analgesic that may help.

   A. Acute sedation _____

   B. Long-term management of anxiety _____

   C. Analgesics

      1. Hemodynamically stable _____

      2. Unstable _____

We'd like to get the patient to level 2 or 3 on the Ramsay Scale.

DOWN IN THE VALI

Everything to do with the ventilator, circuit, and the airway, of course. I won't bore you with the details—just highlight some things that might be important on your board exams.

78. Chest cuirass and ponch-type negative-pressure ventilators are still used in some settings. Hypoventilation can result from what two problems?

   A. _____

   B. _____

79. Positive-pressure ventilation has long been associated with barotrauma. List three of the clinical signs of pneumothorax.

   A. Chest motion _____

   B. Percussion note _____

   C. Breath sounds _____

80. Tension pneumothorax is life-threatening in a ventilated patient. How and where is this treated?
   A. How?

   B. Where in the chest?

81. What is volutrauma and how is it prevented?

82. Air-trapping in ventilator patients can result in what condition?

_____

83. Oxygen toxicity may damage lung tissue. Every effort should be made to reduce the F_{IO_2} to what value?

_____

84. List three ways to reduce the risk of ventilator-associated pneumonias.

A. Positioning _____

B. Nebulizers or MDIs _____

C. Reduce condensates _____

And, of course, the essential antiinfection procedure . . .

CHAPTER HIGHLIGHTS

Fill in the blanks, thanks.

85. Positive physiologic effects of PPV include improved _____ and ventilation, and decreased

_____ of breathing.

86. No single _____ pattern has been demonstrated to be more physiologically effective than another.

87. Research indicates better ventilator synchrony and gas exchange with the _____ flow

pattern than the _____ flow pattern.

88. _____-triggering appears to be a better choice than _____-triggering when it is available on the ventilator.

89. PEEP is applied to restore _____ in restrictive disease and _____ the airways in obstructive disease.

90. PEEP allows the RCP to decrease the _____, thereby avoiding the complications of _____ toxicity.

91. Positive pressure ventilation is detrimental to the $\dot{V}/\dot{Q}$ ratio primarily by shifting _____ to areas that are less _____.

92. PPV may decrease venous _____ and cardiac _____.

93. PPV may cause hepatic and gastrointestinal malfunction primarily due to decreased _____ of those _____ beds.

CASE STUDIES

Case 1, Part 1

A trauma patient is stabilized after a motor vehicle accident. He is intubated and transported to the ICU, where you place him on a ventilator. As soon as you put him on the machine, his blood pressure falls dramatically.

94. What should you do (right away!)?

_____

95. What is the most likely cause of hypotension in a trauma patient who has been placed on positive-pressure ventilation? _____

Case 1, Part 2

Two days later, the patient has developed poor lung compliance and hypoxemia associated with noncardiogenic pulmonary edema (ARDS). He is being ventilated on VC-CMV, 12,900, +15 cm H_2O PEEP, and FIO_2 70%. Blood gases show pH 7.37, $PaCO_2$ 38, and PaO_2 55. Peak inspiratory pressure is 60 cm H_2O, and plateau pressure is 50 cm H_2O.

96. There are two serious problems here. Identify them.

A. Serious problem No. 1 _____

B. Serious problem No. 2 _____

97. What change(s) in ventilator strategy would you suggest?
    A. Problem No. 1

    B. Problem No. 2

Not much, actually. Nothing new, that is. Of course you need to be able to recognize the harmful effects of PPV. If the patient develops a pneumothorax, you would assess, recognize, and recommend treatment. Chapter 40 reviews each of the common modes of ventilation, and the board exams are quite clear that you should be familiar with them, as I mentioned in Chapter 39. Let's move on.

FOOD FOR THOUGHT

98. If the newest modes of ventilation are not proven to alter patient outcomes, why should we use them?

99. Patients on ventilators have a really high incidence of GI bleeding. Why is GI bleeding such a big deal to RTs?

- One place you might look is www.ards.org. This sight has information in lay terms and has some application if you'd like to learn more about managing this condition.
- For a more scientific approach, there is ARDSNet at www.ardsnet.org.
- Or you can get general info at www.emedicine.com/emerg/topic788.htm.

Oh, I could go on and on. but you are getting sleepy, very sleepy, now you will go to sleep, and when you wake up you will remember the physiology of ventilator support.

44 Initiating and Adjusting Ventilatory Support

Paralyze resistance with persistence.
Woody Hayes

A long time ago, in an ICU far, far away, we used a one-size-fits-all approach to mechanical ventilation. It was easier that way, but we did not realize how this could harm the patient. Chapter 44 is one of the best and most important chapters in Egan's because it details a clear-cut plan for initiating and managing the ventilator in terms of what's wrong with the patient (i.e., custom-made ventilation). The concept of pathophysiology-based mechanical ventilation is so important the NBRC included an article on the concept in their newsletter. So, whether you are talking about board exams or clinical practice, it's the way to go.

FIRST THINGS FIRST

I'll share my approach and you can see if it works for you. First, I read the chapter and highlighted key points with one of those fluorescent yellow markers. It took 2 hours and four cups of coffee. Next, I mapped out a plan. Looks like this:

- **Step One.** Decide whether to use positive or negative pressure. Easy because negative pressure is pretty much used for long-term neuromuscular problems and chest wall disorders. Only used in the hospital if the patient brings it in.
- **Step Two.** Full ventilator support, or partial support? I'll pick full support if the patient is apneic or paralyzed by drugs, or exhausted from struggling to breathe. I'll remember to use this for a short period of time to avoid muscle atrophy. Partial support is good for patients with a drive to breathe, those being weaned, or to minimize adverse effects of positive pressure.
- **Step Three.** Select volume or pressure control. Volume control works pretty well and is especially good when you want to control minute ventilation and $Paco_2$. Pressure control is great when you need to keep the pressures low to prevent lung injury with ARDS or ALI. PC is also good when you want to let the patient control the flow and volumes. It's more comfortable and flexible.
- **Step Four.** Pick a mode. Assist-control (CMV) and SIMV are the most common and best understood of all the modes. Pressure support is almost always added to SIMV to help reduce work of breathing.
- **Step Five.** Select settings for ventilation. Rate, volume, Fio_2, and PEEP should be set according to pathophysiology. Alarm settings are pretty standardized.
- **Step Six.** Assess the patient after you initiate your choices. Make changes to meet your goals for the patient. Comfort and synchrony, gas exchange and hemodynamics. That's what you want to look at.

WORD WIZARD

I feel really bad about all these acronyms . . . lucky for you we already covered every one of these babies. Besides, I'm saving my strength for vocabulary in Chapter 45.

CASE STUDIES

We're nearing the end of this book. At this point, I think you would benefit from less traditional workbook questions and fill-in problems. Let's go right to the cases and find out if you understand how to initiate and adjust ventilatory support. I found five basic types of lungs and 10 specific disorders that make up almost every case of mechanical ventilation.

Table 44-7 on page 1060 is dynamite! It covers most of the bases. Your five basic types of lungs are

- Normal lungs—like a young OD patient: 8 to 10 ml/kg for tidal volume
- Normal lungs—like a neuromuscular patient: 10 to 12 ml/kg for tidal volume

- Obstructed lungs—like acute exacerbation of COPD or asthma: 8 to 10 ml/kg for tidal volume
- Stiff lungs—like ARDS/ALI: 6 to 8 ml/kg for tidal volume. Can go lower to keep pressures down.
- Kids get 8 to 10 for tidal volume depending on age; on boards, usually 10.

Let's get to work! You will need Tables 44-6, 44-7, and 44-8 to help with the cases. Boxes 44-8 and 44-15 are good, too. You will also need information from other chapters, like airway management, acid-base, and monitoring and management!

Case 1

A 5 foot 5 inch, 60-kg (132-lb) young woman attempted suicide by drug overdose. She is unconscious and breathing slowly and shallowly. The emergency physician elects to intubate this patient.

1. What size ET tube would be appropriate for an adult female?
   - A. 6.0-mm inside diameter
   - B. 7.0-mm outside diameter
   - C. 7.5-mm inside diameter
   - D. 8.0-mm inside diameter

2. In the emergency setting, how will you assess proper tube placement?
   - I. Auscultate the chest.
   - II. Auscultate the epigastrium.
   - III. Attach an exhaled O_2 monitor.
   - IV. Observe chest wall motion.
     - A. I and II
     - B. I and III
     - C. II, III, and IV
     - D. I, II, and IV

After the intubation is completed, a small amount of white secretions are suctioned from the airway. The physician requests a room air ABG at this point. Results show

pH	7.25
$Paco_2$	60 mm Hg
Pao_2	55 mm Hg
HCO_3^-	26 mEq/L

Vital signs are	
HR	115
BP	125/75
RR	26
Temp	37

A chest film is taken, which reveals the tip of the endotracheal tube to be 4 cm above the carina with no sign of a pneumothorax.

3. What action would you recommend in regard to the ET tube placement?
   - A. Advance the tube 2 to 3 cm.
   - B. Withdraw the tube 2 to 3 cm.
   - C. Maintain current placement.
   - D. Remove the tube and insert a laryngeal mask airway.

4. The ABG results are interpreted as _____.
   - A. metabolic acidosis with severe hypoxemia
   - B. respiratory acidosis with moderate hypoxemia
   - C. partially compensated respiratory alkalosis with mild hypoxemia
   - D. partially compensated metabolic alkalosis with moderate hypoxemia

The patient is transported to the ICU. The physician requests that you initiate mechanical ventilation.

5. Calculate ideal body weight. My preferred formula for women is 105 + 5 (height − 60). The answer will be in pounds, and you need to divide by 2.2 to convert to kilograms. Box 44-8 uses 45.5 + 2.3 (height in inches − 60) to get the answer in kilograms. The answers will be slightly different but this won't change outcomes.
   A. 45 kg
   B. 59 kg
   C. 65 kg
   D. 130 kg

6. Which of the following volumes would you recommend?
   A. 400 ml
   B. 600 ml
   C. 720 ml
   D. 1000 ml

7. What mode and rate would you select?
   A. VC-IMV, 18
   B. VC-CMV, 12
   C. VC-IMV, 6
   D. VC-CMV, 8

8. What type of humidification system would you recommend for this patient?
   A. heated wick humidifier set at 35°C
   B. HME
   C. heated passover humidifier
   D. bubble humidifier

One week later, Ms. Robertson is alert and weaning is initiated. When the rate is decreased to 5, however, the patient's spontaneous respiratory rate rises to 30 and tidal volumes drop to 200 ml.

9. To help resolve this problem you might recommend initiation of _____.
   A. CMV
   B. AC
   C. PSV
   D. APRV

Case 2

Paramedics bring a 5 foot 2 inch, 50-kg (110-lb) 65-year-old woman with a history of COPD to the emergency department for treatment of dyspnea. She is wearing a nasal cannula set at 2 L/min. ABGs are drawn. Results show:

pH	7.30
$Paco_2$	70 mm Hg
Pao_2	45 mm Hg
HCO_3^-	34 mEq/L

Vital signs are
HR	100
BP	100/70
RR	34
Temp	39

Noninvasive positive pressure breathing is attempted with bilevel ventilation, but the patient is unable to tolerate the mask and fights the system. A decision is made to intubate and initiate mechanical ventilation. Ms. Peral is given a small amount of sedation and intubated nasally with a 6.5-mm ID tube. Settings are:

Mode	VC-SIMV
Rate	10
V_T	400 ml
FIO_2	28%
PEEP	0
Peak flow	20 LPM
Flow pattern	Decelerating ramp
Sensitivity	1.5 cm H_2O below baseline

10. How long should you wait before drawing an ABG to assess the results of these settings?
    A. 5 minutes
    B. 20 minutes
    C. 40 minutes
    D. 60 minutes

11. What is the maximum desirable plateau pressure during mechanical ventilation?
    A. 15 cm H_2O
    B. 25 cm H_2O
    C. 30 cm H_2O
    D. 40 cm H_2O

During your first ventilator check the following observations are made.

PIP	40 cm H_2O
Plateau	35 cm H_2O
Set rate	10
Total rate	30
Exhaled V_T	425 ml
Spontaneous V_T	100 ml
I:E ratio	1:1.5

12. What high pressure alarm limit should you set?
    A. 35 cm H_2O
    B. 45 cm H_2O
    C. 50 cm H_2O
    D. 65 cm H_2O

13. What value should you set for the low minute ventilation alarm?
    A. 3.5 L
    B. 6.0 L
    C. 7.2 L
    D. 8.0 L

14. Which of the following would result in a lower work of breathing for this patient?
    I.   addition of 100 ml mechanical deadspace
    II. initiation of PSV at 5 cm H_2O
    III. changing to flow-triggering 2 L/min
    IV. addition of 10 cm H_2O PEEP
        A. I and II only
        B. II and III only
        C. I and III only
        D. II, III, and IV

15. What action should you take to increase the I:E ratio?
    A. Increase the peak flow.
    B. Increase the tidal volume.
    C. Increase the set rate.
    D. Increase the FIO_2.

16. What I:E ratio would provide sufficient time for exhalation and prevent auto-PEEP in this COPD patient?
    A. 1:1
    B. 1:2
    C. 1:4
    D. 1:10

A 5 foot 6 inch woman who weighs 100 kg (220 lb) is in the ICU following surgery for multiple injuries sustained in a motor vehicle accident. She has an arterial line and a pulmonary artery catheter in place. Her chest radiograph shows bilateral infiltrates consistent with ARDS. The ET tube is in good position.

Current ventilator settings are

Mode	Volume-controlled CMV
V_T	1000
Rate	12
FIO_2	0.70
PEEP	5 cm H_2O
Peak flow	60 L/min, decelerating ramp
Sensitivity	1.0 cm H_2O below baseline

17. What is this patient's approximate ideal body weight?
    A. 50 kg
    B. 60 kg
    C. 80 kg
    D. 100 kg

18. What initial tidal volume would you recommend to prevent further lung injury?
    A. 480 ml
    B. 600 ml
    C. 720 ml
    D. Maintain current setting

The following data are obtained:

HR	110, NSR with occasional PVCs
BP	110/75 mm Hg
SpO_2	88%
PA	38/8 mm Hg
PCWP	12 mm Hg
CO	5.8 L/min
SvO_2	59%

19. With regard to the patient's oxygenation, what action would you recommend?
    A. Increase the FIO_2.
    B. Increase the PEEP.
    C. Add mechanical deadspace.
    D. Maintain current settings.

A PEEP trial is conducted with the following results.

PEEP	Cstat	PaO_2	CO
5	22	57	5.8
10	25	66	5.7
15	30	72	5.9
20	25	77	5.2
25	22	85	4.8

475

20. What PEEP level would you recommend?
    A. 5
    B. 10
    C. 15
    D. 20
    E. 25

Ms. Cooler continues to deteriorate over the next 2 days. Her compliance and Pao_2 have decreased, while PIP has increased to 60 cm H_2O to maintain a normal $Paco_2$.

21. Which of the following ventilator modes could be considered as alternatives?
    I.   pressure-control CMV
    II.   SIMV volume control
    III. APRV
    IV.   CSV-CPAP
        A. I and III only
        B. II and III only
        C. II and IV only
        D. I and IV only

22. Which of these techniques are used with ARDS to reduce lung injury or improve oxygenation?
    I.   expiratory retard
    II.   prone positioning
    III. permissive hypercapnia
    IV.   unilateral lung ventilation
        A. I and II
        B. II and III
        C. I and IV
        D. III and IV

Case 4

A respiratory student who fell down the stairs while reading *Egan's* suffered a closed-head injury. The student is 5 feet 5 inches tall and weighs 60 kg. ICP and blood pressure are elevated. She is being ventilated with these settings.

Mode	VC-CMV
Rate	12
V_T	600
Fio_2	.30
PEEP	0

Blood gases on these settings are

pH	7.40
$Paco_2$	40
Pao_2	55
HCO_3^-	24

23. This blood gas should be interpreted as _____.
    A. normal with moderate hypoxemia
    B. respiratory alkalosis with mild hypoxemia
    C. compensated respiratory acidosis with severe hypoxemia
    D. compensated metabolic alkalosis with moderate hypoxemia

24. With regard to the oxygenation, what change would you suggest?
    A. Increase the PEEP.
    B. Increase the rate.
    C. Change to APRV.
    D. Increase the Fio_2.

476

25. With regard to the ventilation, what change would you suggest?
    A. Increase the rate.
    B. Increase the tidal volume.
    C. Change to SIMV.
    D. Add mechanical deadspace.

26. What is the formula for calculating the rate needed to produce a desired change in $Paco_2$?
    A. $Paco_2$ measured × set rate ÷ $Paco_2$ desired
    B. $Paco_2$ desired × set rate ÷ $Paco_2$ measured
    C. $Paco_2$ measured × $Paco_2$ desired ÷ set rate
    D. $Paco_2$ measured × Pao_2 measured ÷ set rate

27. What rate would you suggest for this patient if the desired $Paco_2$ is 30 mm Hg?
    A. 8
    B. 10
    C. 14
    D. 16

28. How long should you maintain a head injury patient in a hyperventilated state? (Hint: Try Chapter 43.)
    A. 2 to 4 hours
    B. 6 to 8 hours
    C. 12 to 24 hours
    D. 24 to 48 hours

Case 5

A 5 foot 7 inch 27-year-old woman who weighs 140 lb with a long history of asthma including previous intubation and mechanical ventilation presents in the ED with high-pitched, diffuse wheezing. She is barely able to talk due to her dsypnea. She has not responded to two consecutive SVN treatments with 5 mg of albuterol and 0.5 mg of Atrovent. Peak flows are not measurable and SpO_2 is 92% on 2 L via nasal cannula. She is using her accessory muscles to breathe and has some intercostal retractions on inspiration. She is started on IV SoluMedrol, continuous bronchodilator therapy, and ECG monitoring. One hour later, she is lethargic and breath sounds are virtually absent. You draw an ABG with the following results:

pH	7.29
$Paco_2$	55 mm Hg
Pao_2	64 mm Hg
HCO_3^-	24 mmol
Sao_2	90%

29. What action would you recommend at this time?
    A. continuation of present therapy
    B. oral intubation with 7.5 ET tube and mechanical ventilation
    C. trial of NIPPV via bilevel mask ventilation
    D. tracheostomy and mechanical ventilation

30. The emergency physician elects to move the patient to the MICU as soon as she is stabilized. You assist in the transport. In the ICU, you are asked to set up the ventilator. You would select:
    A. VC-SIMV 14, 400, 0.40 Fio_2, +3 PEEP, +5 PSV
    B. VC-CMV 12, 750, +5 PEEP, 0.40 Fio_2
    C. APRV high PEEP 30, low PEEP 20, 0.60 Fio_2, 1 second release time
    D. CPAP (CSV) +10 PEEP, 0.30 Fio_2

31. What pharmacologic agent is recommended at this time?
    A. inhaled corticosteroids
    B. sedation with midazolam
    C. paralysis with tubocurarine
    D. respiratory stimulus with doxapram

32. Bronchodilator therapy is also indicated. How will you need to adjust the dosage for administration to a ventilated patient?
    A. Give the standard dose.
    B. Increase the dose to 2 to 4 times normal amount.
    C. Decrease the dose by half the normal amount.
    D. Give the standard dose intravenously.

33. Which of the following are major concerns when ventilating severe asthmatics?
    I. pulmonary barotrauma
    II. development of auto-PEEP
    III. ventilator asynchrony
    IV. high airway pressures
        A. I and II
        B. I, III, and IV
        C. II, III, and IV
        D. I, II, III, and IV

34. An appropriate peak flow and flow pattern for this patient would include
    A. 40 L/min with a decelerating flow waveform
    B. 20 L/min with a square flow waveform
    C. 100 L/min with a sinewave flow pattern
    D. 50 L/min with an accelerating flow waveform

35. What alteration to the mode of ventilation might be useful to prevent barotrauma and improve comfort?
    A. addition of mechanical deadspace
    B. using a heated humidifier
    C. switching to pressure control
    D. utilizing inverse ratio ventilation

Case 6

A 6 foot, 176-lb 66-year-old man has been brought to the SICU following coronary artery bypass graft surgery. He has no history of lung disease. He is intubated with a No. 8 oral ET tube. The anesthesiologist asks you to select ventilator settings.

36. What tidal volume is appropriate for this postoperative patient?
    A. 500 ml
    B. 650 ml
    C. 800 ml
    D. 950 ml

37. Why should you add a small amount of PEEP to the system?
    A. to prevent auto-PEEP
    B. to prevent atelectasis
    C. to prevent cardiogenic pulmonary edema
    D. to prevent barotrauma

38. What is your primary goal for this patient?
    A. Prevent ventilator-associated barotrauma.
    B. Prevent ventilator-associated pneumonia.
    C. Control air-trapping.
    D. Wean and extubate as quickly as possible.

Okay, we did six of the common situations you need to be able to manage. The other three are:

Unilateral Lung Disease

39. What position is useful in this type of patient? What special form of ventilation can be used?

    A.   Position

    B.   Special form of ventilation

Neuromuscular Disorders

40. What adjustment to tidal volume might be made?

CHF

41. When your patient is in CHF, he or she has pulmonary edema. What adjustment may help improve oxygenation and work of breathing? What are the choices besides intubation?

WHAT DOES THE NBRC SAY?

The Examination Matrix is quite clear on this subject. You should be able to:
- Initiate and adjust ventilators when settings are specified (and when they're not)
- Initiate and adjust all the primary modes like CMV and IMV
- Select appropriate tidal volume, minute volume, and respiratory rate

You should also know when to modify
- Mode
- Tidal volume
- F_{IO_2}
- Inspiratory plateau
- PEEP and CPAP levels
- Pressure support and pressure control
- Alarm settings
- Mechanical deadspace
- Mean airway pressure
- Inverse ratio ventilation

If you can understand and apply the material in this chapter, you are well on your way to passing your boards and becoming a great therapist!

FOOD FOR THOUGHT

42. What are the two most common ventilator strategies currently in use in the United States?

43. What are the common ventilator modes (and adjuncts like PEEP, PSV, etc.) where you are training or working?

44. How can you determine correct pressure and inspiratory time when you switch from volume-controlled to pressure-controlled ventilation?

One way to approach this on the Internet is to search for the specific diseases you are interested in "mechanical ventilation of COPD patients."

- I found this overview at www.ahrq.gov/clinic/epcsums/copdsum.htm.
- Or you might try www.emedicine.com/emerg/topic788.htm.
- Of course, this is only a summary. To get the real info, you will need to get the journal *Respiratory Care* for March and April 2002. They held a 2-day conference on mechanical ventilation with the world's greatest experts! I can't think of a better way for you to supplement the material in Chapter 44 than to read these two journals. You can't go wrong with this one.
- Or you can do a general search on "ventilator management." One site I found was ventworld.com. They have some case studies at www.ventworld.com/education/casestudies.asp.
- Finally, you might consider another way to use the computer to learn. Most of the schools have good collections of clinical simulations on CD-ROM. These are great ways to study, learn, and test your knowledge. Oh, yeah, good for getting ready for the Clinical Simulation Exams, too!

45 Noninvasive Positive Pressure Ventilation

Thou knows't the mask of night is on my face.
William Shakespeare

Noninvasive positive-pressure ventilation (NPPV) by mask has been used in home care for many years, especially in the treatment of sleep-disordered breathing. Other forms of noninvasive ventilation like rocking beds and pneumobelts have been around since the 1930s. In the 1970s and 1980s, we ventilated many a patient with IPPB and mask to try to avoid intubation. But it was not until 1989 that serious efforts were made to use NPPV as a means of treating acute respiratory failure. Increased technology in NPPV ventilators and advances in mask designs have enabled the modern respiratory therapist to put noninvasive ventilation on the front lines of acute respiratory care in the management of COPD, asthma, and cardiogenic pulmonary edema. NPPV is even used in the chronic care setting to relieve symptoms of hypoventilation and improve quality of life.

WORD WIZARD

Chapter 45 has a few new or strange words you might not recognize. We've been looking for less invasive ways to help people breathe since the first invasive airway management with tracheostomy tubes was performed 350 years ago. In the 1930s a rubber inflatable device called a _____ was strapped to the abdomen to help patients with _____ disease to help move the diaphragm. Later, a _____ bed was designed to help with weaning. Motion _____ was a hazard of the bed. Negative pressure ventilators like the _____ lung were used to treat polio patients but were large and bulky. A chest _____ covers only the chest and looks like a turtle shell. Positive pressure devices became popular in the 1980's. _____, or inspiratory positive airway pressure helps to inflate the lung during inspiration. Positive pressure devices can be used at home to treat nocturnal _____, or they can be used in place of more invasive methods in the ED or the ICU.

GOALS AND INDICATIONS

1. Four important goals of NIPPV in the acute care setting are to

   A. Avoid _____

   B. Improve _____

   C. Decrease _____

   D. Relieve _____

2. In the acute care setting, NIPPV is indicated for nine conditions. Name at least five.

   A. _____

   B. _____

   C. _____

   D. _____

   E. _____

483

3. NIPPV is also indicated for the chronic care setting. List three conditions:

A. _____

B. _____

C. _____

4. All COPD patients should be evaluated for NPPV as an alternative to what two therapies?

_____

5. Patients with status asthmaticus suffer a high degree of complications when intubated and mechanically ventilated. What were the results of Meduri's study on NPPV in treating status asthmaticus?

_____

6. Compare mask CPAP to mask ventilation in the treatment of acute cardiogenic pulmonary edema. When does NPPV outperform CPAP? Which one is first-line therapy?

_____

7. NPPV should be used for what group of patients with community-acquired pneumonia?

_____

8. Should NPPV be used to treat hypoxemic respiratory failure? How much time do you have?

9. List four other indications for noninvasive ventilation in the acute care setting.

A. _____

B. _____

C. _____

D. _____

10. What three criteria does the "Rule of Thumb" say should be met before implementing NPPV in acute respiratory failure?

A. _____

B. _____

C. _____

SELECTION AND EXCLUSION CRITERIA

11. How is the need for ventilatory assistance established?

A. Respiratory rate _____

B. Dyspnea _____

C. $Paco_2$ _____

D. pH _____

E. P/F ratio _____

12. A lot of patients might benefit from NPPV but are excluded because we know it won't work for them. Name at least four of these criteria.

A. _____

B. _____

C. _____

D. _____

Bottom line: The acute respiratory failure must be reversible within a few days!

13. Once you put the patient on the noninvasive ventilator there are some predictors of success that can be measured. Give the values for:

A. Respiratory acidosis _____

B. pH _____

C. Improvement in gas exchange _____

D. RR and HR _____

TOOLS OF THE TRADE

Masks

You get to play with a lot of masks in noninvasive ventilation: nasal, full-face, and total face.

14. Which type of mask is better tolerated? Which one makes a better seal?

_____

15. How can you pick the right mask size—besides plain ol' trial and error?

_____

16. The oral mask has a lot of potential problems. List at least four.

A. _____

B. _____

C. _____

D. _____

17. Despite all the problems with face masks, what huge advantage do they have in the critical care setting?

_____

Ventilators

Positive-pressure ventilators to ventilate critically ill patients via ET usually need a sealed system to operate. Noninvasive ventilators are made to work with leaks. It will help if you understand the following terms:
- CPAP—breathing at an elevated baseline pressure during inspiration and exhalation
- EPAP—elevated pressure at exhalation
- IPAP—elevated pressure during inspiration

Figure 45-14 reproduced here shows a picture of these three concepts.

FIGURE 45-1 *A,* CPAP of 5 cm H_2O with a patient breathing spontaneously and the resulting tidal volume. *B,* Patient-triggered breath during NPPV with pressure support of 5 cm H_2O (IPAP of 10 cm H_2O) and PEEP (EPAP) of 5 cm H_2O and the resulting tidal volume. *C,* Pressure support has been increased to 10 cm H_2O (IPAP 15 cm H_2O). The corresponding increase in tidal volume is evident. *D,* Pressure support is again 5 cm H_2O but PEEP (EPAP) has been increased to 10 cm H_2O. Thus, the IPAP is still 15 cm H_2O. The corresponding decrease in tidal volume is evident.

18. What happens to tidal volume when you increase the EPAP without increasing the IPAP?

_____

19. What are some of the problems with using standard critical care ventilators to deliver mask ventilation? What new mode may help?

START ME UP

Once you've chosen a ventilator and a mask that fits, you have to select mode and settings just like you did for invasive mechanical ventilation.

20. How should you position the patient?

_____

21. How should you prepare the patient for the experience?

22. Give initial settings for use with a noninvasive ventilator

    A. IPAP/ventilatory pressure: _____

    B. EPAP/PEEP: _____

23. What pressure could open the esophagus?

    A. Esophagus opens at _____

    B. Put in an NG tube and _____

24. You won't be setting a tidal volume, but you still want a good one. What volume would you like to achieve? Which control do you increase if the volume is too low?

    A. Goal: _____

    B. Adjust: _____

Chapter **45** **Noninvasive Positive Pressure Ventilation**

25. What two adjustments can be made to improve oxygenation?

Table 45-1 on page 1109 gives a clear overview of what controls to manipulate to get the results you need. You have to do a little fine-tuning to make this work. Don't forget to encourage and reassure the patient.

26. See if you have the basic idea.

    A. Increase _____ to increase tidal volume.

    B. Increase _____ to improve oxygenation and FRC.

    C. Set the rate at _____ and increase the rate to decrease _____.

27. While you can initiate NPPV anywhere, what unit should the patient be in while they are on NPPV?

WHAT COULD GO WRONG?

28. Use Table 45-2 on page 1110 to help you find out what could go wrong and how to fix it!

	Side Effect	Occurrence	Remedy
Masks			
A.	Discomfort		
B.	Claustrophobia		
C.	Skin breakdown		
Flow			
D.	Congestion		
E.	Sinus pain		
F.	Dryness		
G.	Air leaks		
Bad stuff			
H.	Aspiration		
I.	Low blood pressure		
J.	Pneumothorax		

This subject is not a big part of the exams because it is relatively new. I expect to see a growing number of questions in the future. Here's what the matrix says you should know:

- CPAP devices—mask, nasal, or bi-level
- Patient breathing circuits—noninvasive ventilation
- Mechanical ventilation—adjust noninvasive positive pressure ventilation

They don't tell you much, do they? So, for the exams, it's really three things:

- Do you know when to recommend a trial of NIPPV?
- Can you state the initial vent settings?
- What should you change if O_2 is low? If CO_2 is high?

Questions 29-31 refer the following scenario. Circle the best answer.

A 70-year-old patient with COPD does not wish to be intubated and has an advanced directive supporting his wishes. The patient is admitted to the Medical ICU in respiratory failure. ABGs reveal: pH 7.25 $Paco_2$ 66 Pao_2 50.

29. What mode of therapy would the respiratory therapist recommend in this situation?
    A. nasal cannula at 6 L/min
    B. nonrebreathing mask at 10 L/min
    C. continuous positive airway pressure
    D. noninvasive positive pressure ventilation

30. NPPV is initiated on spontaneous mode with IPAP of 8 cm H_2O and EPAP of 2 cm H_2O. ABG;'s reveal: pH 7.29 $Paco_2$ 58 Pao_2 52 HCO_3 30. The respiratory therapist should recommend what change in regard to the carbon dioxide levels?
    A. Increase the respiratory rate setting.
    B. Increase the tidal volume setting.
    C. Increase the IPAP.
    D. Increase the EPAP.

31. What should the RT recommend to improve oxygenation?
    A. Increase the respiratory rate setting.
    B. Increase the tidal volume setting.
    C. Increase the IPAP.
    D. Increase the EPAP.

INFORMATION AGE

Of course, the Internet is good for this subject because it is hot, hot, hot. You could Google the term "NPPV" and get 80,000 hits in less than a second, BUT . . . you'll have too much information.

- A great source is our own *Respiratory Care*. Go to AARC.org and you'll want to look for the November 2000 issue, which is devoted to the subject of NPPV at the end of life. You'll find a lot more as you go along through the *Respiratory Care* journal.
- University Hospital in Newark, NJ, has the Center for Noninvasive Ventilation: www.theuniversityhospital.com/ventilation/index.html.

46 Monitoring and Management of the Patient in the Intensive Care Unit

> *The best monitor is a knowledgeable, observant and dedicated healthcare professional.*
>
> Donald F. Egan, MD

You didn't think I'd finish this book without a quote from Dr. Egan, did you? Truer words were never spoken. ICU monitoring has reached a level of complexity that is as dazzling as it is expensive. The amount of data available to the critical care clinician is staggering. The key to success in this endeavor is to combine appropriate information gathering with sound clinical assessment. You can't learn that from a book! What you can do is learn the basics: normal values, waveforms, terms, and most common problems and situations you will encounter. When you go out into the clinical setting you can learn to apply this new information. I'm going to make you work hard in this chapter, but then you are near the end of the book and you need to put this all together.

WORD WIZARD

Match these key terms to the definitions that follow.

Terms	Definitions
1. _____ afterload	A. pressure the ventricle has to contract against
2. _____ Swan-Ganz catheter	B. pressure stretching the ventricle at the onset of contraction
3. _____ Q_S/Q_T	C. unreal events seen on monitors often caused by movement
4. _____ Apache score	D. popular system for measuring neurologic impairment
5. _____ V_D/V_T	E. hemodynamic monitoring device placed in the pulmonary artery
6. _____ capnography	F. amount of wasted ventilation per breath
7. _____ preload	G. noninvasive measurement of carbon dioxide
8. _____ capnometry	H. popular acute illness index
9. _____ Glasgow Coma Scale score	I. measuring carbon dioxide at the airway
10. _____ artifacts	J. physiologic shunt

RESPIRATORY MONITORING

Quick, memorize Table 46-1 on page 1129! Just kidding, you probably already know this stuff. Right?

11. Gas exchange at the lung is best monitored by what test? What test is best for immediate continuous assessment of oxygenation?

    A. Gas exchange _____

    B. Continuous _____

12. Tissue oxygenation depends on seven factors. That's a lot more complicated than just measuring one number like blood oxygen saturation. List four of these factors and give the correct abbreviation.

A. _____

B. _____

C. _____

D. _____

13. What is the most serious clinical limitation of using pulse oximetry to assess the respiratory status?

_____

14. Pulse oximetry is affected by lots of factors. Name four. (See Box 46-2 on page 1120.)

A. _____

B. _____

C. _____

D. _____

15. What is the value for normal oxygen consumption? _____

16. State the Fick equation for cardiac output (Q_T—this bad boy might show up on your boards).

_____

17. Pao_2/Fio_2 ratio is the most reliable index of gas exchange. What is the normal ratio? What ratio suggests ALI? ARDS?

A. Normal _____

B. ALI _____

C. ARDS _____

18. The most accurate and reliable measure of pulmonary oxygenation efficiency is direct calculation of shunt. State the classic shunt equation.

$Q_s/Q_T =$ _____

19. What two blood gas samples are needed to calculate shunt?

    A. _____

    B. _____

Be sure to check out the Murray Lung Score in Box 46-3 on page 1122. It is a simple, inexpensive way to quantify lung dysfunction.

MONITORING VENTILATION

20. What is the gold standard for assessing the adequacy of ventilation?

    _____

21. Efficiency of ventilation is assessed by measuring physiologic dead space. State the modified Bohr equation. (Another testing favorite!)

    $V_D/V_T =$ _____

22. List the normal and critical values for deadspace–to–tidal volume ratio.

    A. Normal   _____   _____

    B. Critical is >_____ and predicts failure to wean.

23. What is the formula for measuring minute ventilation? (Wow, this chapter is packed with things you might expect to see on your road to credentialing.)

    _____

24. What is the difference between arterial and end-tidal CO_2 in normal subjects?

    _____

25. Capnometry is extremely useful in two emergency situations. Name them.

    A. _____

    B. _____

26. What test has to be done to validate the CO_2 value of the capnometer?

    _____

27. Name the parts of the normal capnograpnic tracing seen here.

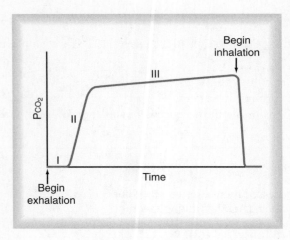

Time-based capnograph.

A. I _____

B. II _____

C. III _____

MONITORING CHEST WALL MECHANICS

28. The pressure volume curve is a ventilator graphic that can show compliance and lower inflection points. The lower inflection point may help you set what ventilator parameter?

_____

29. The upper inflection point may point out what problem?

_____

Compliance

30. Compliance shows stiffness of the lungs. What is the formula for calculating compliance? (Be sure to subtract PEEP.)

C = Change in _____ / change in _____ or (V_T/P_{plat} − PEEP)

31. What is normal compliance?

_____

32. Low compliance on a patient with ARDS may drop to what values?

_____

Resistance

33. What is the formula for calculating airway resistance?

   Raw = _____

34. What is normal airway resistance? What's normal for a ventilated patient?

   A. Normal _____

   B. Ventilated patients _____

35. Effects of what therapy can be measured by resistance changes?

   _____

Peak and Plateau Pressures

36. What is the safe maximum value for peak pressure? _____

37. What are the maximum safe plateau pressures? _____

When peak pressures rise, it is due to either increased resistance or decreased compliance. Take a look at the peak and plateau pressures. When they move up together, the problem is compliance. When the peak pressure goes up and the plateau stays the same, the problem is airway resistance. Box 46-7 on page 1125 gives common clinical conditions that alter compliance and resistance.

Auto-PEEP

Auto-PEEP occurs when lungs don't empty well (obstructive disease) or when there is a high minute ventilation (ARDS). It causes all kinds of problems from difficulty in triggering the ventilator to hemodynamic compromise.

38. What ventilator maneuver unmasks auto-PEEP?

   _____

Work of Breathing

Research hospitals have several methods of measuring work of breathing including the use of esophageal balloons.

39. The simplest way to monitor work of breathing is to monitor the patient's _____

   breathing rate, _____, and the f/V_T ratio.

40. What score for rapid shallow breathing index is a good predictor of weaning success?

   _____

Please note that higher values are used in older patients.

MONITORING MUSCLE STRENGTH

41. What two values are measured at the bedside?

   A. _____

   B. _____

42. What is a normal VC? What VC indicates poor muscle strength?

    A. Normal _____

    B. Poor _____

43. What are the benefits of measuring MIP compared to VC?

    A. _____

    B. _____

44. How long should you measure MIP? _____

45. Why should you use one-way valves when you measure MIP?

MONITORING THE PATIENT–VENTILATOR SYSTEM

Most hospitals require ventilator checks every 2 hours. You need to record a number of values, assess the patient, and evaluate the information gathered so you can make any necessary changes.

46. Briefly discuss the five areas you need to check.

    A. Airway _____

    B. Vent settings _____

    C. Gas exchange _____

    D. Respiratory mechanics _____

    E. Alarms _____

47. Ventilator graphics allow rapid determination of a number of variables. Look at Box 46-8 and list five of the parameters you can check.

    A. _____

    B. _____

    C. _____

    D. _____

    E. _____

48. Table 46-2 on page 1133 tries to explain how to do a patient–ventilator system check. The check is one of the most frequent and common activities that RTs perform. I'll list some key steps and you explain.
   A. Before entering the room

   B. Explain

   C. Observe

   D. Drain

   E. Airway

Chapter **46** **Monitoring and Management of the Patient in the Intensive Care Unit**

F. Inspect

G. Auscultate

H. Note pressures (at least three)

I. IMV

J. Graphic artistry

MATHEMATICS

I'll stop you right there. A lot of important math problems were presented in the last section of Chapter 46. Before we go on to the dreaded *hemodynamics* section, I want to make sure you can do the voodoo. You can look back at the text or just read along. Practice will help you gain understanding.

Shunt

You will at best have to recognize the classic shunt equation. At worst, be able to calculate it (even though we use computers in the clinical setting). Let's see if you can estimate shunt using the formula from *Egan's*.

Let's do it together first.

A patient is breathing 100% oxygen. The PaO_2 is 200. What is the estimated shunt?

- $PAO_2 = (760 - 47) \times 1.0 - PaCO_2$ (assume 40). Say 673 for PAO_2.
- Now plug the numbers into the formula. $673 - 200 = a$ 473–mm Hg difference between A and a!
- If there is a 5% shunt for each 100–mm Hg difference, the estimated shunt is $473/100 \times 5$ or 24%.

Your turn.

49. A patient is breathing 100% oxygen. P_B is 747 (conveniently), $PaCO_2$ is 47 (goodie), and PaO_2 is 300. Estimate the shunt.

   A. $PAO_2 =$

   B. $A - a =$

   C.   Shunt =

Fick

Fick was *the* fizziologist. You can use his equation to calculate cardiac output or oxygen consumption. This isn't used much in the clinical setting but it can be on your boards.

Let's do one together.

What is cardiac output for a patient who has a $\dot{V}O_2$ of 250, a CaO_2 of 19, and a CvO_2 of 14?

Plug the numbers into the formula:

- Q_T (total perfusion or cardiac output) $= \dot{V}O_2/CaO_2 - CvO_2 \times 10$ or . . .
- $Q_T = 250/19 - 14 \times 10 = 250/5 \times 10 = 250/50 = 5$ L/min

Your turn.

50. What is cardiac output for a patient who has an oxygen consumption of 200 ml/min, an arterial content of 20 vol%, and a venous content of 16 vol%?

   A.   Formula _____

   B.   Calculation _____

   C.   Answer _____

You could rearrange this to calculate oxygen consumption if you knew the cardiac output. For example, what is the oxygen consumption for a patient who has a cardiac output of 4 L/min, CaO_2 of 17, and CvO_2 of 13?

$$\dot{V}O_2 = 4 \times 17 - 13 \text{ or } 160 \text{ ml/min. You can keep on rearranging all you like.}$$

Minute Ventilation

That was fun, now try an easy one. Exhaled minute ventilation is respiratory rate $\times$ tidal volume. $V_E = f \times V_T$. For example, a patient has a respiratory rate of 12 and a tidal volume of 500, so the exhaled minute ventilation is 6000 ml, or 6 L.

51. What is the V_E for a patient who has a respiratory rate of 8 and a tidal volume of 400?

   A.   Formula _____

   B.   Calculation _____

   C.   Answer _____

What about a patient who has ventilator breaths and spontaneous breaths (SIMV)?

52. A patient has a set rate of 6 and a machine volume of 700. The patient has 10 spontaneous breaths at 300 ml. What is the total V_E?

Bohr

$V_D/V_T = (PaCO_2 - PECO_2)/PaCO_2$. First we'll calculate the physiologic deadspace–to–tidal volume ratio, and then we'll use it in combination with minute volume.

For example: W

What is the deadspace–to–tidal volume ratio for a patient who has an arterial CO_2 of 40 and an exhaled CO_2 of 30?

$$40 - 30/40 = 10/40 \text{ or } 25\% \text{ Normal}$$

Your turn.

53. Calculate V_D/V_T for a patient who has an arterial CO_2 of 40 and an exhaled CO_2 of 20.

A. Formula _____

B. Calculation _____

C. Answer _____

Now let's combine this with the minute volume equation to calculate *alveolar* minute ventilation. Let's use respiratory rate of 12, tidal volume of 500, $PaCO_2$ of 40, and $PECO_2$ of 30.

- The new formula says: $V_A = f(V_T - V_D)$.
- Deadspace is 25%. So multiply the tidal volume by 0.25 to get the deadspace volume. $500 \times 0.25 = 125$ ml.
- Now plug in the numbers. $V_A = 12(500 - 125)$ or $12 \times 375 = 4500$ ml.

54. Calculate alveolar minute ventilation for a patient who has a rate of 10, tidal volume of 500, arterial CO_2 of 40, and end-tidal CO_2 of 28.

A. Formula _____

B. Calculation _____

C. Answer _____

Expect some combination of this material on your board exams!

Compliance

Like deadspace, compliance calculations are simplified on the board exams. We'll do it both ways here.

First, static effective compliance the simple way.

A patient has an exhaled volume of 600 ml. The plateau pressure is 35 and the PEEP is 5.

$$\text{Compliance is } 600/35 - 5 \text{ or } 600/30 = 20 \text{ ml/cm } H_2O$$

Your turn.

55. Calculate static effective compliance for a patient who has an exhaled volume of 1000, plateau pressure of 35, and PEEP of 10.

   A. Formula _____

   B. Calculation _____

   C. Compliance _____

In clinical practice it may be important to subtract the compressed volume with some ventilaors. A comparison will make this clear. The patient in question 54 had a volume of 600 and compliance of 20. But, if the PIP was 40 cm H_2O and the circuit expansion factor is 5 ml/cm H_2O, then the volume lost to expansion is 200 ml (factor × PIP)! The new compliance calculation is

$$(600 - 200)/(35 - 5) \text{ or } 400/30 = 13 \text{ ml/cm } H_2O$$

You try:

56. Calculate compliance for a patient who has a tidal volume of 800, PIP of 50, plateau of 35, and PEEP of 5. The circuit factor is 4 ml/cm H_2O.

   A. Formula _____

   B. Calculation _____

   C. Compliance _____

Some ventilators compensate for tubing compliance and you don't need to do this step!

Resistance

A look at the difference between PIP and plateau is useful for clinical estimates of airway resistance as well. First, you need to use a square or constant flow pattern on most modern ventilators. Next, you need to determine the flow rate in liters per second, not liters per minute.

Here is an example:

Calculate resistance for a patient who has a PIP of 50 cm H_2O, plateau of 40 cm H_2O, and flow rate of 60 L/min.

60 L/min converts to L/sec this way: 60 L/min ÷ 60 sec/min = 1 L/sec. Now calculate:

$$PIP - plateau \div flow = 50 - 40 \div 1 = 10 \text{ cm } H_2O/L/sec$$

Now your turn.

57. Calculate airway resistance for a patient who has a peak pressure of 50 cm H_2O, plateau pressure of 40 cm H_2O, and flow rate of 30 L/min.

   A. Convert flow to liters per second _____

   B. Resistance formula _____

   C. Calculation _____

   D. Airway resistance is _____

If you are doing patient care, you may not have to calculate to see that resistance or compliance have changed. Look at the difference between peak pressure and plateau pressure. If the difference has increased and all else is stable, then the resistance has also increased. Some ventilators will perform compliance and resistance calculations for you. The manual calculations will give slightly different answers than the ventilator. Policy will determine the way you do the numbers at any particular hospital.

   Remember, if the patient is actively breathing spontaneously, it will be very difficult to make accurate calculations. These are really intended for full ventilatory support.

ASSESSMENT OF HEMODYNAMICS

We're here at last. The dreaded hemodynamics. Strikes terror into the hearts of respiratory care students every-where . . . but it will be okay. Well, break it down into small pieces: indications, complications, normal values, equipment, waveforms. You can do it! Let's start with invasive arterial monitoring.

Arterial lines

58. Identify the two main sites for arterial cannulation in adults.

   A. _____

   B. _____

59. What are the two indications for an indwelling arterial line?

   A. _____

   B. _____

60. List the normal values for these systemic arterial parameters. Check Table 46-3.

   A. Systolic _____

   B. Diastolic _____

   C. Mean _____

When the arterial line doesn't agree with manual measurements, the manual method is safer. One problem may be that the pressure transducer is not at the level of the heart. A transducer that is above the heart results in *lower* pressures on the monitor.

   Another problem may be a "dampened" tracing. This means the waveform is flattened out. Clots and air bubbles in the system are common causes of a dampened tracing.

Equipment

One more area you need to become familiar with is the basic parts of the system. Take a look at this picture.

Use of pressurized IV fluid bag and Intraflow flush device for optimal maintenance of arterial catheter patency. Stopcocks may be placed on each side of the flush device for room air reference and blood sampling. (From Schroeder JE, Daily EK: Techniques in bedside hemodynamic monitoring, St. Louis, 1976, Mosby.)

Starting at the top, you see a **pressurized IV bag** that may also contain heparin to help reduce the chance of clotting. The main thing is the pressure. Without it, blood from the patient could back up into the system, and we wouldn't be able to **flush,** or wash out blood, back into the artery. The **transducer** converts the arterial pressure wave form to an electronic signal that can be sent to the amplifier and displayed on the monitor.

Special **stiff,** or **noncompliant IV tubing** connects from the transducer and continuous flush device to the catheter that is in the artery. This tubing prevents the arterial pressure wave from being damped as it passes up to the transducer (just like when ventilator tubing expands as a breath passes through it we lose some in the expansion).

There now, that wasn't too bad.

PULMONARY ARTERY PRESSURE MONITORING

Flow-directed, balloon-tipped, pulmonary artery catheter . . . oh, let's just call it a "Swan."

Dr. Swan and Dr. Ganz are credited with developing this nifty tube for looking at the pressures inside the heart and lungs. So many people still call it a "Swan" or "Swan-Ganz" catheter. Pulmonary artery catheter (PAC) is more generic. Pulmonary artery monitoring **is** a complex subject, but you can make it much simpler if you start by learning certain basic pieces of information. (You can also pass your boards . . .)

61. Name six conditions that suggest insertion of a PAC.

A. _____

B. _____

C. _____

D. _____

E. _____

F. _____

62. Measurement of PCWP is especially helpful in separating your noncardiogenic (ARDS) and cardiogenic pulmonary edemas (CHF). What value for PCWP suggests ARDS?

_____

63. Let's look at the catheter itself. Identify the labeled parts.

Quadruple-channel pulmonary artery catheter.

A. _____

B. _____

C. _____

D. _____

E. _____

F. _____

G. _____

H. _____

I. _____

Pneumopnugget

A picture is not the best way to learn this, but it's OK. Either get a catheter from one of your instructors or look at one in the ICU that is in a box, then in a patient. You really should learn the parts of this baby.

64. Now label the following four waveforms.

A, Position of pulmonary arterial catheter in heart. *B,* As monitored by pressure tracings.

Pneumopnugget

These are the four patterns seen on insertion and during normal monitoring. Just like in ECGs, there are abnormal patterns, too, but don't worry about them yet. Each of the normal waveforms corresponds to an anatomical location. So if, for example, the catheter is supposed to be in the pulmonary artery but you see a right ventricular waveform, you know something is wrong (maybe it is pulled back too far). Or, if the waveform appears wedged when it isn't supposed to be, perhaps the catheter has migrated too far forward.

65. List the normal values for these parameters. (See Table 46-3 on page 1140.)

A. Central venous pressure (CVP) _____

B. Right atrial pressure (RA) _____
C. Pulmonary artery

   1. Systolic _____

   2. Diastolic _____

D. Pulmonary artery wedge pressure (PWP, PCWP, PAWP) _____

WHAT DOES IT ALL MEAN?

Interpretation of PAC readings is a pretty complex subject. I want you to learn some of the basics, so I will deliberately be simplifying. Right atrial pressure (RAP) and CVP are often used interchangeably. CVP represents preload to the right side of the heart. It can be a good indicator of the fluid volume status of the patient. It could also tell us if there is a backup in the system between the right atrium and the left atrium. Like pulmonary hypertension, a blood clot, heart failure, or a defect in the tricuspid valve. The wedge pressure does much the same for the left side. Under normal circumstances it shows us the left ventricular preload. Considered along with CVP, it helps decide about the fluid balance. If both CVP and PWP are low, you should consider hypovolemia.

505

Here is where the RT must really think. Because both values are measured inside the chest, and positive pressure ventilation increases intrathoracic pressure, it is possible for the ventilator to affect the readings. The pressure tracings will move up and down with positive pressure breaths, so you may be able to detect this by watching the tracing increase and decrease as the ventilator cycles. But PEEP makes a constant increase in pressure, and PEEP levels above 10 cm H_2O, especially in hypovolemic patients, can artificially elevate the values, especially the wedge pressure. A high value means the patient has too much fluid, so someone might conclude the patient needs to lose some fluid when really he or she is dry! A complete explanation of what to do about this would keep us here a long time, but here are some ideas:

1. Measure pressure values from the PAC at end exhalation. You will need to run off a printed strip to do this, since the digital values on the monitor are averaged.

2. Do not take the patient off the ventilator to measure values, especially if the patient is on a high level of PEEP.

3. Correct the PAC values if the patient is on a high level of PEEP. This is not simple—remember that the degree of pressure transmitted depends on lung compliance as well . . . so learn more about this before you try it.

You can use the catheter to look at other things besides overall fluid balance. Diagnosis of certain conditions is aided by information from the PAC. Table 46-4 on page 1142 provides a look at some of these conditions. For example, compare ARDS to left ventricular failure. The pulmonary artery pressure may increase in both conditions, the radiograph shows infiltrates, and breath sounds may reveal crackles. Both patients have hypoxemia and decreased lung compliance. But, the failing left ventricle causes the wedge pressure to go up, where ARDS does not. Combine this with patient history and other assessments, and you get the big picture. Certain other values can be measured besides pressure, so let's look at those next.

66. List the normal values for these parameters. (See Table 46-3 on page 1140.)

A. Cardiac output (CO) _____

B. Cardiac index (CI) _____

C. Systemic vascular resistance (SVR) _____

D. Pulmonary vascular resistance (PVR) _____

With the Swan, cardiac output is measured via thermodilution. This is very helpful information, especially in the administration of drugs that support cardiac function, or if you want to know if changes in the ventilator are affecting the heart. The problem is that cardiac output is not personal enough. For example, you would expect a Sumo wrestler to have a bigger cardiac output than an elderly woman, but both would be technically within the normal range at 5 L/min of output. If you divide the output by the body surface area, you derive cardiac index, and this is more useful, because everyone should have the same range for cardiac index. Anyone who drops below 2.5 is in trouble!

Another useful calculation is vascular resistance. It's just like airway resistance (PIP − plateau/flow), only now we want to know how much pressure drop occurs when we push the blood through the vessels. Let's look at the pulmonary vascular resistance formula, because you might have to calculate this on your boards.

$$PVR = MPAP - PAWP/CO$$

If we have a patient with a mean pulmonary artery pressure of 12 mm Hg, CVP of 4 mm Hg, and cardiac output of 4 L/min, we get 12 − (4/4) = 2 mm Hg/L/min for the resistance. Sometimes this number is multiplied by 80 to convert it to dynes. Either way, PVR is normally quite low.

67. What common respiratory problem results in vasoconstriction, or elevated vascular resistance in the pulmonary vessels? (Hint: It's the first one on the list under PVR in Table 46-3.)

_____

506

68. Calculate PVR for a patient who has a mean pulmonary artery pressure of 15 mm Hg, CVP of 3 mm Hg, and CO of 5 L/min.

Sometimes you need to be able to calculate mean arterial pressure so you can work the resistance problem. Remember that MAP = systolic pressure + (2 × diastolic)/3.

69. Calculate mean pulmonary artery pressure if systolic pulmonary artery pressure is 25 mm Hg and diastolic pulmonary artery pressure is 10 mm Hg.

By now, your brain must be getting tired. **Remember** to learn the basics and normal values. When you are looking at the data, think about where in the heart or lungs the pressure is being measured. That will help give you a clue about what part of the system has become abnormal. To increase your expertise you will have to go to the clinical setting and look at the patient data from the PAC and learn interpretation at the bedside.

NEUROLOGIC MONITORING

70. Why are the pupils of interest in assessing neurologic status?

_____

71. Why shouldn't you check a patient's gag reflex?

_____

72. Name one of the breathing patterns that suggests a neurologic deficit.

_____

73. Describe the patient that goes with the ICP values below.

   A. 10 to 15 mm Hg _____

   B. 15 to 20 mm Hg _____

   C. 30 to 35 mm Hg _____

74. The Glasgow Coma Scale is a popular tool used to assess acute neurologic deficits. What do the following scores mean?

A. 9 to 13 _____

B. <8 _____

TROUBLESHOOTING THE PATIENT–VENTILATOR SYSTEM

75. Troubleshooting revolves around what two general problem areas? (See Box 46-12.)

A. _____

B. _____

76. Use Table 46-7 to help you identify common problems.

	Clue	Possible Problem	Corrective Action
A.	Sudden increase in PIP	1.	
		2.	
B.	Gradual increase in PIP	1.	
C.	Sudden decrease in PIP	1.	
		2.	
D.	Decreased minute/tidal volume	1.	
		2.	
E.	Increased minute or tidal volume	1.	
		2.	

77. Use Box 46-12 to help you identify four patient-related causes of sudden respiratory distress.

A. _____

B. _____

C. _____

D. _____

78. List four ventilator-related causes of sudden respiratory distress.

A. _____

B. _____

C. _____

D. _____

79. Regardless of the source of the problem, what is always the first priority?

_____

508

80. If there is any doubt as to the cause or solution of a problem, what action should you take? (See Box 46-13.)

81. How can you check the patency of the artificial airway?

82. Sedation and paralysis may be needed outside of the normal sedation humanely given in the ICU. Some patients cannot tolerate the ventilator without medication. The key is to avoid oversedation and troubleshoot all the physiologic stuff like hypoxia first. Give examples of drugs in the following classes:

A. Tranquilizing agents

   1. _____

   2. _____

   3. _____

B. Narcotic analgesics

   1. _____

   2. _____

C. Neuromuscular blocking agents

   1. Long-term (nondepolarizing) _____

   2. Short-acting (depolarizing) _____

D. Sedative/hypnotics and miscellaneous

   _____

The flavor of the month for this one is propofol (Diprivan). We like to call this stuff "milk of amnesia." Looks like milk. Rapid acting and has a short half-life so it's easy to get out of the system when the nurses turn off the IV! Amidate, or etomidate, is a great drug for managing the airway that has some advantages over the paralyzing agent Anectine.

WHAT DOES THE NBRC SAY?

The issue of hemodynamics in the board exams is a bit tricky. Hemodynamics used to be a heavy hitter, with 10 or more questions on the Written Registry. The last revision of the exams removed most of this material. Now you see only a few questions and they are less technical in regard to equipment and focus more on identifying clinically important material that all ICU staff need to understand. Because whole textbooks are devoted to hemodynamic monitoring or ventilator management, *Egan's* cannot possibly give you everything you need. It is a great place to start, and it clearly

509

summarizes the main points. Chapter 46 will make an excellent reference when you go to prepare for the tests. Here are some sample questions. Circle the best answer.

83. A 42-year-old patient with a cervical spine injury is being mechanically ventilated in control mode. As you enter the room, the low pressure alarm is sounding. The patient is connected to the ventilator, but you do not see his chest moving. Your first action would be to _____.
    A. manually ventilate the patient with the resuscitation bag
    B. check the alarm settings
    C. observe the exhaled volumes
    D. manually ventilate the patient with the mechanical ventilator

84. After insertion of a Swan-Ganz catheter via the left subclavian vein, a patient's compliance quickly drops. The high pressure alarm on the ventilator is activated. Breath sounds are absent over the left chest and the trachea is deviated to the right side. The patient appears extremely anxious. What action should the RCP take?
    A. Use a capnometer to assess ventilation noninvasively.
    B. Recommend administration of Versed.
    C. Call for a portable chest radiograph.
    D. Recommend chest tube insertion.

85. A 38-year-old woman with a diagnosis of myasthenia gravis is being mechanically ventilated. As you enter the room, the high pressure alarm is sounding. The patient appears anxious. Auscultation reveals coarse bilateral rhonchi. What action should you take at this time?
    A. Manually ventilate the patient.
    B. Check the alarm setting.
    C. Recommend sedation.
    D. Suction the patient.

86. An 89-year-old woman with emphysema is being mechanically ventilated. The high pressure and high rate alarms are being activated. Breath sounds are clear. Pulse oximetry and vital sign values are within normal limits. Hemodynamics are normal. ABGs are stable. The patient is very agitated and her respiratory rate is 32. What are your recommendations?
    A. Administer Versed.
    B. Increase the alarm limit.
    C. Suction the patient.
    D. Call for a portable chest radiograph.

87. The data below are reported for a patient:
    PCWP   25 mm Hg
    PAP   40/24 mm Hg
    CI   1.9 L/min/m^2

    These data suggest which of the following?
    A. noncardiogenic pulmonary edema
    B. cardiogenic pulmonary edema
    C. pulsus paradoxus
    D. hypovolemia

88. When properly placed, the distal tip of the Swan-Ganz catheter will be located in the _____.
    A. left atrium
    B. right atrium
    C. right ventricle
    D. pulmonary artery

Questions 89 through 91 refer to the following situation:

A patient is intubated and placed on the ventilator after she develops respiratory failure following a hip replacement surgery. The following values are recorded:

Pa_{CO_2}	50 mm Hg
Pa_{O_2}	60 mm Hg
Fi_{O_2}	0.40
PE_{CO_2}	10 mm Hg
Tidal volume	800 ml
Respiratory rate	20

89. These data indicate a deadspace–to–tidal volume ratio of _____.
   A. 20%
   B. 40%
   C. 60%
   D. 80%

90. What is the exhaled minute volume?
   A. 8.0 L
   B. 12.0 L
   C. 16.0 L
   D. 20.0 L

91. What is the alveolar minute volume?
   A. 3.2 L
   B. 11.2 L
   C. 12. 8 L
   D. 16.0 L

92. The following information is recorded for a patient:

$\dot{V}_{O_2}$	200 ml/min
Ca_{O_2}	16 vol %
$C\bar{v}_{O_2}$	12 vol %

What is the cardiac output?
   A. 2.0 L/min
   B. 3.0 L/min
   C. 4.0 L/min
   D. 5.0 L/min

93. The hemodynamic data below are recorded for a patient who is being mechanically ventilated.

Cardiac output	3.5 L/min
PAP	16/8 mm Hg
PWP	4 mm Hg
CVP	2 mm Hg
HR	125/min

These data probably indicate _____.
   A. hypovolemia
   B. pulmonary hypertension
   C. fluid overload
   D. pulmonary embolism

Well, I could go on like this forever, but I think you get the picture.

FOOD FOR THOUGHT

There was an editorial in the journal *Respiratory Care* a few years ago entitled something like this: "The pulmonary artery catheter—it goes in through your arm and you pay through the nose." I want you to think about three questions

511

in relationship to this idea. First, do you think it is important to use top of the line technology in every setting? Second, if your loved one was ill, what would you want for them? Third, do you think the average person understands the complexity of "the high cost of medicine?"

INFORMATION AGE

- Ventworld has some interesting items: www.ventworld.com. Hemodynamics, blood gas, and shunt calculators and cases galore. Have fun exploring the virtual anesthesia textbook or the H-H equation.

47 Discontinuing Ventilatory Support

I'm losing.
Reported as the last words of Frank Sinatra

It's relatively easy to initiate mechanical ventilation, and some patients are equally easy to get back off again. Unfortunately, there is still no magic number that tells you a patient will be successfully weaned or removed from support. You will have to customize the job for each patient. Sometimes this task takes all our skills and resources to accomplish. Sometimes, it can't be done!

WORD WIZARD

Gosh, it looks like you already know all the key terms in this chapter. Take a break from the acronyms and let's move on to the three basic methods of weaning.

FIRST THINGS FIRST

1. What's the difference between weaning and discontinuing ventilator support?

   A. Wean _____

   B. Discontinue _____

2. What are the three basic methods for discontinuing?

   A. _____

   B. _____

   C. _____

3. Regardless of the reason for initiating mechanical ventilation, what has to happen before you can get the patient

   off the ventilator? _____

REASONS FOR VENTILATOR DEPENDENCE

4. Patients may need mechanical ventilation for apnea, ventilatory failure, or hypoxemia. They may remain dependent because of what four factors?

   A. _____

   B. _____

   C. _____

   D. _____

5. State the four factors that determine total ventilatory workload.

   A. _____

   B. _____

   C. _____

   D. _____

6. What do fever, shivering, agitation, trauma, and sepsis have in common?

   _____

7. List two causes of increased deadspace ventilation.

   A. _____

   B. _____

8. Name four common causes of decreased lung compliance.

   A. _____

   B. _____

   C. _____

   D. _____

9. Name three causes of decreased thoracic compliance.

   A. _____

   B. _____

   C. _____

10. State three causes of increased airway resistance.

   A. _____

   B. _____

   C. _____

11. Why are artificial airways implicated in increased airway resistance?

   _____

12. Give examples of conditions that adversely affect ventilatory capacity. Check out Box 47-2 on page 1156 for some clues.

    A. CNS drive

       1. _____

       2. _____

       3. _____

       4. _____

    B. Muscle strength

       1. _____

       2. _____

       3. _____

       4. _____

13. Once ventilatory muscles are fatigued, how long should they be rested prior to any attempt at weaning?

    _____

Ok, so now you have this giant shopping list of things that could make removal from the ventilator difficult. Sometimes one thing, like reduced drive to breathe from drugs, is the problem. That's easy to solve. You can give an antidote (like Narcan for heroin or morphine), cleanse the blood (dialysis, for example), or just wait for the effects to wear off (anesthesia, for instance). Or, you might run into something a little more complicated. Like a depressed COPD patient with congestive heart failure (CHF) who has a small ET tube, bronchospasm, malnutrition, CO_2 retention, and electrolyte disorders along with the lung infection that put him on the ventilator in the first place! That's a plate full of issues to be resolved prior to weaning. See Box 47-3: Factors Contributing to Ventilator Dependence on page 1157 if you need this to get more complicated.

PATIENT EVALUATION

Careful, systematic assessment is an especially important part of your approach to ventilator discontinuance.

14. What is the first thing you should evaluate whether you are considering weaning or taking the patient off the ventilator? The single most important thing.

    _____

15. What are the four questions you should ask?

    A. _____

    B. _____

    C. _____

    D. _____

Once the patient is stable and things are looking up, you can take a look at the weaning indexes. I told you (see Chapter 41, Table 41-2) these things would return to haunt you! Do they work? Like everything else, they sometimes work. Even though indexes have limitations, we still need to gather the information because it helps quantify the patient's overall status.

16. Your board exams will expect you to identify these classic criteria for weaning from mechanical ventilation. Remember that no one criterion mandates that you wean or don't wean! Use Table 47-1 to help out with this question.

Measurement	Critical Value
A. Pa_{CO_2}	
B. pH	
C. VC (ml/kg)	
D. Spontaneous V_T	
E. Spontaneous rate	
F. V_E	
G. MVV	
H. MIF (NIF, MIP)	
I. V_D/V_T	
J. $P(A - a)O_2$ on 100%	
K. P/F ratio	
L. Pa_{O_2}	
M. Qs/Qt	
N. F_{IO_2}	
O. f/V_T	
P. Compliance	

Another giant menu to memorize, then apply to clinical. (IF it seems overwhelming, break it down into small pieces; learn a few at a time. Then chant this mantra "I want to be a really good RT, I want to be a really good RT . . .")

17. Describe the breathing patterns that may cause problems with weaning or discontinuance.

18. Physical assessment of respiratory muscles may be useful. Describe what you are looking for in this area.

19. Rapid shallow breathing index may be the best overall predictor of weaning outcomes. Calculate the index for a patient who has a spontaneous rate of 25 with a spontaneous volume of 350 ml. What are the criteria for success?

   A. Calculation _____

   B. Criteria _____

20. How could you modify the criteria to be a better predictor with elderly patients?

   _____

21. What do you have to do with the ventilator patient to get the RSBI?

22. Give the Pa_{O_2} and F_{IO_2} values that should be met prior to weaning.

   A. Pa_{O_2} _____

   B. F_{IO_2} _____

23. What is the effect of excessive carbohydrate administration?

   _____

24. Identify the critical values for confirming cardiovascular stability? (Refer to Table 47-2 on page 1161.)

Measurement	Values Inconsistent With Weaning
A. Heart rate	_____
B. Systolic pressure	_____
C. Diastolic pressure	_____
D. Hemoglobin	_____
E. Cardiac index (CI)	_____

25. Describe the three ways that renal function may affect weaning.

A. _____

B. _____

C. _____

26. Describe the ideal CNS status you'd like to see.

27. How is ability to be weaned different from ability to be extubated?

28. Because many factors are associated with success, weaning indexes are becoming more popular. What is a weaning index? Which one is the most useful?

_____

PREPARING THE PATIENT

A quick glance at Box 47-6 on page 1163 should amuse you or scare you. More than 60 factors to improve before attempting to discontinue the ventilator. The RT should start by optimizing those parts of the patient's medical condition over which they have direct control, and focus on psychological and environmental factors they can influence.

29. Name two drug therapies the RT can utilize to reduce airway resistance.

A. _____

B. _____

30. How else can the RT improve conditions in the airway?

_____

31. What time of day should weaning activities be conducted? _____

32. What percentage of patients may develop "ICU psychosis" or other psychological disturbances after a few days in the unit? _____

33. How could the RT help the patient get adequate sleep?

_____

34. Describe the environmental considerations that may improve patient well-being.

_____

35. What three methods does *Egan's* identify for helping patients communicate?

A. _____

B. _____

C. _____

WEANING METHODS

When the original problem is resolving, the indexes look good, and you've optimized as many factors as possible, you must get down to the business of discontinuing the ventilator. Rapidly or slowly, you have several methods to choose from.

36. List the three basic methods of discontinuing support.

A. _____

B. _____

C. _____

37. Instead of putting the patient on a T-piece with an aerosol, you could use one of the spontaneous (CSV) ventilator modes. Name these two modes and suggest appropriate levels of support.

A. _____

B. _____

38. Describe the specific advantage of using the ventilator instead of the T-tube.

_____

39. What is the typical minimum length of time for a spontaneous trial when you are going for rapid discontinuance?

_____

40. How should you position the patient prior to the trial breathing period?

_____

Rapid discontinuance works really well on patients who have been on the ventilator for a short period of time (e.g., a postoperative patient, an OD who is now awake, that sort of thing). Wouldn't it be nice if more patients fell into this category? For the more difficult customer, you basically have three choices: T-piece, SIMV, or SBT.

41. Describe the T-piece (T-tube) trial for gradual weaning (see Box 47-8).

_____

42. What F_{IO_2} is ideal for T-piece weaning?

_____

43. What happens at night? _____

44. Describe the variation of this method where the patient is kept on the ventilator.

45. What are the biggest drawbacks to T-piece weaning?

46. Compare T-piece to IMV weaning.

47. Why do you think IMV (SIMV) is such a popular weaning method in the United States?

48. What are the typical initial settings when SIMV is used for full ventilatory support?

    A. Tidal volume   _____

    B. Respiratory rate   _____

49. What is the typical amount the rate is adjusted at any one time in SIMV weaning?

_____

50. When is partial support an unwise ventilator strategy?

51. Describe pressure support ventilation (PSV).

_____

52. What is PSV max? _____

53. From what level of PSV may a patient be extubated?

_____

54. *Egan's* gives a formula for estimating the level of pressure support needed to overcome work of breathing. Calculate the level needed for a patient who has a PIP of 50 cm H_2O, plateau pressure of 30 cm H_2O, a ventilator flow rate of 60 L/min, and a spontaneous inspiratory flow rate of 30 L/min. (You can look at the Mini Clini "Setting Pressure Support" for help.)

    A. Formula _____

    B. Calculation _____

    C. Answer _____

If you're just trying to overcome work of breathing through the ET tube, it's a lot easier to use the "tube compensation" modes found on newer ventilators. The machine does the calculating for you. Other times you want to set PSV to achieve a desired tidal volume, either in units of ml or ml/kg. Another way to set PSV is to increase the pressure until spontaneous rate drops to a desirable level.

SPONTANEOUS BREATHING TRIALS

Spontaneous breathing trial (SBT) is the hottest of the hot for ventilator discontinuance! Remember, this should be done formally and systematically by the therapist. The first SBT is a brief screening trial. Box 47-10 gives a step-by-step procedure for you.

55. How long is the first SBT? _____

56. The patient must meet two of the following three criteria to continue:

    Assessment   **Criteria for Success**

    A. Spontaneous V_T _____

    B. MIP   _____

    C. Respiratory rate   _____

57. The formal SBT is at least _____ minutes and no longer than _____ minutes.

58. The SBT must be performed with a T-piece or, if they stay on the vent, with PSV of _____ cm H_2O or CPAP of ≤ _____ cm H_2O.

59. Monitor the patient during the trial. You should stop the SBT if distress occurs.

    Assessment   **Signs of Serious Distress**

    A. Mental status   _____

    B. Respiratory rate   _____

    C. Heart rate   _____

    D. Blood pressure   _____

    E. Spo_2 _____

    If they fail the SBT, put them back on the ventilator with FULL SUPPORT for 24 hours.
    Try to figure out why they failed and fix the problem (for example, more aggressive bronchial hygiene). IF they PASS the SBT, keep them off the ventilator for a little while longer and consider extubation!

60. When should you repeat the SBT if the patient fails the first trial?

    _____

61. Describe mandatory minute ventilation (MMV).

    _____

62. What specific patient population would be at risk when using MMV?

63. MMV systems compare spontaneous minute ventilation to desired minute ventilation. How do they adjust the ventilation delivered by the machine?

_____

64. What is the main advantage of flow-triggering over pressure triggering?

_____

65. VS, VAPS, ASV, etc. are new methods of approaching ventilation. What is the basic idea behind these modes?

_____

66. Discuss the role of NIPPV in weaning.

Table 47-4 on page 1176 of your text summarizes the pros and cons of the various weaning methods. That was a long section, but we're not done yet. Charge up your laptop and crank up your Ipod so we can go on.

MONITORING THE PATIENT

67. What are the two easily monitored and reliable indicators of patient progress during weaning?

A. _____

B. _____

68. What is the single best index of ventilation?

_____

69. What is the simplest way to monitor oxygenation during weaning?

70. Give the expected and excessive changes for each of the following parameters. Check out Table 47-6 if you get lost.

Parameter	Expected	Deleterious
A. Respiratory rate		
B. Pa_{O_2}		
C. Pa_{CO_2}		
D. Heart rate		
E. Blood pressure		

The NBRC will expect you to know these changes well. So do your instructors. (So does the patient!)

EXTUBATION

Weaning and extubation are separate issues. We know this, but other clinicians may not be as clear, so the RT has to be a strong advocate in the decision to remove or maintain the artificial airway. Failed extubation may be hazardous to your patient's health. A study published in the July 1999 issue of *Respiratory Care* indicated that a failure rate (patient requiring reintubation) of 10% to 20% was acceptable in the medical ICU population. In the surgical ICU (uncomplicated postoperative patients), a failure rate of less than 5% is OK. Failure rates above 20% probably mean you are not assessing the patients carefully enough. Failure rates below 10% probably mean you are keeping the patient on the ventilator too long!

71. What is the important thing to remember about the presence of the artificial airway in terms of weaning? What can be done about it? (See Table 47-7 on page 1178.)

_____

72. What is the minimum ability required for personnel performing routine extubation?

_____

73. What is the minimum ability required for personnel performing high-risk extubation?

_____

74. What are common patient complaints following extubation?

75. Describe the cuff leak test (see Box 47-16).

76. Identify the appropriate treatment for postextubation stridor.

   A. Mild _____

   B. Moderate _____

   C. Severe _____

77. What patients are at risk for aspiration following extubation? How can you minimize the risk?

   _____

FAILURE TO WEAN

As much as we all want to get the patient off the vent, it doesn't always work.

78. Identify two common causes of weaning failure for each of the following areas.
   A. Oxygenation

      1. _____

      2. _____

   B. Ventilation

      1. _____

      2. _____

   C. Cardiovascular

      1. _____

      2. _____

79. The ICU is no place for the long-term ventilator patient. It's too expensive, and the staff are not usually trained to deal with the issues. What are the alternate care sites?

   _____

80. Table 47-8 is a monster! Identify strategies for each of the following problems.

Problem   Management Strategy

A. Anemia   _____

B. Tube-related WOB   _____

C. Bronchospasm   _____

                         _____

D. Secretions   _____

                         _____

E. Dyspnea   _____

                         _____

F. Muscle fatigue   _____

                         _____

G. Hemodynamics   _____

                         _____

H. Infection   _____

I. Metabolic   _____

                         _____

J. Nutrition   _____

K. Exercise   _____

                         _____

L. Psychological   _____

                         _____

                         _____

M. Sleep   _____

                         _____

                         _____

N. Pain   _____

                         _____

Many of these techniques are useful once the patient is removed from the ICU and placed in an alternate site. A skilled, multidisciplinary approach is needed for the chronic ventilator patient. In the end, some patients will remain on the machine for life.

81. Who should be involved in the decision to terminate life support?

_____

82. Who does *Egan's* suggest perform the actual termination?

_____

CASE STUDIES

Case 1

A 61-year-old woman is placed on the ventilator for respiratory failure for CHF and COPD. Twenty-four hours later, the physician asks for your recommendation regarding weaning. Breath sounds reveal coarse crackles in both bases. Pedal edema is present as well. The following information is obtained.

Spontaneous RR	28
Spontaneous V_t	0.2 L
MIF	−18 cm H_2O
VC	0.6 L
HR	116
BP	90/60
pH	7.33
$Paco_2$	35 mm Hg
Pao_2	65 (on Fio_2 0.5)
Cardiac index	2.3

83. What is your assessment of her respiratory status?

84. Has the primary problem been resolved?

85. What is the rapid shallow breathing index?

86. Explain your recommendation regarding initiating weaning? If you recommend weaning, also recommend the method.

A 61-year-old man is placed on the ventilator following open-heart surgery. Twelve hours later, the patient is awake and the physician asks for your recommendation regarding weaning. The following information is obtained:

Spontaneous RR	14
Spontaneous V_T	0.2 L
MIF	−35 cm H_2O
VC	1.2 L
HR	116
BP	90/60
pH	7.37
$Paco_2$	35 mm Hg
Pao_2	85 (on Fio_2 0.35)

87. What is your assessment of his respiratory status?

88. Has the primary problem been resolved?

_____

89. What is the rapid shallow breathing index?

_____

90. Explain your recommendation regarding initiating weaning? If you recommend weaning, also recommend a technique.

A 61-year-old is placed on the ventilator following an acute episode of Guillain-Barre syndrome. At 21 days later, the patient is regaining strength and movement in his limbs. The physician asks for your recommendation regarding weaning. The following information is obtained:

Spontaneous RR	22
Spontaneous V_T	0.22 L
MIF	−20 cm H_2O
VC	1.0 L
HR	116
BP	90/60
pH	7.38
$Paco_2$	37 mm Hg
Pao_2	70 (on Fio_2 0.40)

91. What is your assessment of his respiratory status?

_____

92. Has the primary problem been resolved?

_____

93. What is the rapid shallow breathing index?

_____

94. Explain your recommendation regarding initiating weaning? If you recommend weaning, also recommend a technique.

A 5 foot 2 inch, 50-kg, 80-year-old woman has been on the ventilator for 2 days following open-heart surgery due to hemodynamic instability. The vitals are now stable. The physician wants you to conduct a spontaneous breathing trial. You suction the patient and sit her up for trial. Pretrial respiratory rate is 22, MIP is –45 mm Hg, and spontaneous volume is 400 ml. She is placed on a T-piece for 3 minutes with 40% oxygen. After 3 minutes, the f is 25, MIP is –40, and V_T is 420.

95. What would you recommend at this time?

_____

96. What is the RSBI? _____

97. How long does she need to succeed on the trial before you would consider extubation?

_____

WHAT DOES THE NBRC SAY?

I guess it's clear from the amount of questions I've put in this chapter that weaning and discontinuance are important topics. But is weaning really specified in the exam matrices? The Examination Matrix states that you should "Initiate and modify weaning procedures" and "wean or change weaning procedures and extubation." The key to understanding this subject is in the ways mechanical ventilation is applied. Modes like PSV, SIMV, IMV, CPAP, and PEEP are frequently cited in different areas of these test preparation tools. This makes it difficult to know exactly how many questions on weaning will be on an individual test. It could vary from a few (two or three) to many (five to seven)!

Here are some examples for your thinking pleasure. Circle the best answer.

98. Which of the following would you evaluate prior to initiating T-piece weaning?
   I. Pao_2
   II. Gag reflex
   III. Spontaneous respiratory rate
   IV. Urine output
      A. I and II only
      B. I and III only
      C. II and IV only
      D. III and IV only

99. A patient being assessed for readiness to wean has the following values:

pH	7.36
$Paco_2$	42 mm Hg
Pao_2	67 mm Hg (Fio_2 40%)
MIP	–25 cm H_2O
Pulse	105
Respirations	20
VC	12 ml/kg

   What action should the RT recommend at this time?
   A. Initiate a T-piece trial.
   B. Continue with mechanical ventilation.
   C. Initiate breathing exercises to strengthen ventilatory muscles.
   D. Repeat the vital capacity maneuver.

100. Which of the following indicates a readiness to wean?
    A. spontaneous rate of 28
    B. spontaneous tidal volume of 200 ml
    C. negative inspiratory force of 18 cm H_2O
    D. minute volume of 8 L/min

101. An alert patient is being mechanically ventilated. Settings are:

Mode	SIMV
Rate	2
Tidal volume (set)	800
F_{IO_2}	0.30
PEEP	5 cm H_2O

    ABG results 30 minutes after initiating these settings are:

pH	7.37
Pa_{CO_2}	38 mm Hg
Pa_{O_2}	75 mm Hg

    What should the RT recommend at this time?
    A. Increase the set rate to 4.
    B. Discontinue mechanical ventilation.
    C. Decrease the PEEP to 0 cm H_2O.
    D. Decrease the F_{IO_2} to 0.21.

102. A 70-year-old, 70-kg (154-lb) patient with a history of COPD is being mechanically ventilated. The patient is alert, but making no spontaneous efforts.

Mode	AC
Rate	12
Tidal volume (set)	800
F_{IO_2}	0.40
PEEP	3 cm H_2O
pH	7.51
Pa_{CO_2}	38 mm Hg
Pa_{O_2}	95 mm Hg
HCO_3^-	36 mEq/L

    Which of the following should the RT recommend?
    I. Change to SIMV mode.
    II. Decrease the F_{IO_2}.
    III. Decrease the set rate.
    IV. Decrease the PEEP.
        A. I and II only
        B. I and III only
        C. I, II, and III only
        D. I, III, and IV only

103. A patient is being ventilated in the SIMV mode with a rate of 8, volume of 800, and F_{IO_2} of 0.40. ABG results show:

pH	7.47
Pa_{CO_2}	33 mm Hg
Pa_{O_2}	88 mm Hg
HCO_3^-	23 mEq/L

    What action should the RT recommend in response to these findings?
    A. Increase the tidal volume.
    B. Increase the F_{IO_2}.
    C. Change to AC mode.
    D. Reduce the rate.

104. A patient on SIMV experiences difficulty each time you try to reduce the rate below 6. The patient becomes tachypneic with a rate of 28 and a spontaneous volume of 200. Which of the following modifications would be *least* useful in this situation?
   A. adding pressure support ventilation
   B. T-piece weaning
   C. trial of extubation
   D. changing to flow-by or flow triggering

It's not too difficult to wean patients on paper if you know your *values!* Watch out for COPD patients who are being overventilated or overoxygenated by the machine.

FOOD FOR THOUGHT

Your book mentions weaning indexes but doesn't really mention the details. Here's the scoop. Simplified Weaning Index (SWI) and CROP are two of the better methods.

$$SWI = \frac{f_{mv}(PIP - PEEP)}{MIP} \cdot \frac{PaCO_2 mv}{40}$$

$$CROP = \frac{C_{dyn} \cdot MIP \cdot \frac{PaO_2}{PAO_2}}{f}$$

105. What is the single best approach to weaning?

_____

INFORMATION AGE

- David Walker, MA, RRT, RCP, presents an overview of this subject at http://home.earthlink.net/~firstbreath/ventxt. htm.
- For some expert information on long-term ventilation, you might like to try Barlow Hospital. Their site is at www. barlow2000.org.
- The Society of Critical Care Medicine will give you a set of evidence-based weaning guidelines originally published in *Chest* magazine in December 2001: www.sccm.org/.
- Or for better fun you can go directly to the American College of Chest Physicians (ACCP) Web site and check out all the guidelines: http://www.chestnet.org/education/guidelines/currentGuidelines.php.
- The U.S. government's version is found at www.ahrq.gov/clinic/tp/mechtp.htm.

This is a very rich, hot topic on the Internet.

Neonatal and Pediatric Respiratory Care

Any sufficiently advanced technology is indistinguishable from magic.
Arthur C. Clarke

If you actually knew me, you'd understand that I really don't like taking care of sick babies or kids. I have always been an adult care practitioner. Not that I haven't bagged my fair share of babies, or treated croup, or cystic fibrosis, or even epiglottitis . . . when I had to.

In general, I leave kids to those who like to care for them. On my boards, however, neonatal and pediatrics were my best areas. I knew that I was clinically weak, so I made an extra effort to know the subject well. Whether you dream of working with this special population, or in a community hospital where you will need the skills and knowledge periodically, or just want to do well on your boards, you will find Chapter 48 is just what the doctor ordered. It's a comprehensive and comprehensible overview of the care and feeding of little ones who can't breathe. I'll warn you right now that this is a very long chapter, packed with a huge amount of information, so make an extra large pot of coffee for this one. (If you need a refresher on fetal lung development and anatomic differences between kids and adults, you'll find it in Chapter 8.)

WORD WIZARD

I guess you've noticed that I think medical terminology is important and that I like crosswords. Here's a final puzzle to help you build up your baby talk (on p. 534).

FETAL ASSESSMENT

1. Assessment of the newborn begins with maternal history. Identify three conditions that are likely to result in a baby that is small for its gestational age. (Refer to Table 48-1 on page 1186.)

   A. _____

   B. _____

   C. _____

2. Identify five maternal factors likely to lead to premature delivery. (Refer to Table 48-1 on page 1186.)

   A. _____

   B. _____

   C. _____

   D. _____

   E. _____

3. What maternal metabolic condition is likely to result in an infant who is large for its gestational age?

   _____

ACROSS

1. Four part cardiac disorder
5. Baby hemoglobin
6. This hole connects the right and left atria
9. Persistent hypertension
10. Premature babies are prone to this breathing pattern
13. Inflammation of the small airways
16. Mysterious fatal disorder of newborns
17. ——————— fibrosis, a lethal genetic disorder

DOWN

2. Common obstructive disease of children
3. Short for 65 roses
4. Rapid breathing that comes and goes
7. Life-threatening infection of airway cartilage
8. Fetal doo-doo
11. Flaring means distress
12. Neutral thermal environment
13. Lung disease in IRDS and ventilator survivors
14. Viral upper airway infection that results in a barking cough
15. Infant respiratory distress syndrome

4. The fetus can be assessed by a variety of methods. Briefly describe each of the following tests. Think "When would I recommend this test?" and you'll be thinking like an RT!

   A.   Ultrasonography

   B.   Amniocentesis

   C.   Fetal heart rate monitoring

   D.   Fetal blood gas analysis

5. What L/S ratio indicates lung maturity? When does this usually occur?

_____

6. What is the relationship between fetal scalp gases and arterial blood gases?

_____

7. When are Apgar scores taken? _____

8. You *simply must* learn the Apgar scoring system. (Refer to Table 48-2 on page 1188.)

	Sign	0	1	2
A.	Heart rate			
B.	Respiration			
C.	Muscle tone			
D.	Reflex			
E.	Color			

Hint: You could make up some kind of mnemonic to help you remember the five signs like "Heart Rate Must Really Count."

9. What term is used to describe the following weeks of gestation?

   A. Before 38 weeks _____

   B. 38 to 42 weeks _____

   C. After 42 weeks _____

10. Name the two common systems used for assessing gestational age based on physical characteristics and neurologic signs.

   A. _____

   B. _____

11. Explain the abbreviations and identify the weights that correspond to the following terms.

	Abbreviation	Full Name	Weights/Percents
A.	VLBW		
B.	LBW		
C.	AGA		
D.	LGA		
E.	SGA		

12. Why does anyone care about birth weight and gestational age?

13. State the normal range for a full-term infant's vital signs.

    A. Heart rate _____

    B. Respiratory rate _____

    C. Blood pressure _____

14. Describe the usual way to take an infant's heart rate. Where do you place the stethoscope?

    A. Method _____

    B. Stethoscope placement _____

15. Infants in respiratory distress typically exhibit one or more of these five signs. Explain the significance of each sign.

    A. Nasal flaring _____

    B. Cyanosis _____

    C. Expiratory grunting _____

    D. Retractions _____

    E. Paradoxical breathing _____

16. What scoring system is used to grade the severity of underlying lung disease?

    _____

17. What are the two usual sites for obtaining blood gas samples in infants according to Chapter 48?

    A. _____

    B. _____

18. Name two noninvasive methods used for assessment.

    A. _____

    B. _____

19. List the ABG values for preterm and term infants at birth. (Refer to Table 48-4 on page 1192.)

	Parameter	Preterm (1 to 5 hours)	Normal Term (5 hours)	Normal Preterm Infants (5 days)
A.	pH			
B.	Paco$_2$			
C.	Paco$_2$			

RESPIRATORY CARE TECHNIQUES

Back to Basics

20. Considering the hazards, we need to agree on the safe limits for oxygen therapy. Give the accepted ranges for these parameters.

    A. Paco$_2$ _____ to _____

    B. Fio$_2$ <_____%

    C. Spo$_2$ _____ to _____

21. Hyperoxia is associated with ROP and BPD in some infants. What do these acronyms stand for?

    A. ROP: _____

    B. BPD: _____

22. Name two other factors associated with ROP. (Refer to Box 48-1 on page 1193.)

    A. _____

    B. _____

23. What is meant by the "flip-flop phenomenon?"

24. How could oxygen cause heart problems to worsen in some newborns?

25. Compare the use of the following oxygen delivery devices. (Refer to Table 48-5 on page 1194.)

	Device	Age	Advantage	Disadvantage
A.	AEM			
B.	Cannula			
C.	Incubator			
D.	Hood			
E.	Tent			

26. Name four conditions where secretion retention is common in children.

    A. _____

    B. _____

    C. _____

    D. _____

27. Identify one other situation where bronchial hygiene therapy may be useful.

28. Because infants can't cough on command, how will you get the mucus out once it is mobilized?

29. How long should you wait after feedings to perform postural drainage on infants and small children?

    _____

30. How can you help prevent hypoxemia during head-down positioning?

Chapter 48   Neonatal and Pediatric Respiratory Care

31. Give up the hazards of overheating or underheating gases administered to newborns.
    A. Overheating

        1. _____

        2. _____

    B. Underheating

        1. _____

        2. _____

        3. _____

32. How is application of the nasal cannula different for adults and kids in terms of humidification?

33. Identify three reasons why continuous nebulization is usually avoided in infants.

    A. _____

    B. _____

    C. _____

34. How would you deliver a bronchodilator to a newborn? (Refer to Table 48-6 on page 1196.)

35. How would you deliver an MDI to an infant?

36. What is the dosage range for albuterol delivered by SVN? (Refer to Table 48-7 on page 1198.)

_____

37. What is the dosage range and frequency for racemic epinephrine?

A. Dose _____

B. Frequency _____

38. What is the dosage and treatment schedule for nebulized budesonide?

A. Dose _____

B. Treatment schedule _____

39. Identify the correct ET size and suction catheter size for these kids. (Refer to Table 48-8 on page 1199.)

	Age/Weight	ET Internal Diameter (ID)	Length (Oral)	Suction
A.	<1000 g			
B.	1000 to 2000 g			
C.	2000 to 3000 g			
D.	>3000 g			
E.	2 years			
F.	6 years			

If this seems silly, don't laugh; parts of question 20 will appear on your board exams!

40. State the two formulas for calculating tube diameter and length. (Refer to Table 48-8 on page 1199.)

A. Tube ID No. 1 _____ Tube ID No. 2 _____

B. Tube length oral No. 1 _____ Tube length nasal No. 2 _____

41. What is the consequence of placing an ET tube that is too small in an infant?

42. Estimate the correct tube size for a 4-year-old using the first formula in question 21.

43. Estimate the correct tube size for a child who is 122 cm (48 inches) tall.

_____

44. Which laryngoscope blade is usually used for infant intubation?

_____

45. What is the main difference between infant or pediatric ET tubes and adult ET tubes?

_____

46. What are the recommended vacuum pressures for suctioning infants and children?

A. Infants   _____

B. Children _____

47. How should you preoxygenate newborns to avoid hyperoxia? (This procedure is very different than it is in adults!)

48. What is the duration of suctioning for newborns? How does this compare to adults?

NEONATAL RESUSCITATION

49. What is the first step of resuscitation immediately after delivery?

_____

50. What action should be taken if meconium is visible in the larynx?

_____

51. Identify the criteria for initiating chest compressions after delivery.

_____

ADVANCED FUN AND GAMES

52. Play with baby's FRC by applying CPAP. What is the specific indication for CPAP? Give the blood gas values.

A. Indication   _____

B. Blood gas values   _____

53. Name four signs of respiratory distress that suggest using CPAP. (Refer to Box 48-5 on page 1201.)

A. _____

B. _____

C. _____

D. _____

54. Discuss adjustment of CPAP in infants.
    A. Start at

B. Adjust in increments of

55. CPAP is usually administered to an infant via what type of delivery system? What about kids?

A. Baby   _____

B. Kids   _____

HIGH-FLOW NASAL CANNULA

Most cannulas work but only at low flows due to humidification issues. New humidifiers allow you to go higher.

56. What is the range of flow given for the new cannulas?

_____

Chapter **48** **Neonatal and Pediatric Respiratory Care**

57. You know you have respiratory failure and the need to ventilate when:

    A. $Paco_2$ < _____

    B. $Paco_2$ > _____

58. You suspect you need to ventilate with these pulmonary diseases.

    A. _____

    B. _____

    C. _____

    D. _____

59. Give the range of tidal volumes for infants. _____

60. Identify the inspiratory time ranges that should be set for these age groups.

    A. Neonates _____

    B. Older children _____

61. Ventilator rates should be adjusted to maintain what range of $Paco_2$?

    _____

62. What PEEP levels are usually used in neonates? _____

63. Why would it be common to observe lower exhaled than inhaled volumes in pediatric patients? Hint: Think about

    the type of airway used. _____

64. Describe how to reduce the following parameters during weaning.
    A. Fio_2

    B. PEEP

65. List at least five things you should consider prior to extubating a baby.

A. _____

B. _____

C. _____

D. _____

E. _____

HIGH FREQUENCY VENTILATION

66. List four clinical indications for initiating low–lung volume high-frequency ventilation (HFV).

A. _____

B. _____

C. _____

D. _____

67. Identify the two common characteristics of HFV.

A. V_T _____

B. Rate _____

68. What are the two most common types of HFV?

A. _____

B. _____

69. Oxygenation in HFV is adjusted through increases in mean airway pressure and F_{IO_2}, just like in adults. CO_2 elimination depends mainly on what factor? How is this different than standard adult ventilator therapy?

70. How would you wean a patient from HFV?

JUST SAY NO

Nitric oxide (NO) is an FDA-approved drug. When you inhale this gas, it's called iNO. NO selectively vasodilates pulmonary vessels surrounding the functional alveoli.

71. What effect does NO have on oxygenation?

72. Two big problems exist with NO inhalation. Explain.
    A. Rebound pulmonary hypertension

    B. Altered hemoglobin

You can read more about this gas in Chapter 38: Medical Gas Therapy.

EXTRACORPOREAL MEMBRANE OXYGENATION

Hours of Boredom, Moments of Terror

A friend of mine who performs extracorporeal membrane oxygenation (ECMO) describes her job as pretty routine until something goes wrong. One of my students, who is a flight attendant, says the same thing about her job! ECMO is a fascinating and vital form of therapy where RTs play a leading role. Over 16,000 neonates have been treated with ECMO with a 78% survival rate.

73. What does ECMO do?

74. Describe the two basic forms of ECMO.
    A. VA

B. VV

75. Give three examples of neonatal conditions where ECMO is being used after conventional medical therapies fail.

A. _____

B. _____

C. _____

WHAT DOES THE NBRC SAY?

The exam matrices make detailed references to the material in Chapter 48, but they point out that most neonatal/pediatric stuff is on the Registry Examinations not the Certification Exam. Here's a partial list:

- Perinatal data
  - Maternal history
  - Perinatal history
  - Apgar scores
  - Gestational age
  - L/S ratio
  - Preductal and postductal oxygenation studies
- Equipment
  - Oxygen hoods and tents
  - Specialized ventilators: high frequency

The Clinical Simulation Examination Matrix makes it clear that you will have one pediatric and one neonatal problem. That material is covered in Chapter 34.

While Chapter 48 covers some of this information, you would be wise to consider taking a neonatal resuscitation program (NRP) and pediatric advanced life support (PALS) course before you take the boards. Here are some sample multiple choice questions. Circle the best answer.

76. Which of the following tests would be useful in determining lung maturity?
    A. sweat chloride
    B. L/S ratio
    C. fetal hemoglobin
    D. pneumogram

77. Calculate the Apgar score for a crying infant who has a heart rate of 120, actively moves, sneezes when a catheter is put in the nose, but has blue extremities.
    A. 5
    B. 6
    C. 7
    D. 9

78. The simplest way to apply CPAP to treat hypoxemia in an infant is to use _____.
    A. nasal prongs
    B. nasal mask
    C. full face mask
    D. oxygen hood

Chapter 48 **Neonatal and Pediatric Respiratory Care**

FOOD FOR THOUGHT

If you choose to work in this field, it would be a good idea to take the Neonatal/Pediatric Specialist Examination to test your knowledge and demonstrate your competence in this specialty area.

INFORMATION AGE

Whole books are written on this subject and you're going to need one to cover neonatal and pediatric respiratory care in depth. If you like the Internet, I'll make these suggestions:

- Virtual Children's Hospital is a good site: www.vh.org/pediatric. It has been partially dismantled, but lots of the files are still available.
- Another good source is www.lungusa.org/diseases.

For pediatric life support you can find good material at http://www.geocities.com/nyerrn/er/pals.htm.

49 Patient Education and Health Promotion

Quit worrying about your health. It will go away.
Robert Orben

Teaching can be very satisfying—when learning is taking place! (I should know . . . .) It's equally frustrating to try to learn when teaching is disorganized or the objectives are unclear. (You should know . . . .) Client and community education really go to the far ends of the spectrum. It is tremendously rewarding to help someone quit smoking; learn to be more independent; or to teach children how to manage their asthma. These are REAL victories in the battle for better health! On the other hand, you can go nuts trying to get your message across to some people. Chapter 49 provides you with valuable ideas on how to develop, conduct, and measure the outcomes of a health education program. You can use this information in school, with patients, in the community, and in teaching co-workers. Let's go do some educating!

WORD WIZARD

Teacher Talk
I want to make sure you have a good grasp of the key terms in this chapter before you apply them. Write out the definition for each of these terms. You can use the chapter or the glossary.

1. Affective domain _____

2. Cognitive domain _____

3. Health education _____

4. Health promotion _____

5. Psychomotor domain _____

PATIENT EDUCATION

Respiratory care practitioners have always been on-the-spot instructors at the bedside, but the role of RT as formal educator has increased dramatically in the past few years as health care delivery methods and settings have changed.

Overview
6. What are the top five causes of death in the United States?

A. _____

B. _____

C. _____

D. _____

E. _____

549

7. Why is educating the public about these illnesses so important?

_____

_____

WHAT'S IN A DOMAIN?

8. Why should you consider developing written objectives for patient teaching? (Isn't that just something teachers do to look good?)

_____

_____

9. How can you state an objective in measurable terms?

A. Begin with a . . . _____

B. Write an action . . . _____

C. Add a condition . . . _____

D. Write a standard . . . _____

10. Give an example of an objective for each of the following learning domains. (Oh, go ahead, take one out of *Egan's*.)

Domain	Objective
A. Cognitive	_____
B. Affective	_____
C. Psychomotor	_____

11. Which of the learning domains (*domain* is a French word that means "realm, estate, or property") should be evaluated before you proceed with patient education?

_____

_____

12. Maslow's hierarchy of needs (pretty useful if you apply it . . .) explains why a dyspneic patient will not be very receptive to learning a new skill. How can you assess readiness to learn?

_____

_____

13. What is the key to motivating patients to learn?

_____

_____

14. What is the key to teaching psychomotor skills? How can you confirm that a patient or family member has learned a new skill?

_____

_____

15. Give an example from the text of how to relate psychomotor skills a patient uses every day to help make the transition from everyday life to therapy.

_____

F.A.T. T.I.P.S*

Now that you've reviewed some important ideas about teaching, let's take a look at:

CRYSTAL CLEAR CLASSROOM COMMANDMENTS
I.   Meet immediate patient needs *first*.
II.   Create an educational setting.
III.   Include hearing, seeing, touching, writing, speaking.
IV.   Keep sessions short.
V.   Repeat, repeat, repeat!
VI.   Allow plenty of time to practice skills.
VII.   Spend time preparing for the session.
VIII. Organize your materials and presentation.
IX.   Personalize and customize the learning experience.
X.   Be enthusiastic!!!
If you think about your own learning experiences, you will have no difficulty believing in these powerful ideas for improving your teaching abilities. (Make a copy and mail them to someone!)

*Forget academic theory; this is practical stuff.

Teaching Children

16. How is teaching children different from teaching adults? How is it the same? (Refer to Boxes 49-1 and 49-2 on page 1224 of your text.)

17. Where could you find resource materials to help in teaching children with asthma? (Check out the Mini Clini!)

_____

18. What suggestions are given for rewarding performance?

Evaluation

19. What process answers the question "Has the patient learned?" When should you begin to develop this process?

20. Describe some of the ways you can tell if a patient has met affective domain objectives.

HEALTH EDUCATION

Naturally, RTs are expected to be role models who demonstrate healthy behaviors in public. Imagine giving a patient information about nicotine intervention when you smell like cigarettes yourself! Role models aren't enough, however, to achieve large-scale improvements in public health.

21. The primary goal of health education is to _____ people's _____.

22. Learning activities must incorporate values and beliefs of the learner. What four factors need to be considered in this area?

   A. _____

   B. _____

   C. _____

   D. _____

23. How do the personal characteristics of the educator impact on learning?

24. State the four central, preventable causes of the major causes of death in the United States.

   A. _____

   B. _____

   C. _____

   D. _____

25. Compare the standard medical approach to health in the United States with the public health model.

26. Give goals and examples of each of the following levels of prevention.

Level	Goal	Example
A. Primary	_____	_____
B. Secondary	_____	_____
C. Tertiary	_____	_____

27. Give examples of projects where RTs can participate in organized health promotion activities targeted at primary, secondary, or tertiary goals.

   A. Primary _____

   B. Secondary _____

   C. Tertiary _____

28. Besides the hospital, name four other settings where RTs would be likely to function as individual counselors or public health advocates.

   A. _____

   B. _____

   C. _____

   D. _____

CASE STUDIES

Your text has several perfectly good cases in the form of "Mini Clinis," so let's do something else.
Suppose you had to teach your classmates how to use a peak flow meter. Write three objectives
for this topic for each domain using behavioral terms.

29. Cognitive domain

   A.

   B.

   C.

30. Affective domain

   A.

   B.

   C.

31. Psychomotor domain
    A.

    B.

    C.

32. How long would your teaching session last?

    _____

33. Give examples of how you would involve the following senses in your session?

    A. Hearing _____

    B. Seeing _____

    C. Touching _____

    D. Writing _____

    E. Speaking _____

34. Give an example of how you would measure learning for each domain.

    A. Cognitive _____

    B. Affective _____

    C. Psychomotor _____

Not much. Oh, you should be able to educate a patient. Here's an example.

35. The best way to ensure that a patient learned to properly administer a bronchodilator via MDI is to _____.
    A. ask the patient to answer questions regarding inhaler use
    B. give the patient appropriate literature regarding MDI use
    C. ask the patient to demonstrate how to use the inhaler
    D. have the patient explain when he is to use the MDI

FOOD FOR THOUGHT

36. Why do you think the public should be educated about the risk factors for the top five causes of death? After all, a lot of RTs are employed taking care of patients who have ignored these risk factors.

37. How is teaching other caregivers different from teaching patients or family members?

_____

INFORMATION AGE

A lot of times I am looking for teaching materials that have already been designed by others. No point in reinventing the wheel, right? Here are some places where you can find material that is ready to use.
- COPD resources: www.aarc.org/klein/. The AARC of course!
- Asthma: www.breatherville.org/breatherville.htm. A great asthma site!
- Lung disease in general: www.lungusa.org/. The American Lung Association. You can also go to your local chapter.
- Go to National Jewish at: http://nationaljewish.org.
- Our college library subscribes to "MD Consult," an Internet information service that also allows you to download and customize patient teaching sheets. You can find similar items if you don't have MD Consult, all you have to do is go online.

The Internet is at its finest in this area. I can get material on any subject from teaching tracheostomy care to ARDS. Literally anything.

50 Cardiopulmonary Rehabilitation

No one is useless in this world who lightens the burden of another.

Charles Dickens

Alvan Barach first recommended reconditioning programs for COPD patients over 40 years ago. Unfortunately, it was not until recently that these programs began in earnest around the nation. When I worked in home care in the 1980s, it was often up to the individual therapist to try to provide and encourage these concepts for individual patients. Now there are many well-established inpatient and outpatient programs to meet the physical and psychosocial needs of our patients with chronic lung disease.

While there are many good textbooks and patient teaching aids available, you will find that Chapter 50 provides an excellent overview of the subject. Even if you don't work in rehabilitation, you will be in a position to identify patients who can benefit from these services, and can play a key role in improving the quality of your patients' lives. You may also wish to participate in one of the Better Breather's Clubs founded by the American Lung Association, local health care organizations, or chapter of the American Association for Respiratory Care.

WORD WIZARD

You can build impressive mental muscles by adding these words to your vocabulary. Match the following terms and acronyms to their definitions.

Terms and Acronyms	Definitions
1. _____ ADL	A. physical activities designed to strengthen muscles and improve O_2 utilization
2. _____ Borg scale	B. measure of an individual's ability to perform common tasks
3. _____ CORF	C. point where there is insufficient O_2 to meet the demands of energy metabolism
4. _____ Karvonen's formula	D. measure of an individual's perception of breathing difficulty
5. _____ METS	E. cardiac goal for aerobic conditioning based on 65% of maximum O_2 consumption
6. _____ OBLA	F. ratio of CO_2 production to O_2 consumption
7. _____ reconditioning	G. Medicare-approved facility that provides ambulatory rehab services
8. _____ respiratory quotient	H. common method used to calculate target heart rate for exercise
9. _____ target heart rate	I. indirect measure of physiologic work performed during exercise stress testing

DEFINITIONS AND GOALS

Pulmonary rehabilitation is not the same animal as other types of rehab, although it can contain some of the same elements.

10. What is meant by the general term "rehabilitation?"

11. The definition of pulmonary rehabilitation is really long. Please put it into your own words.

12. What are the two general goals of pulmonary rehabilitation?

    A. _____

    B. _____

SCIENTIFIC BASIS FOR PULMONARY REHABILITATION

Exercise physiology plays an important role in our understanding of the benefits of reconditioning, but physiology alone is not sufficient to achieve desired outcomes in patients with COPD.

13. How do social sciences play a role in establishing ways to improve the patient's quality of life?

14. Why is MVV a useful pulmonary function test in regard to assessing physical activity?

15. How can you estimate MVV using simple spirometry?

    _____

16. Identify the three general ways that reconditioning will increase exercise tolerance.

    A. _____

    B. _____

    C. _____

17. Compare the roles of psychosocial and physical methods in terms of outcomes of rehabilitation.

18. Describe the two-way relationship of physical reconditioning and psychosocial support.

PULMONARY REHABILITATION PROGRAMS

Program designs may vary, but the desired outcomes and basic components are similar.

19. Why is it so important to have specific objectives for the program goals?

20. State five accepted benefits of exercise reconditioning. (Refer to Table 50-1 on page 1239.)

A. _____

B. _____

C. _____

D. _____

E. _____

21. Research literature clearly shows that rehabilitation has proved benefits. List a few of the top items under "unproved"—this is what rehabilitation can't accomplish!

A. _____

B. _____

C. _____

22. Name three common goals (not objectives) for rehab programs.

    A. _____

    B. _____

    C. _____

23. Who manages the overall care in a program and screens the prospective patients?

_____

24. What is the first step in patient evaluation for a pulmonary rehab program?

_____

25. Name four tests that should be included with the physical examination.

    A. _____

    B. _____

    C. _____

    D. _____

26. Two tests are usually conducted to assess cardiopulmonary status. State two purposes for these tests.
    A. Exercise evaluation

        1. _____

        2. _____

    B. Pulmonary function testing

        1. _____

        2. _____

27. List two contraindications and two complications of exercise testing.
    A. Contraindications
        1.

        2.

B. Complications
    1.

    2.

28. Identify four physiologic parameters that should be monitored during exercise testing.

    A. _____

    B. _____

    C. _____

    D. _____

29. Name two types of patients that are usually excluded from selection for rehab.

    A. _____

    B. _____

30. State the four general groups of patients included in pulmonary rehab programs.

    A. _____

    B. _____

    C. _____

    D. _____

31. What are the benefits of grouping patients together on the basis of severity and overall ability?

32. Give one benefit and one drawback of the open-ended program model.

    A. Benefit _____

    B. Drawback _____

33. Give one benefit and one drawback to the traditional closed design.
    A. Benefit

    B. Drawback

34. Describe two ways to set target heart rate for patient exercise.

    A. Formula _____

    B. Estimate _____

35. Describe a typical walking exercise program. What is our minimum walk time?

36. What is the basic concept behind ventilatory muscle training?

37. Briefly discuss the following high-priority program educational components.
    A. Breathing control

    B. Stress management

    C. Medications

    D. Diet

38. What is the ideal class size for a rehab program? What external factor affects this ideal?

39. Give specific examples for each of the following sources of program reimbursement.

    A. Nongovernment health insurance

    _____

    B. Federal and state health insurance

    _____

    C. Ancillary insurance _____

    D. Other options _____

40. What is/are the most likely cause(s) of lack of measurable improvement within a pulmonary rehab program?

41. Potential hazards do exist. Give one from each category:

    I.   Cardio   _____

    II. Blood gas   _____

    III. Muscular   _____

    IV. Miscellaneous   _____

CASE STUDIES

Case 1

An alert 55-year-old man with long-standing asthma and COPD is admitted for acute exacerbation of his illness following a "chest cold." This is the fourth admission for this patient in the past 3 months. He tells you that he has had to quit his job and take early retirement because of his lung problems.

42. What concerns does this situation raise?

43. Explain the benefits of entering a rehab program to this patient.

Case 2

A 57-year-old woman with chronic bronchitis is enrolled in your pulmonary rehab program. During walking exercises, she complains of dyspnea and will not continue with the walk.

44. What assessments would be useful in this situation?

45. Give several possible methods for modifying the exercise program to improve this patient's compliance.

WHAT DOES THE NBRC SAY?

In the case of pulmonary rehabilitation, the Examination Matrix is very specific:
1. Explain planned therapy and goals to patient in understandable terms to achieve optimal therapeutic outcome.
2. Educate patient and family in disease management.
3. Counsel patient and family concerning smoking cessation.
4. Instruct patient and family to assure safety and infection control.

You will only see about two multiple choice per examination (CRT and WRE). The Clinical Simulation Matrix includes identical items but also specifically mentions that you may encounter a case of a patient with COPD who needs pulmonary rehabilitation. This means that rehab is a small but very important part of the credentialing process. Here are a few representative questions. Circle the answer.

46. A COPD patient has enrolled in a pulmonary rehabilitation program. The patient should be informed that the program will help provide all of the benefits *except* _____.
    A. increased physical endurance
    B. improved PFT results
    C. increased activity levels
    D. improved cardiovascular function

47. During an exercise test a patient is able to reach a maximum heart rate of 120. His resting heart rate is 70. What target heart rate would you recommend for this patient during aerobic conditioning?
    A. 70 beats per minute
    B. 85 beats per minute
    C. 100 beats per minute
    D. 115 beats per minute

48. Which of the following tests would be useful in assessing ventilatory reserve during exercise testing?
    A. forced vital capacity
    B. maximum voluntary ventilation
    C. body plethysmography
    D. single breath nitrogen washout

FOOD FOR THOUGHT

All through *Egan's* we find references to the Borg Scale (must be something to do with Star Trek!). This scale is a valuable tool that can be easily used at the bedside or in the rehab setting.

49. Describe the Borg Scale. _____

50. What are the units of measurement on the scale?

_____

51. What is the value of this instrument?

INFORMATION AGE

- A good place to start is the home page of the American Association of Cardiovascular and Pulmonary Rehabilitation: www.aacvpr.org.
- You could look at the program at National Jewish: www.nationaljewish.org/disease-info/diseases/copd/mgmt/pulm-rehab/index.aspx.
- Postgraduate Medicine Online has a good overview: www.postgradmed.com/issues/1998/04_98/celli.htm.
There are lots more sites. The Internet is a very useful resource for the topic of pulmonary rehabilitation!

Respiratory Care in Alternative Settings

Problems are only opportunities in work clothes.
Henry J. Kaiser

Egan's had to end with a beginning, and Chapter 51 introduces you to a fast-growing segment of the respiratory industry. As health care is being redefined on many levels, the work setting for our profession is moving outside the boundaries of the traditional medical center concept. Alternative care settings provide special challenges for the respiratory therapist (RT), particularly the new graduate.

WORD WIZARD

Acronyms.alt

No matter what else you got out of this book, you're bound to have a brain full of odd letter combinations. Don't worry, be happy. This is the last of the acronyms. (I promise!) Write out the meanings.

1. CMS _____

2. DME _____

3. HCFA _____

4. NPPV _____

5. SAHS _____

6. SIDS _____

7. SNF _____

8. TTOT _____

RECENT TRENDS

9. What is the most common alternative site for health care?

_____

10. What was the overall effect of the PPS system? How has the BBA impacted RTs?

    A. PPS

    B. BBA

11. What were the results of the Muse study?

DEFINITIONS AND GOALS

12. Name the four areas of subacute or alternate care.

    A. _____

    B. _____

    C. _____

    D. _____

13. What is subacute care?

14. Name some of the most common respiratory care services provided in alternate settings.

   A. _____

   B. _____

   C. _____

   D. _____

15. What is the most common age groups receiving subacute care?

   _____

16. State at least three of the benefits of respiratory home care.

   A. _____

   B. _____

   C. _____

   Now give up three typical disease states that need our help.

   D. _____

   E. _____

   F. _____

STANDARDS

17. Why does government play a major role in setting standards for the regulation of postacute care?

   _____

18. What is the purpose of the Medicare Provider Certification Program?

19. Who is responsible for accreditation of companies that provide home care services?

   _____

20. What are the two types of accreditation for respiratory home care?

   _____

21. Why do many RTs prefer working in the postacute care setting?

22. Compare traditional and alternative settings in terms of the following areas (Table 51-1).

Area	Traditional	Alternative
A. Diagnostic tests	_____	_____
B. Equipment	_____	_____
C. Supervision	_____	_____
D. Patient assessment	_____	_____
E. Work schedule	_____	_____
F. Time constraints	_____	_____

DISCHARGE PLANNING

23. Explain the role of the following practitioners in the postacute care team. (Refer to Table 51-2 on page 1260.)

    A. Utilization and review _____

    B. Social services _____

    C. Physical therapy _____

    D. Physiatrist _____

    E. DME supplier _____

24. How can you confirm that a nonprofessional caregiver is able to perform care?

    _____

25. Discuss items in the home environment that must be assessed prior to discharge. Check out Box 51-1 if you get stuck.
    A. Accessibility

B. Equipment

C. Environment

OXYGEN THERAPY

Ok, this is it—The big one! Oxygen is the most common mode of RT used outside the hospital and the one that is tested the most, too!

26. Why do so many people use home oxygen in the United States?

_____

27. State two of the documented benefits of home oxygen therapy.

A. _____

B. _____

28. Describe the six elements that must be included in a home oxygen prescription.

A. _____

B. _____

C. _____

D. _____

E. _____

F. _____

29. The AARC Clinical Practice Guideline for Oxygen in the Home clearly states the indications for oxygen outside the acute care hospital. You MUST know this, so cough it up!

   A.   Adults, etc. >28 days Pao_2 ≤ _____ mm Hg, or Sao_2 ≤ _____

   B.   Cor pulmonale, CHF, or critical >56% Pao_2 ≤ _____ mm Hg, or

   Sao_2 ≤ _____.

   C.   Ambulation, sleep, or exercise if Sao_2 falls below _____%.

   Seriously; only these patients will qualify for O_2 outside the hospital in most cases. You are expected to know these criteria for your boards, so you can discharge patients and advise the staff. Remember, the home care folks cannot qualify the patients because it is a conflict of interest.

30. What are the two primary uses of compressed oxygen cylinders in the alternative setting?

   A.   E cylinder _____

   B.   H cylinder (or M) _____

31. How do flowmeters used in alternative settings differ from those used in the hospital?

   _____

32. Let's compare the advantages and disadvantages of the oxygen supply systems available for use in alternative settings (see Table 51-3). If you can get this down, you will be a really useful RT who can participate in discharge planning and actually help your patients and your organization.

System	Advantage	Disadvantage
A. Cylinders		
1.	_____	_____
2.	_____	_____
B. Liquid		
1.	_____	_____
2.	_____	_____
C. Concentrator		
1.	_____	_____
2.	_____	_____

33. Liquid oxygen is weighed to determine the amount available. If a patient was using 3 L/min with a 100-lb system that was one-fourth full, how many hours would the gas last? (See Table 51-4 on page 1266.)

34. Explain how an oxygen concentrator works. KISS.

35. What is the typical range of oxygen percentage a concentrator will supply?

    A. 1 to 2 L/min _____

    B. 3 to 5 L/min _____

36. What effect will the concentrator have on a patient's electrical bill? (Remember that money is a BIG issue for fixed-income elderly who are ill.)

    _____

37. Describe some of the methods for avoiding communication problems with patients receiving home oxygen

    therapy. _____

38. In addition to providing a backup supply, what other precautions should be taken in terms of concentrator power supply?

39. List at least four areas that should be evaluated when checking a home patient's oxygen concentrator.

    A. _____

    B. _____

    C. _____

    D. _____

40. When a patient is placed on an oxygen conserving device, how would you determine the correct liter flow to use?

41. What actions should a patient who is wearing transtracheal oxygen take if he believes the catheter isn't working properly?

42. In theory, how would a demand flow oxygen conserving system benefit the patient?

43. What are the two main drawbacks to demand flow systems?

44. In what situations should a patient or caregiver be instructed to alter the prescribed flow setting?

45. State the three main problems associated with insertion of the transtracheal catheter (see Box 51-4).

   A. _____

   B. _____

   C. _____

46. Describe the basic methods for avoiding complications of transtracheal catheters.

47. Give examples for each of the three main groups of patients who are placed on ventilators in the alternative care setting (see Table 51-5 on page 1272).
   A. Nocturnal ventilation

   1. _____

   2. _____

   3. _____

   B. Continuous mechanical ventilation

   1. _____

   2. _____

   3. _____

   C. Terminally ill

   1. _____

   2. _____

48. Identify the three common settings where ventilatory support is delivered outside the hospital.

   A. _____

   B. _____

   C. _____

49. Invasive long-term ventilation is always provided via what type of airway?

   _____

50. Describe the emergency situations a family must be able to deal with in caring for a home ventilator patient.

51. Identify at least three situations where NIPPV is partly contraindicated.

   A. _____

   B. _____

   C. _____

52. Identify at least three situations where NIPPV is absolutely contraindicated.

    A. _____

    B. _____

    C. _____

53. What options exist for patients who do not want invasive ventilation and cannot use NIPPV?

54. What options are available on invasive positive-pressure ventilator systems during power failures, or if a patient

    wishes to be mobile? _____

55. What is the biggest challenge associated with NIPPV?

    _____

56. Identify the three basic types of negative pressure ventilators.

    A. _____

    B. _____

    C. _____

OTHER MODES OF POSTACUTE RESPIRATORY CARE

57. What is the primary use of bland aerosols in the postacute setting?

58. What is the major problem with delivery of bland aerosols?

    _____

59. What are the two limits on Medicare reimbursement for compressor-driven SVNs in the alternate setting?

A. _____

B. _____

60. How can you prevent bacterial growth on suction catheters that are used repeatedly?

_____

61. State three common clinical problems or patient complaints associated with SAHS.

A. _____

B. _____

C. _____

62. What is the primary treatment for this condition?

_____

63. When should nasal masks be replaced?

_____

64. Discuss solutions to the common complaint of nasal dryness?

65. What infant condition suggests the use of apnea monitoring? How long do they need the monitor?

A. Condition _____

B. Duration of monitoring _____

PATIENT ASSESSMENT AND DOCUMENTATION

66. Describe the main areas you would check during initial screening of a patient following admission to a postacute care facility.

67. What areas would be important to assess **besides** the usual vital signs and evaluation of the respiratory system?

68. How often should a member of the home care team perform a follow-up evaluation for patients receiving respiratory care treatments? What factors should be considered in determining the frequency of visits?

EQUIPMENT DISINFECTION AND MAINTENANCE

69. Describe the process for cleaning a home nebulizer (for example):

A. _____

B. _____

C. _____

D. _____

70. Describe the guidelines for using water in humidifiers and nebulizers.

71. What is the most important principle of infection control in the home setting?

PALLIATIVE CARE

72. According to the World Health Organization, palliative care involves control of what two debilitating symptoms?

    A. _____

    B. _____

73. What is hospice?

CASE STUDIES

Case 1

A 70-year-old with COPD is discharged with an order for home oxygen. The room air blood gas prior to discharge is:

pH	7.47
$Paco_2$	33 mm Hg
Pao_2	62 mm Hg
Sao_2	92%

Medicare returns the CMN as disapproved on the basis that this patient does not meet the criteria for saturation of Po_2 for home oxygen.

74. Make an argument for keeping the patient on oxygen based on your knowledge of respiratory physiology. You won't find a clear answer in the text. (This is a real case and we did get reimbursement! Hint: What does the low $Paco_2$ and high pH indicate?)

Case 2

A home care patient whom you are seeing uses an oxygen concentrator. He calls you (late at night, of course) to say that he doesn't think he is getting an adequate amount of flow from his cannula.

75. What are some possible causes of this problem?

76. What would you suggest Steve do at this time?

Case 3

An active 49-year-old with α_1-antitrypsin deficiency is to be discharged with home oxygen. The prescription is for 2 L/min continuous oxygen.

77. What system would you recommend for this patient to use at home?

78. What about a portable system?

WHAT DOES THE NBRC SAY?

Home care is included in the rehabilitation section of the examination matrix. You can expect only a few questions. Usually these relate to cleaning or home oxygen. Here are some representative questions. Circle the answer.

580

79. A patient with a tracheostomy is to receive humidification via a nebulizer in his home. With regard to water for the nebulizer, which of the following would be the most appropriate choice for the home setting?
   A. Sterile distilled water should be obtained from the DME provider.
   B. Tap water is sufficient for the home setting if the nebulizer is cleaned properly.
   C. Bottled water can be used as long as it is distilled.
   D. Tap water that is boiled may be used for up to 24 hours.

80. Which of the following actions would an RT perform during the monthly check of a home oxygen concentrator system?
   I.   replacement of the silica pellets in the sieve bed
   II. analysis of the F_{IO_2} delivered by the concentrator
   III. filter replacement
   IV. evaluation of the concentrator's electrical system
       A. I and II
       B. II and III
       C. II and IV
       D. III and IV

81. A patient who is wearing a transtracheal oxygen catheter suddenly becomes dyspneic. The first action the patient should take would be to _____.
   A. call the physician
   B. clean the catheter
   C. increase the oxygen flow to the catheter
   D. remove the catheter and proceed to the emergency department

82. A patient who is using oxygen at home occasionally needs to go out for health care appointments. What type of portable system would you recommend for this patient?
   A. E cylinder with standard flowmeter
   B. E cylinder with conserving device
   C. small liquid oxygen reservoir
   D. Patients can go out for short periods without supplemental oxygen.

83. A respiratory care practitioner determines that a cuirass-type negative pressure ventilator is now reading a pressure of −20 cm H_2O, when it should be cycling at −35 cm H_2O. The patient is in no distress, but the measured tidal volume is 200 ml lower than the desired volume. The practitioner should _____.
   A. begin manual ventilation of the patient
   B. check for leaks in the system
   C. increase the vacuum setting
   D. increase the amount of air in the cuff

FOOD FOR THOUGHT

Concentrators have changed dramatically in the last few years.

84. Discuss the special features of these two high-tech sieves.
   A. Respironics Millenium M10

B. Inogen One

INFORMATION AGE

A wide variety of information is available to enhance your knowledge of respiratory home care, rehabilitation, and palliative care.

- You might want to look at the Web site of a national company like Linde: www.linde-gastherapeutics.com or Apria www.apria.com.
- If you're looking for patient resources, Assist Guide is the most comprehensive national Web site. Here you can find resources for any home or senior need in almost any state: www.agisnetwork.com.
- Your Lung Health is a superb site: www.yourlunghealth.org/healthy_living/living/resp_home_care.
- I think palliative care is pretty hot stuff for our profession. The November and December 2000 *Respiratory Care* journal has two full issues devoted to palliative care! I highly recommend that you check this out online at AARC. org.
- Pulmonary rehabilitation is equally important. Check out the Web site of the American Association of Cardiovascular and Pulmonary Rehabilitation: www.aacvpr.org.
- You might also look to National Jewish at www.nationaljewish.org/medfacts/pulmonary.html.